Practical Casebook
Child Health Nursing for
GNM and Post Basic BSc Nursing Students

Name of the Student : ....

Register No./Enrollment No. : ....

Course/Year : ....

Batch : ....

Name of the Institute : ....

Practical Casebook
Child Health Nursing for GNM and Post Basic BSc Nursing Students

(According to the Newly Revised INC Syllabus)

Second Edition

Sudhakar A
MSc (N), MBA (HM)
PGDC (NICU and ICU), LLB, PhD (Pedia)
Academic Dean/Principal
Popular Institute of Medical Foundation
Popular College of Nursing and Paramedical Institute
Varanasi, Uttar Pradesh, India

Foreword
Awadhesh Kumar Kaushik

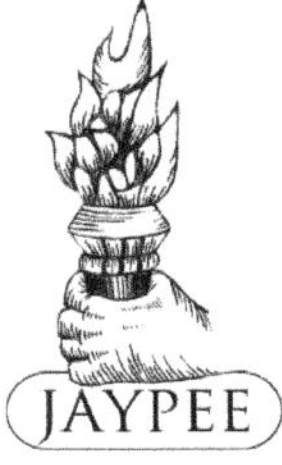

JAYPEE BROTHERS MEDICAL PUBLISHERS
The Health Sciences Publisher
New Delhi | London

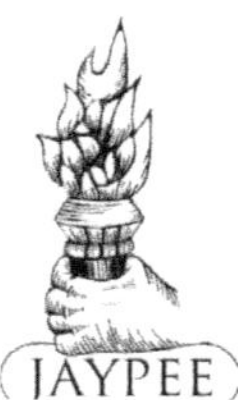 **Jaypee Brothers Medical Publishers (P) Ltd**

Headquarters

Jaypee Brothers Medical Publishers (P) Ltd
EMCA House, 23/23-B
Ansari Road, Daryaganj
New Delhi 110 002, India
Landline: +91-11-23272143, +91-11-23272703
+91-11-23282021, +91-11-23245672
Email: jaypee@jaypeebrothers.com

Corporate Office

Jaypee Brothers Medical Publishers (P) Ltd
4838/24, Ansari Road, Daryaganj
New Delhi 110 002, India
Phone: +91-11-43574357
Fax: +91-11-43574314
Email: jaypee@jaypeebrothers.com

Overseas Office

J.P. Medical Ltd
83 Victoria Street, London
SW1H 0HW (UK)
Phone: +44 20 3170 8910
Email: info@jpmedpub.com

EU GPSR Authorised Representative

Logos Europe, 9 rue Nicolas Poussin
17000, La Rochelle, France
Phone: +33 (0) 6 67 93 73 78
E-mail: Contact@logoseurope.eu

Website: www.jaypeebrothers.com
Website: www.jaypeedigital.com

Inquiries for bulk sales may be solicited at: jaypee@jaypeebrothers.com

Practical Casebook: Child Health Nursing for GNM and Post Basic BSc Nursing Students

First Edition: 2016

Second Edition: **2023**

ISBN: 978-93-5465-621-7

Dedicated to

My Daughter's Ms Jayani Sree SS
and
Ms Navanya Sree SS

Message

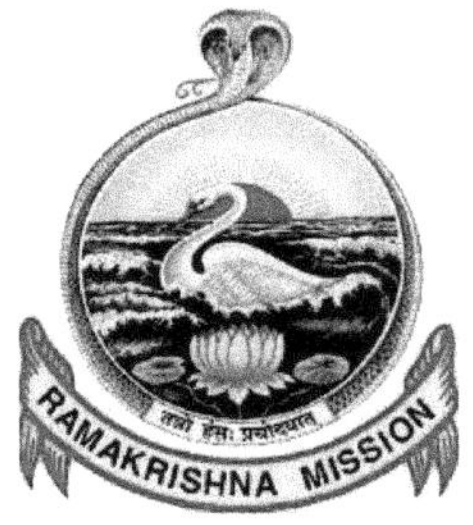

Vivekananda Polyclinic and Institute of Medical Sciences

Ramakrishna Mission Sevashrama
Vivekananda Puram, Lucknow,Uttar Pradesh - 226 007

Phones: (0522) 232 8942, 232 1277, Fax: (91522) 232 9624
E-mails: rkmvplko@gmail.com; rkml@ramakrishnalucknow.org

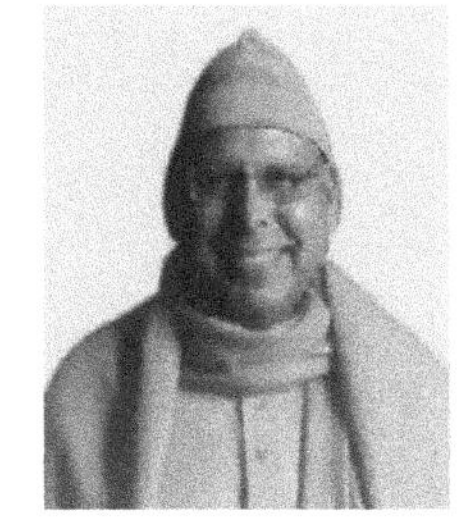

Message to the Nursing Students

"Who Serves Jiva (Creatures), Serves God Indeed"—Swami Vivekananda

Sri Ramakrishna, the Spiritual Preceptor of Swami Vivekananda, taught to the world that God can be worshipped not only with eyes closed, but also with eyes open by way of serving the needy human beings, considering them as living embodiments of the Almighty. Such a holistic attitude transforms our mundane activities into holy worship of the Divine. If the nurses are able to orient their attitude in this manner, then their profession becomes a loving engagement with the Divine and a source of perennial joy and fulfillment.

In order to bring out the best in ourselves, we must transcend the domain of our selfish interests and learn to serve others in a selfless spirit. Swami Vivekananda said, "Unselfishness is God." He further pointed out its practical implications saying, "The best work that you ever did for yourselves was when you worked for others. This life is short, vanities of the world are transient, but ***they alone live who live for others, the rest are more dead than alive***. Be not afraid of anything. You will do marvellous work. The moment you fear, you are nobody. It is fear that is the great cause of misery in the world. It is fear that is the greatest of all superstitions. It is fear that is the cause of our woes and it is fearlessness that brings heaven even in a moment." "All power is within you. Believe in that, do not believe that you are weak. You can do anything and everything, without even the guidance of anyone. Stand up and express the divinity within you."

Swami Vivekananda had great expectations from the youth. He said, "It is the young, the strong and healthy, of sharp intellect that will reach the Lord. This is the time to decide your future while you possess the energy of youth, not when you are worn out and jaded, but in the freshness and vigor of youth. Work—this is the time; for the freshest, the untouched and unsmelled flowers alone are to be laid at the feet of the Lord and such He receives. Rouse yourselves, therefore, for life is short. A far greater work is this sacrifice of yourselves for the benefit of your race, for the welfare of humanity."

This textbook on *Pediatric Nursing*, authored by Sri Sudhakar A, Associate Professor of Vivekananda College of Nursing, Lucknow, not only presents the essential theoretical knowledge of this particular specialty of Nursing but also attempts to provide the requisite practical wisdom towards improved patient care for the children.

I sincerely believe that the inputs contained in this volume, augmented with the aforesaid spirit of service as envisaged by Swami Vivekananda, will definitely provide adequate knowledge, attitude, skills and habits in the nursing students, so as to enable them to carry out their duties and responsibilities as competent professional skilled nurses.

Swami Muktinathananda

Foreword

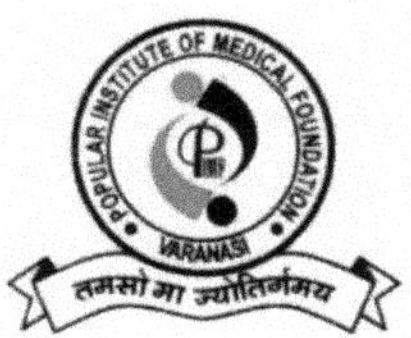

Reg. No. : 092718

Popular Institute of Medical Foundation

Head Office : N-10/60, A-2, DLW Road, (In front of Flyover), Kakarmatta, Varanasi-221004 (U.P.)
Mobile : 9119950022, 7752999777, 9076700105   Fax : 0542-2300506   Email : pimfvns@gmail.com

Foreword Message to the Nursing Scholars

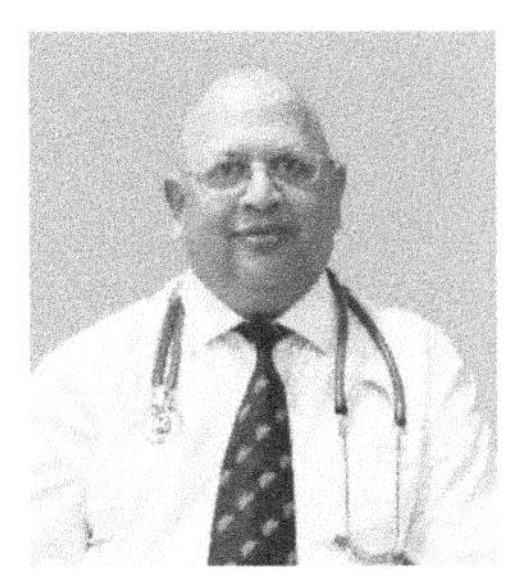

Dear nursing students, life is priceless and good health is our most precious gift! A healthy body and a sound mind help us live a wholesome life, and enjoy all its moments—both big and small. It is the constant backdrop that our wellbeing demands.

The creator has given human beings the most intricate body—one that is most valuable. Our body is the greatest asset we have, but unfortunately most of us don't care and treat it that proper way. We need to value our body, protect and cherish it. Most importantly, we must give our bodies, the respect it so richly deserves. *Popular Hospital* provides the safest, highest quality health care and the best experience possible to our patients. This is what we strive for every day and night.

Our aim is to ensure sentiments of satisfaction and peace consistently, from patient to patient. We continue to do so through our unrelenting efforts to devise processes that revolve around the patients' well-being. Our doctor teams are an integral and vital part of our commitment to deliver exceptional care. Their passion to heal and their constant drive toward higher quality outcomes is unmatched. They are thoroughly professional, approachable and always ready to extend a personal touch. They bring their excellence to speed up the patient's recovery and return to normal life with the least amount of stress.

We are running the *Popular Group of Nursing and Paramedical Institutions* under the Popular Institute of Medical Foundation, Varanasi and Mirzapur.

We are providing comprehensive knowledge, skill and high quality of clinical training to our students with excellent teaching faculty. We are expanding our network to reach across Uttar Pradesh. Its namely as a Popular Hospital, Bachchhao, Varanasi, City Hospital, Varanasi, Popular Hospital, Gopiganj (Bhadohi), Popular Hospital, Mirzapur and we are expanding shortly coming soon are hospitals in Lucknow and New Delhi (in the name of "Popular Hospital and Niraamaya Diagnostic").

This *Practical Casebook on Child Health Nursing for GNM and Post Basic BSc Nursing Students,* 2nd edition authored by Prof Dr Sudhakar A, Academic Dean/Principal of Popular College of Nursing and Paramedical Institute (PIMF), Varanasi and Mirzapur. This pediatric case book covered all the theoretical and practical topics in INC syllabus and this practical case book gives more confidence to students and improves children's health status in hospitals. I strongly suggest that the content of this book will fulfill all the learning expectations of students in the pediatric nursing field without any discomfort. I wish all the nursing students and pediatric nursing fraternity to serve your duty and responsibility with a spirit of knowledge and dedicated manner towards your patients and be a competent professional skilled nurse in future.

Awadhesh Kumar Kaushik
Director/Chairman
Popular Group of Hospitals
Popular Institute of Medical Foundation
Varanasi, Uttar Pradesh, India

Preface to the Second Edition

I am very much honored and delightful to readers of my first edition. I gladly bring it to my readers this Second Edition of Practical Casebook: Child Health Nursing for GNM and Post Basic BSc Nursing Students. This new edition has been updated to reflect the dynamic pediatric health care environment, essential procedures, safety initiatives and upgradation of pediatric nursing practice. As in our previous edition, the concept, content, examples and illustrated diagrams were designed with the goal of assisting the GNM and Post Basic BSc Nursing students and teachers to make the transition to best nurse practitioners.

This edition mainly focused on the necessary updates in practical knowledge and skills needed by the student nurse as an integral member of healthcare industry essential team and nurse manager of holistic child health care. Student practical requirement related learning Issues and nursing care priorities, delegation of child health care, health care quality improvement, biophysiological parameters of pediatric nursing, and advanced clinical procedures are updated in this edition. This edition makes our GNM and Post Basic BSc Nursing students complete their child health nursing clinical requirements within stipulated time duration. This edition focuses on the improvement of current quality and safety issues and initiatives impacting the current healthcare industry. We continue to bring you comprehensive, holistic updated practical information on developing a nursing student career.

This edition made for pediatric nursing students, this Casebook covered all the child health nursing subject related practical requirements with reference materials, as per newly revised INC (Indian nursing council) syllabus. The main concept of this edition is availability of all the practical reference notes and exam point of view content was enriched. This edition will help the students to attend their practical examination with full confident and secure more numbers. A genuine time has been spent in the revision of this Practical Casebook and this edition will help the pediatric nursing students to complete their practical requirement on time without any trouble.

This edition will help the pediatric nursing teachers to monitor and evaluate the students continuously without any burden. This casebook helps the clinician instructed to teach and guide their students in clinical area itself without any further reference. They can evaluate the clinical performance of the students instantly. This edition is user-friendly and techno friendly to teachers and students.

Constructive criticism and comments for further enrichment of this casebook are always heartily welcome. I hope my hard work will be useful to all the pediatric nursing students and clinical nurses. Kindly email me at sudhakarsumith8@gmail.com

"Never stop learning, for when we stop learning, we stop growing, so keep learning".

Sudhakar A

Preface to the First Edition

This practical casebook is meant for the GNM and Post Basic BSc Nursing students. It covers all the child health nursing practical requirements as per the newly revised Indian Nursing Council (INC) syllabus. The main concept of this practical casebook is to minimize the students' writing schedule and make them comfortable in studies.

I decided to take up this project with the spirit of my hard-work schedule to help the pediatric nursing students to complete their requirements on time and without difficulties.

Pediatric nursing students are spending more time in making and filling up the records. In this schedule, our students are wasting a lot of time and they would not get sufficient time to prepare for their board/university examinations. For this reason, most of the students have requested me to do something to get more time for studying rather than writing. Based on their humble request, I decided to reduce their writing burden. At the same time, they should complete their requirements on time without fail. I expect that after using this practical casebook, the pediatric nursing students will improve their independent practice, and good judgment skills in their subject. Also the students can update their knowledge and have positive attitude towards the care of the child health.

I hope this practical casebook will satisfy the GNM and Post Basic BSc Nursing students, child health nursing students and it will fulfill their expectations towards the completion of the practical requirements without delay.

I hope this casebook will be user-friendly and cost-effective for the students and teachers.

Constructive criticism and comments for further enrichment of this casebook are always heartily welcome.

I hope my hard work will be useful to all the pediatric nursing students and clinical nurses.

'Learn comfortably and work with joy and happiness.'

Sudhakar A

Acknowledgments

This is my duty to say sincere gratitude to the Almighty for His love and kind grace in the completion of this book. Here by I credit my lovable thanks to my parents Mr P Anumanthan and Mrs Dhanalakshmi, who helped me succeed in all walks of life.

I feel honored to convey my special thanks and gratitude to our respected Secretary Swami Muktinathananda Ji, Ramakrishna Mission Sevashrama, Lucknow, Uttar Pradesh, India for his special prayer and blessings for the completion of my project successfully.

I feel honored to covey my special thanks and gratitude to our honorable Director Dr AK Kaushik and Managing director Dr. Kiran Kaushik Popular Group of Hospitals and Popular Group of Academics, for their great support and Blessing for the completion of my project successfully.

This is my great job to say thanks to my respected Research Director cum Guide Professor Dr K Revathi, MAHER (Deemed to be University), Chennai, for her special guidance and support to complete my project.

I wish to express my special thanks to our honorable Research Co-Guide Professor Dr Vaijayanthi Mala (MAHER Deemed to be University), Chennai, for her truthful prayers and efforts to complete this project successfully.

This is my great job to say thanks to my principal respected Professor Dr A Jayasudha, Who make me to grand success of this book.

I would like to take the opportunity to thank respected Dr Sathish Kumar Jayapal and Professor Dr Judi Arulappan who have helped and inspired me to take up this project.

I wish to express my special thanks to our honorable Professor DLS Agrahari BHU-IMS College of Nursing, Varanasi for his truthful prayer and efforts to complete this project successfully.

I wish to express my special thanks to my dear close friends Mr Srinivasan, Nursing Officer, AIIMS, Bhubaneswar and Mr Nagaraj, Nursing Officer, Tamil Nadu government for their truthful efforts to make this project success.

I convey my loveable thanks to my dear wife Mrs Syama Sudhakar and my sister-in-law Mrs Hema Anil NS who gave an encouragement to complete this book.

I convey my heartfelt thanks to my dear sweet daughters SS Jayani Sree and SS Navanya Sree for showing enough patience and sacrifices at the time of my project work and also for the contribution of their photographs in this project.

I convey my special thanks to my dear Father and Mother-in-law Mr Sankaran and Mrs Umadevi for their special prayer to complete my project grand success.

I express my deep sense of gratitude and thanks to my brother and Mr A Gajendra Prasad and sister-in-law G Sathya and their children Ms Pooja Hashmi and Mr Bhavan, for rendering emotional support during the hardworking period for preparation of this project.

My sincere thanks are due to all my seniors, colleagues and friends who encourage me to write this clinical book.

I convey my heartfelt thanks to Respected Late Mr Akash Saini, Assistant Area Manager, Jaypee Brothers Medical Publishers who has helped me timely to publish this practical record book successfully.

I am very grateful to the whole team of M/s Jaypee Brothers Medical Publishers (P) Ltd, New Delhi, India, who helped and guided me, Shri Jitendar P Vij (Group Chairman), Mr Ankit Vij (Managing Director), Mr MS Mani (Group President), Dr Madhu Choudhary (Publishing Head–Education), Ms Pooja Bhandari (Production Head), Ms Sunita Katla (Executive Assistant to Group Chairman and Publishing Manager), Ms Samina Khan (Executive Assistant to Publishing Head–Education), Ms Seema Dogra (Cover Visualizer) and their team members, for all their support to work in this project and make it a success. Without their cooperation, I could not have completed this project.

Contents

Student Profile

Name of Student : ....

Register No./Enroll No. : ....

Course/Year : ....

Subject : ....

Batch : ....

Name of Exam Board/University : ....

Name of the Institute : ....

....

Address of the Institute : ....

....

....

....

Signature of Student   **Subject Coordinator/HOD**   **Principal**

OVERALL PRACTICAL EVALUATION OF THE STUDENT

Practical Mark Sheet

S. No.	Requirements Details	Maximum Marks	Minimum Marks	Marks Obtaineds	Remarks Pass/Fail
1.	Growth and Developmental Assessment	50	25		
2.	Medical Care Plan	25	12.5		
3.	Surgical Care Plan	25	12.5		
4.	Medical Case Study	50	25		
5.	Surgical Case Study	50	25		
6.	Case Presentation	50	25		
7.	Health Talk	50	25		
8.	Observation Report	50	25		
9.	**Field Visit**	–	–	–	–
	a. Anganwadi School	25	12.5		
	b. School for Mentally Challenged Children	25	12.5		
	c. School for Blind/Deaf and Dumb Children	25	12.5		
	d. Juvenile Delinquency School	25	12.5		
10.	Drug Study	25	12.5		
11.	Clinical Evaluation	100	50		
12.	Model Practical Exam	100	50		
	Total Marks	**675**	**338**		

Signature of Student   **Subject Coordinator/HOD**   **Principal**

INTERNAL ASSESSMENT MARKS

Internal Assessment Marks: 50

Total Marks obtained by the Student	:................. 40 Marks
Behaviour/Attitude of the Student	:.................. 5 Marks
Attendance Percentage of the Student	:.................. 5 Marks

Students Obtained IA Marks　　　　　　.........../50 Marks

Internal assessment formula:

$$\frac{\text{Total obtained practical marks}}{\text{Total Maximum practical marks}} \times 40$$

Signature of Student　　　　　　**Subject Coordinator/HOD**　　　　　　**Principal**

CHILD HEALTH NURSING

Practical Requirements

University/Board Examiner Evaluation Checklist

II.	Developmental Study (Growth and Developmental Assessment)	Number of Requirements	Signature of Students	Signature of the Teacher
1.	Neonate/Newborn Baby	1		
2.	Infants	1		
3.	Toddler	1		
4.	Preschooler	1		
5.	School Going Children	1		
6.	Adolescents	1		
III.	**Nursing Care Plan**			
1.	Medical Care Plan	1		
2.	Surgical Care Plan	1		
IV.	**Nursing Case Study**			
1.	Medical Case Study	1		
2.	Surgical Case Study	1		
3.	Case Presentation	1		
4.	Health Talk	1		
V.	**Observation Report**			
1.	Care of Baby in Critical Care Units [Preterm Baby]	1		
VI.	**Drug Study**			
VII.	**Field Visit**			
1.	Anganwadi School/Under-Five Clinic	1		
2.	School for Mentally Challenged Children	1		
3.	School for Blind/Deaf and Dumb Children	1		
4.	Juvenile Delinquency School	1		
VIII.	**Clinical Evaluation of the Students**			
1.	Over all Clinical Performance of the Students	1		

Internal Examiner

Mr/Mrs.........................

Date :......./....../...20.......

External Examiner

Mr/Mrs...

Date :.........../.........../20............

Pediatric Case Assessment: Tools and Techniques

1. Anthropometric Measurement Tool

2. Pediatric History Collection Tools

3. Apgar Score

4. Gestational Age Assessment (Ballard Score)

5. Fluid Calculation

6. General Formula Used to Assess the Child Health

7. Dehydration Assessment Tool

8. Administration of Oral, IM, and IV Medication

9. Pain Assessment Scale

10. Baby Bath/Sponge Bath

11. Glasgow Coma Scoring Scale

12. Feeding Children by Katori-Spoon, and Paladai Cup

13. Feeding: Nasogastric, Gastrostomy and Jejunostomy

14. Care of Surgical Wounds: Dressing and Suture Removal

15. Nutritional Assessment

16. Application of Restraints

17. Administration of Oxygen Inhalation by Different Methods

18. Procedure on Bowel Wash

19. Procedure on Insertion of Suppositories

20. Enema

21. Urinary Catheterization and Drainage

22. Care of Baby in Incubator/Radiant Warmer

23. Care of a Child on Ventilator

24. Continuous Positive Airway Pressure

25. Administration of Fluid with Infusion Pumps

PEDIATRIC CASE ASSESSMENT: TOOLS AND TECHNIQUES

Definition of Nursing

Nursing encompasses autonomous and collaborative care of individuals of all ages, families, groups and communities, sick or well and in all settings. It includes the promotion of health, the prevention of illness, and the care of ill, disabled and dying people.
                                                  —World Health Organization (WHO)

Definition of Pediatric Nursing

Pediatrics can be defined as the branch of medical science that deals with the care of the children, from conception to adolescence (birth to 18 years), in health and illness. It is concerned with preventive, curative, and rehabilitative care of children.

Normal Vital Signs

Age groups	Respiration rate/minute	Heart rate	Blood pressure
Neonates/newborn baby	40 breath/mts	140 beats/mts	65/45 mm Hg
1–2 years	30 breath/mts	110 beats/mts	75/50 mm Hg
3–7 years	30 breath/mts	100 beats/mts	90/60 mm Hg
8–9 years	30 breath/mts	90 beats/mts	95/65 mm Hg
10–18 years	20 breath/mts	90 beats/mts	100/70 mm Hg
Adults	18 breath/mts	80 beats/mts	120/80 mm Hg

ANTHROPOMETRIC MEASUREMENT TOOL

Definition

Anthropometric measurement is defined as the study of human body measurements especially on a comparative basis. It is a science which deals with the measurement of the size, weight, and proportions of the human body (Dorland's Medical Dictionary). This procedure will concentrate on noninvasive techniques of determining these parameters.

The term **anthropometric** refers to comparative measurements of the body. Anthropometric measurements are used in nutritional assessments. Those that are used to assess growth and development in infants, children, and adolescents include length, height, weight, weight-for-length, and head circumference (length is used in infants and toddlers, rather than height, because they are unable to stand). Individual measurements are usually compared to reference standards on a growth chart.

Parameters

- Weight measurement
- Height measurement
- Head circumference
- Chest circumference
- Midarm circumference
- Abdominal circumference.

Weight Measurement Technique

- At birth baby weight is 2.5–3 kg
- Double the birth weight by 5 months = 5–6 kg
- Triple the birth weight by 1 year = 7.5–9 kg.

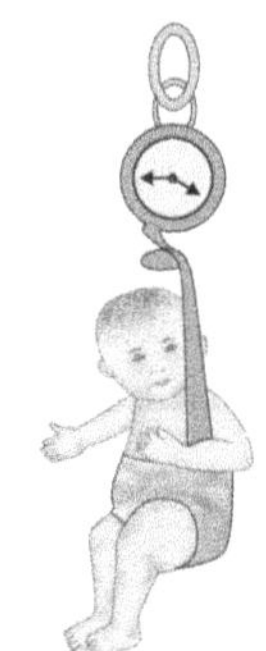

Technique

- Explain the procedures to parents
- Handwash
- Check the weighing machine reading, it should be 'zero' level

- Remove the cloths and place the weight machine (digital and manual)
- While reading the weight use the play materials for accurate reading
- Take the reading and document.

Height Measurement Technique

- At birth baby height is 50 cm (20 inch)
- Average height is 48 to 52 cm (18 to 22 inch)

Formula for pound to weight conversion

$$\Rightarrow \frac{\text{Pound}}{2.2 \text{ kg}}$$

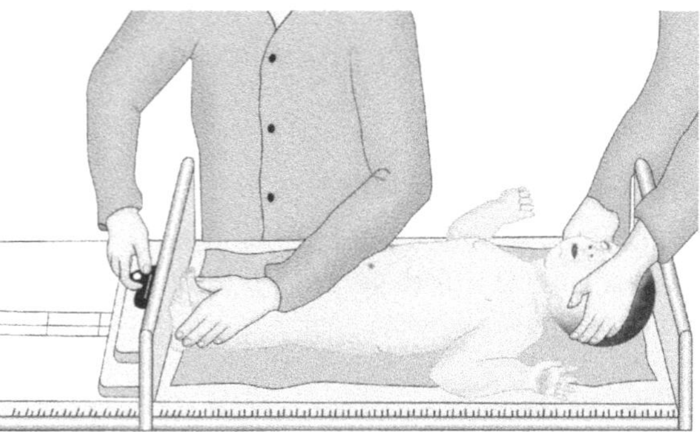

Technique

- Explain the procedures to parents
- Handwash
- Check the infantometer, it should be working condition
- Place the baby in supine position (digital and manual)
- Ask the child to stand in straight position over the height machine
- Before reading the height observe the child position
- Child head, shoulder, buttocks and heel should touch the measurement board
- While reading the weight use the play materials for accurate reading
- Take the reading and document.

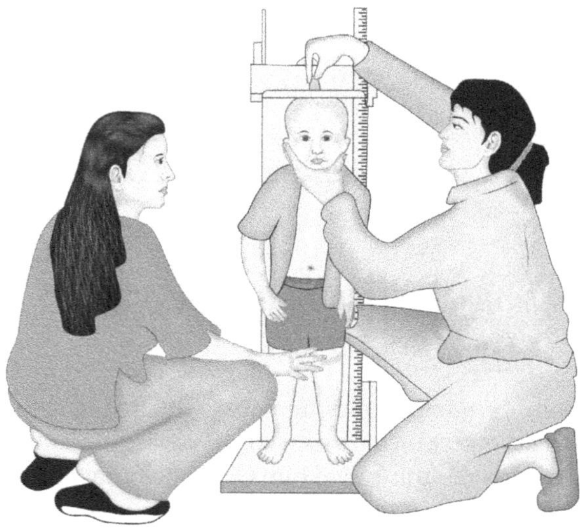

Head Circumference Technique

- At birth baby head circumference is 33–35 cm (13–14 inch)
- Average head circumference is 33–37 cm (13 to 15 inch)
- The 6 month baby head circumference is 42–44.5 cm (16.5–17.5 inch)
- The 1 year baby head circumference is 45–47.5 cm (17.7–17.7 inch)
- During the 1 year there is 12 cm increased in head circumference
- The 1– 5 years of age the child will gain 5 cm
- Adult head size is achieved between 5 to 6 years.

Technique

- Explain the procedures to parents
- Handwash
- Check the inch tape, it should be working condition
- Place the infant baby in supine position over the bed
- Provide the comfort position to child
- Child head should be measures around the skull
- Hold the measurement tape over the occipital, parital bone (above the earlobe) and forehead
- While reading the weight use the play materials for accurate reading
- Take the reading and document.

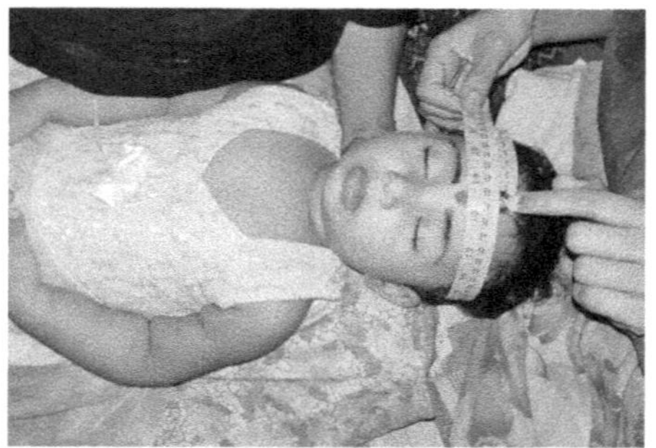
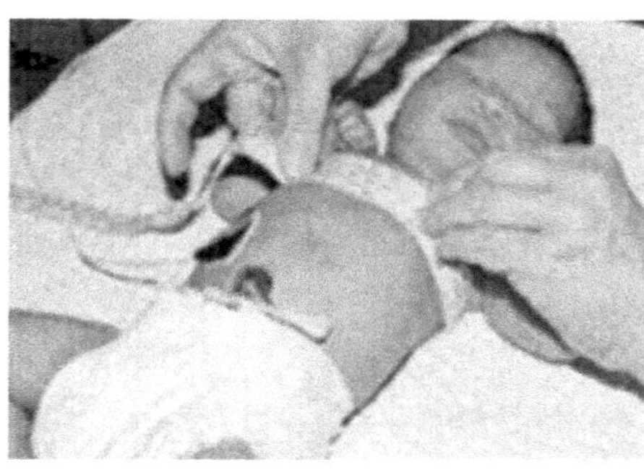
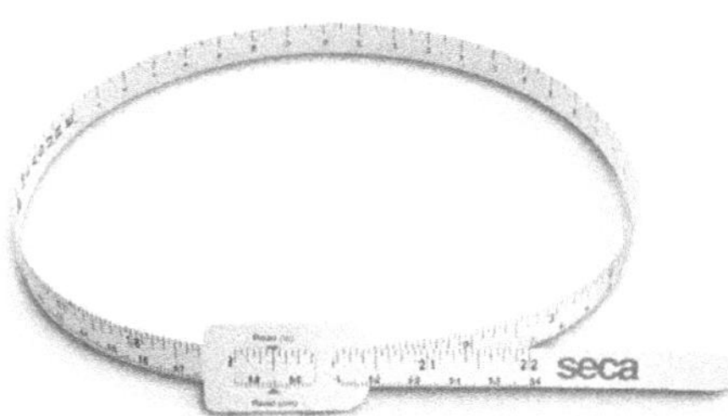

Chest Circumference Measurement Technique

- At birth baby chest circumference is 32–34 cm
- Average chest circumference is 31–33 cm
- At the time of 1 year head and chest will be equal.

Technique

- Explain the procedures to parents
- Handwash
- Check the inch tape, it should be working condition
- Place the infant baby in supine position over the bed
- Provide the comfort position to child
- Child chest should be measures around the thoracic cavity
- Hold the measurement tape around chest between the breast nipples
- While reading the weight use the play materials for accurate reading
- Take the reading and document.

Midarm Circumference Measurement Technique

- During the 1–5 years of age it remains reasonably static between 15–17 cm among healthy child
- It is conventionally measured over the left upper arm, at the point marked midway between acromion process (shoulder) and olecranon process (elbow) with arm bent at right angle to measure
- To ask the child to site or standing position
- Ask child to hold the hand loose and comfortable
- Reading less than 12.5 cm it indicates severe malnutrition
- Reading between 12.5 and 13.5 cm it indicates moderate malnutrition.

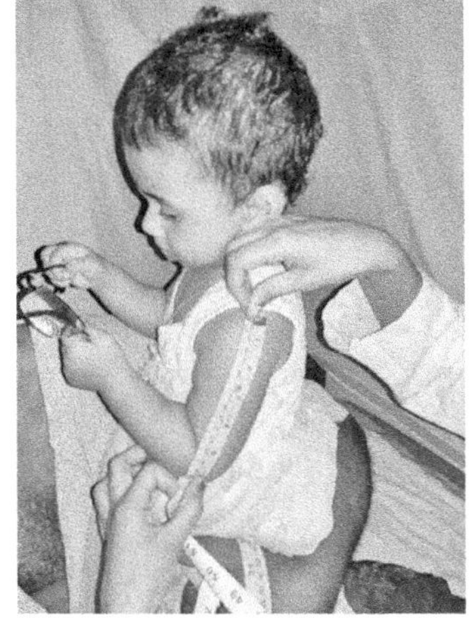

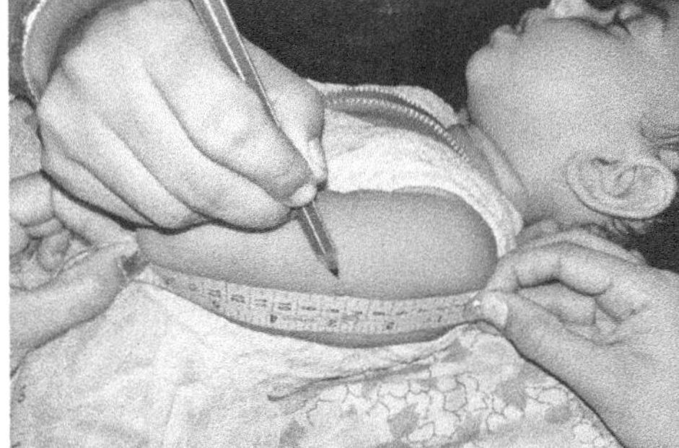

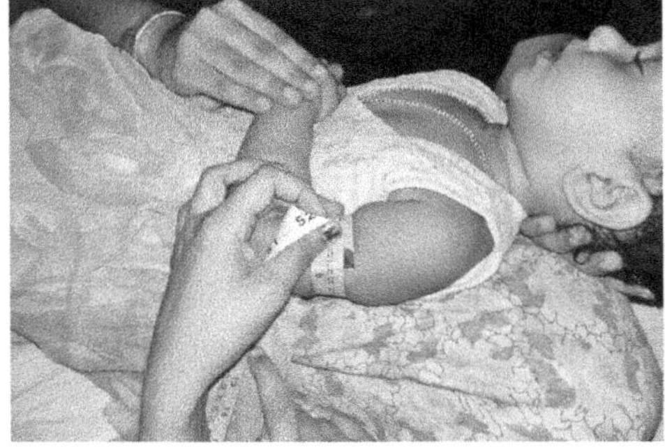

Step 1: Measuring acromion process (shoulder) to olecranon process (elbow) with arm bent at right angle

Step 2: Measuring midway between upper arm

Step 3: Measuring the reading around the midway of upper arm

Abdominal Circumference Measurement Technique

- At birth baby abdominal circumference is 32 cm (12.5 inch)
- Average abdominal circumference is 31–33 cm.

Technique

- Explain the procedures to parents
- Handwash
- Check the inch tape, it should be working condition
- Place the infant baby in supine position over the bed
- Provide the comfort position to child
- Child chest should be measures around the abdomen cavity

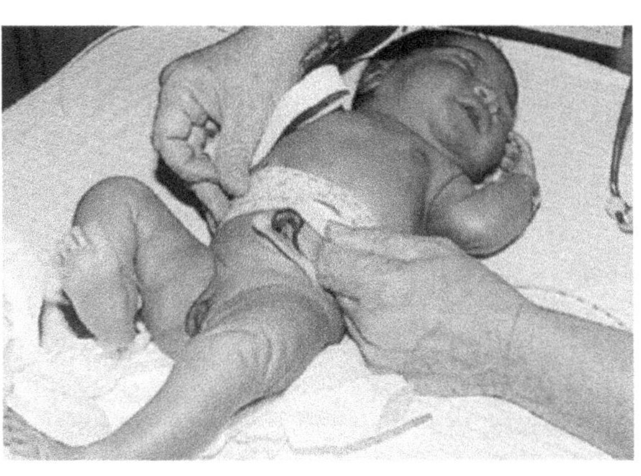

- Hold the measurement tape around abdomen (0.5 cm above the umbilicus)
- While reading the measurement, nurse should use the play materials
- Take the reading and document.

PEDIATRIC HISTORY COLLECTION TOOLS

A collection of complete history on a child parents not only is necessary, but also leads to the correct diagnosis in the vast majority of children. The history usually is obtained from the child parents and the older child, or the caretaker of sick children. After learning the fundamentals of collecting and recording the historical data, the nuances associated with the giving of information must be interpreted.

Aims

- Direct comprehensive examination and investigation of the sick child
- Formulate a correct diagnosis (or form a differential diagnosis)
- Establish the background of a child's illness (psychological, family and social circumstances)
- Explain and maintain a good relationship with the child and parents. This helps child and parent(s) to accord with the advice given by the healthcare professional
- Use the interaction with the child and parent's as part of the therapeutic process
- Use the understanding and knowledge of context and background to tailor pragmatic, appropriate treatment strategies
- Take an overview of the child's previous and current state of health to anticipate or identify any problems which may not be immediately apparent.

Always ask to Parents 'BIFIDA'

B-Birth details and problems

I-Immunization history

F-Feeding problems

I-Infection and exposure details

D-Developmental history

A-Allergic reaction.

The Pediatric Life Threatening Events

The MISFITS

The MISFITS can be guide in managing very young children who admitted in emergency department with serious life-threatening events. The emergency nurse always remembers that while assessing the child must follow 'THE MISFITS', assessment tool.

T	• Trauma
H	• Heart diseases or hypovolemia
E	• Electrolyte disturbance
M	• Metabolic disturbance
I	• Inborn erros of metabolism
S	• Sepsis
F	• Formula dilution or over concentration
I	• Intestinal catastrophe
T	• Toxins
S	• Seizures or CNS abnormalities

APGAR SCORE

APGAR is an essential and emergency test performed on a baby soon after the birth in labour room, 1 and 5 minutes assessment can be performed after the birth. The 1-minute score determines the baby can adjust delivering process. The 5–minute score will help to assess the baby can be adopted the extrauterine life without any difficulty.

The APGAR score was developed in 1952 by an anesthesiologist named Virginia Apgar, it referred to as an acronym for:

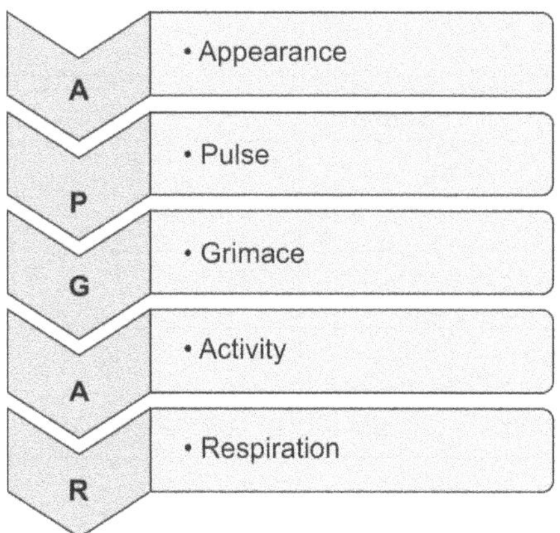

The 'APGAR' Score

The Apgar score Signs		0-Points	1-Points	2-Points	Total Score
A	Appearance (skin Color)	The baby's whole body is completely bluish-gray or pale	Good color in body with bluish hands or feet	Good color all over	
P	Pulse (heart rate)	Absent/no heart rate	Less than 100 beats per minute	At least 100 beats per minute	
G	Grimace (reflex response)	Absent (no response to stimulation)	Grimace during suctioning/stimulation	Grimace and pull away, cough, or sneeze during suctioning	
A	Activity (muscle tone)	Absent of the limp movements	Some flexion of arms and legs	Active motion	
R	Respiration (breathing)	Not breathing	Weak cry; may sound like whimpering, slow or irregular breathing	Good, strong cry; normal rate and effort of breathing	

Severely depressed	0–03
Moderately depressed	04–06
Excellent condition	07–10

GESTATIONAL AGE ASSESSMENT (BALLARD SCORE)

To determine the approximate gestational age of a newborn, you will assess six neuromuscular and six physical characteristics. This assessment, the New Ballard Score, is appropriate for newborns from 20 to 44 weeks of gestation, with the characteristics to assess varying with the stage of maturity. Each parameter scores from minus 2 to 5, with the cumulative score correlating with a gestational age between 26 and 44 weeks.

Timing of the gestational assessment influences the accuracy of its results. For newborns younger than 26 gestational weeks, perform the assessment sooner than 12 hours after birth. For newborns beyond 26 gestational weeks, perform the examination within 96 hours of birth. Overall, it is best to perform the examination within 48 hours of birth. This assessment information is essential because gestation relates directly to the likelihood of complications during the newborn period. Lower scores correlate with prematurity; higher scores correlate with postmaturity. Commercially printed worksheets are available to use when performing this assessment.

Maturational Assessment of Gestational Age (New Ballard Score)

Name of the child: .... IP No.: ....

Date/time of birth: .... Date/time of exam: ....

Age when examined: .... Sex: ....

Birth weight: .... Length: ....

Head circumference: .... Examiner: ....

APGAR score: 1 Minute .... 5 Minutes ....

Neuromuscular Maturity

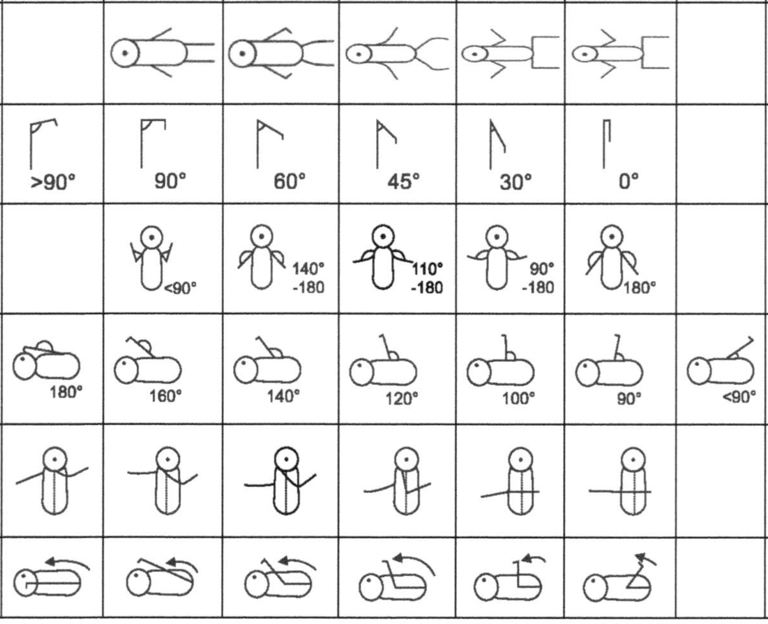

Neuromuscular maturity sign	Score							Record score here
	−1	0	1	2	3	4	5	
Posture								
Square window (wrist)	>90°	90°	60°	45°	30°	0°		
Arm recoil		<90°	140°–180	110°–180	90°–180	180°		
Popliteal angle	180°	160°	140°	120°	100°	90°	<90°	
Scarf sign								
Heel to ear								
Total neuromuscular maturity score								

	Score
Neuromuscular:	
Physical:	
Total:	

Maturity Rating

Score	Weeks
−10	20
−5	22
0	24
5	26
10	28
15	30
20	32
25	34
30	36
35	38
40	40
45	42
50	44

Physical Maturity

Physical maturity sign	Score							Record score here
	−1	0	1	2	3	4	5	
Skin	Sticky, friable, transparent	Gelatinous, red, translucent	Smooth pink, visible veins	Superficial peeling and/or rash, few veins	Cracking, pale areas, rare veins	Parchment, deep cracking, no vessels	Leathery, cracked, wrinkled	
Lanugo	None	Sparse	Abundant	Thinning	Bald areas	Mostly bald		
Plantar surface	Heel-toe 40–50 mm: −1< 40 mm: −2	>50 mm no crease	Faint red marks	Anterior transverse crease only	Creases ant. 2/3	Creases over entire sole		
Breast	Imperceptible	Barely perceptable	Flat areola no bud	Stippled areola 1–2 mm bud	Raised areola 3–4 mm bud	Full areola 5–10 mm bud		
Eye/ear	Lids fused loosely:−1 tightly:−2	Lids open pinna flat stays folded	Sl. Curved pinna; soft; slow recoil	Well-curved pinna; soft but ready recoil	Formed and firm instant recoil	Thick cartilage ear stiff		
Genitals (male)	Scrotum flat, smooth	Scrotum empty, faint rugae	Testes in upper canal, rare rugae	Testes descending, few rugae	Testes down, good rugae	Testes pendulous, deep rugae		
Genitals (female)	Clitoris prominent and labia flat	Prominent clitoris and small labia minora	Prominent clitoris and enlarging minora	Majora and minora equally prominent	Majora large, minora small	Majora cover clitoris and minora		
Total physical maturity score								

FLUID CALCULATION

The understanding of the principles of fluid and electrolyte balance is vital for the maintenance of stable internal environment. This is even more essential infants who have less reserves of body water and electrolytes and in newborn babies who may be deficient of the homeostatic mechanism to protect them against the changes related to abnormal losses. Thus, it is important to assess the nature and magnitude of any disturbance in different clinical situations and at different ages because correction of the imbalance is essential for speedy recovery.

- Very young infants are vulnerable to more water loss because of physiological inability of their renal tubules to concentrate.
- Higher metabolic rate and larger surface area compared to total body weight in young infants favor rapid fluid loss. Unless fluids are adequately replaced in the presence of continued loss dehydration and consequences of dehydration are likely to set in.
- Larger turnover is another problem in young infants. An infant exchanges about one-half of his or her ECF everyday compared to one-seventh in an adult.
- Thirst mechanism is very effective in older children and adults compared to very young infants. In the presence of excessive water loss, young infants do not express their thirst for fluids effectively when there is a negative balance of intake during water loss.

Fluid Measurement Values

1 mL	15 drops
1 Liter	1000 mL (1000 × 15 = 15,000 drops)
1 Tablespoon	15 mL
1 Teaspoon	5 mL
1 ounce	30 mL

Drops Factors

Normal IV set 1 mL   = 16 macro drops

Micro volume 1 mL   = 60 micro drops

Example

40 mL/hr   = 40 × 16

Macro drops = 40 × 16/60 = 12 drops/mts.

Micro drops = 40 × 60/60 = 40 drops/mts.

Formula for Calculation of Daily Fluid Requirements

4:2:1 Method

Body weight	Fluid/hour	Fluid/day
0–10 kg	4 mL/kg/hour	100/kg/day
11–20 kg	40 mL/kg/hour + 2 mL/kg/hour	1000 mL + 50 mL/kg for each kg
Above 20 kg	60 mL/kg/hour + 1 mL/kg/hour	1500 mL + 20 mL for each kg.

Key note

- 4 mL/kg/hr for 1st 10 kg
- Adding 2 mL/kg/hour for second 10 kg
- Adding 1 mL/kg/hour for each kg over 20 kg

* Adding 1st 10 kg 1000 mL/day + (50 mL/each kg/day)

* Adding 1st 20 kg 1500 mL/day + (20 mL/each kg/day)

Example : 1 hour Based/Day Based

Name of the child: Master Raju

Age: 1 year

Actual weight of child: 8 kg

1. Formula: 4 mL/kg/hour

    = 8 × 4 = 32 mL/hour

2. Formula: 100 mL/kg/hour

    = 8 × 100 = 800 mL/day

Example : 2 hours Based/Day Based

Name of the child: Master Suresh

Age: 3 years

Actual weight of child: 15 kg

1. Formula: 40 mL/kg/hour + 2 mL/kg/hour

    = First 10 kg 40 mL/hour (see the note)

    = 5 × 2 = 10 mL + 40 mL

    = 50 mL/hours

2. Formula: 1000 mL + 50 mL/kg for each kg

    = 1000 mL + (50 × 5 = 250 mL) = 1250 mL/day

Example : 3 hours Based

Name of the child: Master Saravanan

Age: 5 years

Actual weight of child: 25 kg

1. Formula: 60 mL/kg/hour +1 mL/kg/hour

    = First 20 kg 60 mL/hour (see the note)

    = 5 × 1 = 5 + 60 = 65 mL/hour

Example : 4 days Based

Name of the child: Master Saravanan

Age: 5 years

Actual weight of child: 25 kg

2. Formula: 1500 mL + 20 mL/kg for each kg

    = 1500 mL + (20 × 5 = 100 mL) = 1600 mL/day

Intravenous fluid (Drops) calculation formula

$$\frac{\text{Total volume of fluid (mL)}}{\text{Total hours} \times 60} \times 15 \text{ Drops}$$

Example

$$\frac{1500 \text{ mL} \times 15 \text{ drops}}{12 \times 60} = \frac{22,500}{720} = \textbf{31.25 drops/minute}$$

GENERAL FORMULA USED TO ASSESS THE CHILD HEALTH

Expected Weight and Height of Normal Children

According to 'Ballpark'

1. Average birth weight is   : 2.5–3 kg
2. Double the birth weight by the 5 months   : 5–6 kg
3. Triple the birth weight by one year   : 7.5–9 kg

According to 'Werch's' Formula

Weight

- At birth   : 2.5–3 kg
- 3–12 months : Age in months + 9/2
- 1–6 years   : Age in years × 2 +8
- 7–12 years   : Age in years × 7–5/2

Height

- At birth = 50 cm/20 inches
- At 1 year = 75 cm/30 inches

2 to 12 years

- Age in years × 6 + 77 (cm)
- Age in years × 2 + 30 (inches)

<table>
<tr><td>

Example: 1

Name of the child: Master Varun

Age	: 5 months
Sex	: Male

Formula : Age in months + 9/2

$$\frac{5+9}{2} = \frac{14}{2} = \textbf{7 kg}$$

</td><td>

Example: 2

Name of the child: Master Raja

Age	: 2 years
Sex	: Male

Formula : Age in years × 2 + 8

= 2 × 2 + 8

= 4 + 8

= **12 kg**

</td></tr>
<tr><td>

Example: 3

Name of the child: Master Kumar

Age	: 8 years
Sex	: Male

Formula: Age in years × 7–5/2

$$\frac{8+7}{2} = \frac{56-5}{2} = \textbf{25.5 kg}$$

</td><td>

Height Example:

Name of the child: Master Shiva

Age	: 5 years
Sex	: Male

Formula: Age in years × 6 + 77 (cm)

= 5 + 6

= 30 + 77 = **107 cm**

</td></tr>
</table>

Malnutrition Assessment Formula

$$\frac{\text{Actual weight of the child}}{\text{Expected weight of the child}} \times 100$$

Classification of Nutritional Status

Nutritional status	Expected weight for age	Presence of edema
Normal	More than 80%	No
Under nutrition	60–80%	No
Kwashiorkor	60–80%	Yes
Marasmus	Less than 60%	No
Marasmus and Kwashiorkor	Less than 60%	Yes

Degree of Malnutrition (According to IAP)

Grade of malnutrition	Weight for age standard (mean)%	Severity
Normal	>80%	Normal
Grade 1	71–80%	Mild
Grade 2	61–70%	Moderate
Grade 3	51–60%	Severe
Grade 4	<51%	Very severe

DEHYDRATION ASSESSMENT TOOL

First assess your patient for dehydration				
	A	**B**	**C**	**D**
Step 1: • Look at general conditions • Eyes • Thirst	Well alert eyes are normal not thirsty and drinks normally	• Irritable and restless • Sunken eyes • Thirsty and drinks eagerly	• Floppy, lethargic or unconscious • Sunken eyes • Drinks poorly or not able to drink	• SHOCK • Unconscious not able to drink
Step 2: Feel—pinch the skin	Goes back immediately	Goes back slowly	Goes back very slowly More than 2 seconds	As in C plus capillary refill more than 3 seconds, cold hands
Step 3: Decide degree of dehydration	No signs or dehydration	Two or more signs means some dehydration	Two or more signs means severe dehydration	SHOCK
Step 4: Treat	Use treatment plan A	Use treatment plan B	Use treatment plan currently	Treat shock very urgently

Signs	Mild	Moderate	Severe
Severe weight loss	Up to 5%	6–10%	More than 10%
Appearance	Active, alert	Irritable, alert, thirsty	Lethargic, looks sick
Capillary filling (compared to your own)	Normal	Slightly delayed	Delayed
Pulse	Normal	Fast, low volume	Very fast, thready
Respiration	Normal	Fast	Fast and deep
Blood pressure	Normal	Normal or low orthostatic hypotension	Very low
Mucous membranes	Moist	Dry	Parched
Tears	Present	Less than expected	Absent
Eyes	Normal	Normal	Sunken
Pinched skin	Springs back	Tents briefly	Prolonged tenting
Fontanel (infant sitting)	Normal	Sunken slightly	Sunken significantly
Urine flow	Normal	Reduced	Severely reduced

Note

- A 10 kg child who is 5% dehydrated will weigh 9.5 kg.
- A 10 kg child who is 10% dehydrated will weigh 9 kg.
- A 5 kg child who is 10% dehydrated will weigh 4.5 kg.

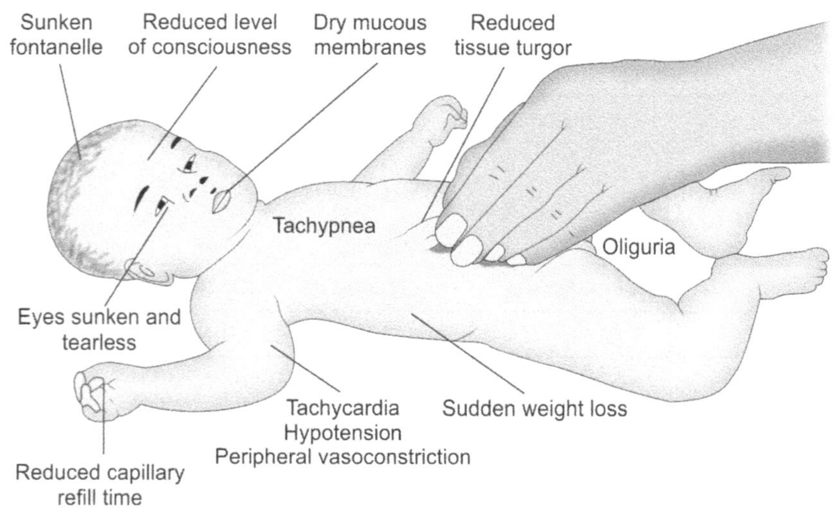

Dehydration assessment technique

Table: Classification of dehydration

Type of dehydration	Abnormality	Possible causes
Isotonic	• Equal loss of water and sodium from extra-cellular volume • Does not cause osmotic water shift from intra-cellular volume	• Gastrointestinal fluid losses (e.g. vomitting, diarrhea)
Hypertonic	• Water loss exceeds sodium loss • Intra-cellular volume is reduced because of osmotic shift of water into extra-cellular volume • Sometimes called intra-cellular dehydration	• Inadequate water intake because of a defective thirst center, unconsciousness, lack of available water or inability to drink • Excessive perspiration loss • Osmotic diuresis (i.e. loss of water due to glucose in urine) • Diuretic therapy with insufficient water intake
Hypotonic	• Sodium loss exceeds water loss • Intra-cellular volume is expanded because of osmotic shift of water from extra-cellular volume into cells • Sometimes called extra-cellular dehydration	• Excessive perspiration or other gastrointestinal fluid losses • Water replacement without sodium replacement • Diuretic therapy with excessive unrestricted water intake

ADMINISTRATION OF ORAL, IM, AND IV MEDICATION

Oral Route Administration

The medicine can be administered orally as liquids, capsules, tablets, or chewable tablets. Because the oral route is the most convenient and usually the safest and least expensive, it is the one most often used. However, it has limitations because of the way a drug typically moves through the digestive tract. For drugs administered orally, absorption may begin in the mouth and stomach. However, most drugs are usually absorbed from the small intestine. The drug passes through the intestinal wall and travels to the liver before being transported via the bloodstream to its target site. The intestinal wall and liver chemically alter (metabolize) many drugs, decreasing the amount of drug reaching the bloodstream.

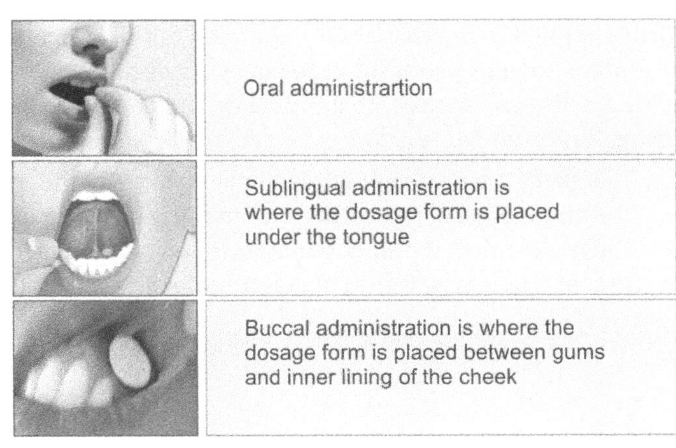

Sublingual and Buccal Routes Administration

A few drugs are placed under the tongue (taken sublingually) or between the gums and teeth (buccally) so that they can dissolve and be absorbed directly into the small blood vessels that lie beneath the tongue. These drugs are not swallowed. The sublingual route is especially good for nitroglycerin, which is used to relieve angina, because absorption is rapid and the drug immediately enters the bloodstream without first passing through the intestinal wall and liver.

Sublingual and Buccal Administration of Drugs

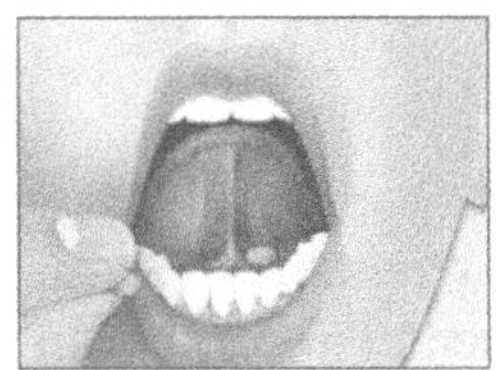

Inhalation Route Administration

A medicine administered by inhalation through the mouth must be atomized into smaller droplets than those administered by the nasal route, so that the drugs can pass through the windpipe (trachea) and into the lungs. Smaller droplets go deeper, which increases the amount of drug absorbed. Inside the lungs, they are absorbed into the bloodstream.

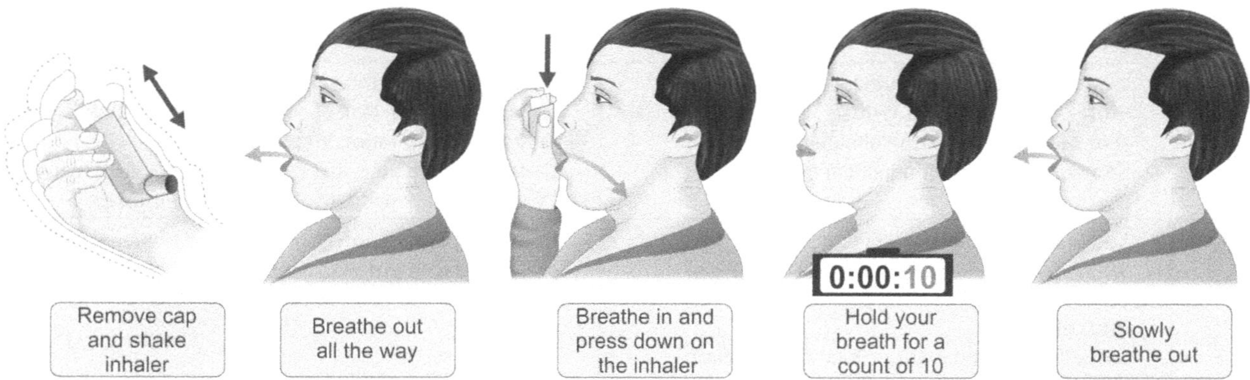

Cutaneous/Topical Route Administration

Drugs applied to the skin are usually used for their local effects and thus are most commonly used to treat superficial skin disorders, such as psoriasis, eczema, skin infections (viral, bacterial, and fungal), itching, and dry skin. The drug is mixed with inactive substances. Depending on the consistency of the inactive substances, the formulation may be an ointment, cream, lotion, solution, powder, or gel (see Topical Preparations).

- The use of eye drops containing beta blockers in the treatment of glaucoma
- The application of topical steroids in the management of dermatitis
- The use of inhaled bronchodilators in the treatment of asthma
- The insertion of pessaries containing clotrimazole in the treatment of vaginal candidiasis.

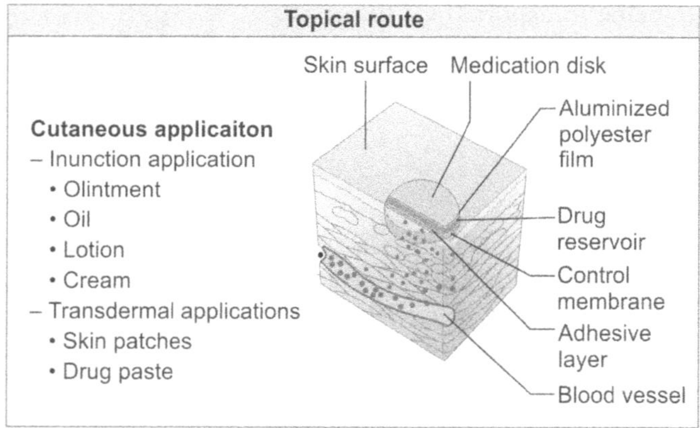

Rectal Administration

The rectal route has considerable disadvantages in terms of patient acceptability and unpredictable drug absorption but it does offer a number of benefits. It offers a valuable means of localized drug delivery into the large bowel, for example the use of rectal steroids in the form of enemas or suppositories in the treatment of inflammatory bowel disease. Antiemetics can be administered rectally for nausea and vomiting and paracetamol can be given to treat patients with a pyrexia who are unable to swallow.

Parenteral Administration

Parenteral drug administration can be taken literally to mean any non-oral means of drug administration, but it is generally interpreted as relating to injection directly into the body, by-passing the skin and mucous membranes. The common routes of parenteral administration are intramuscular (IM), subcutaneous and IV.

Administration by injection (parenteral administration) includes the following routes:

- Subcutaneous (under the skin)
- Intramuscular (in a muscle)
- Intravenous (in a vein)
- Intrathecal (around the spinal cord)

Advantages of Parenteral Administration

- Drugs that are poorly absorbed, inactive or ineffective if given orally can be given by this route
- The intravenous route provides immediate onset of action
- The intramuscular and subcutaneous routes can be used to achieve slow or delayed onset of action
- Patient compliance problems are largely avoided.

Disadvantages of Parenteral Administration

- Requires trained staff to administer
- Can be costly
- Can be painful
- Aseptic technique is required
- May require supporting equipment for example, programmable infusion devices.

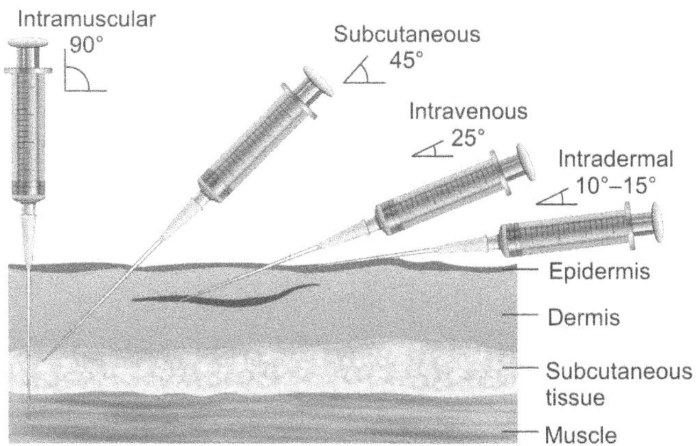

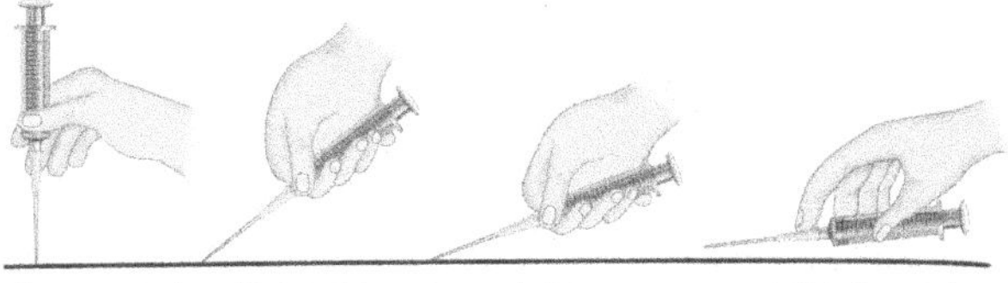

PAIN ASSESSMENT SCALE

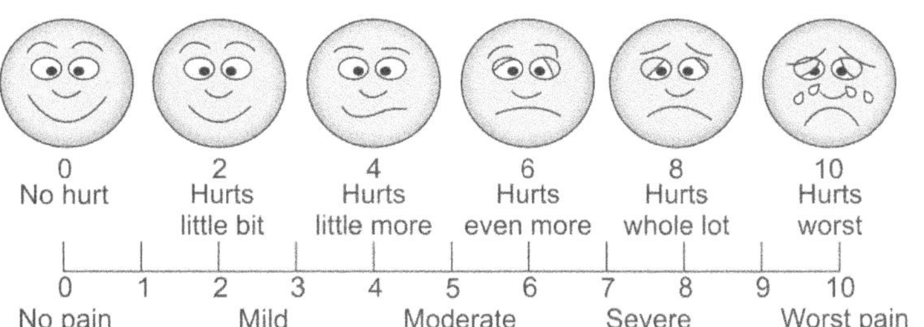

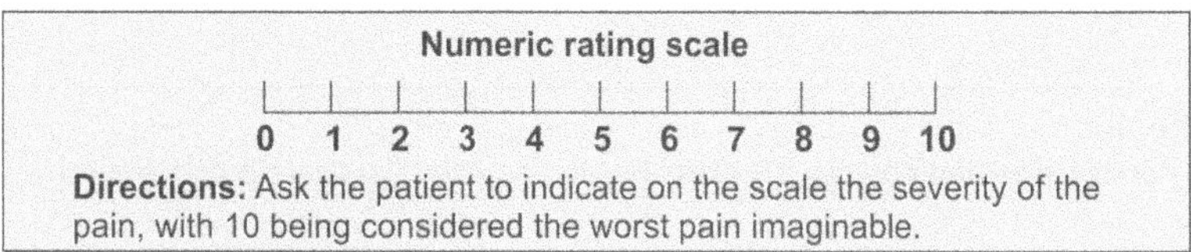

Figure: Pain rating scale used to establish a baseline against which treatment results are judged: the numeric scale is also administered verbally.

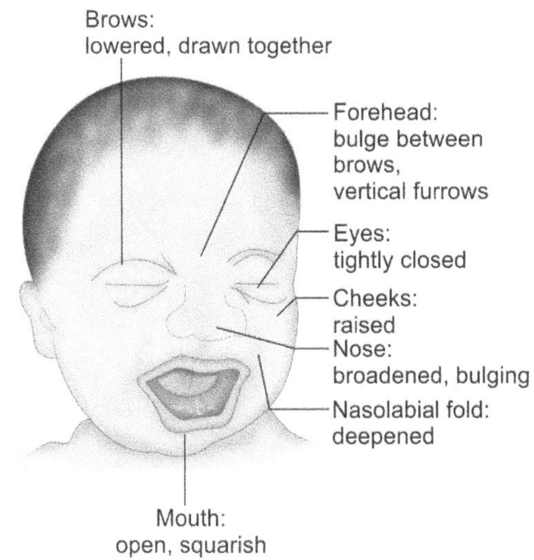

Facial expression of physical distress and pain in the infant

BABY BATH/SPONGE BATH

Introduction

Bathing is the cleaning of the body with soap liquid under the water or the immersion of the body in to water. It may be practiced for personal hygiene, religious ritual or therapeutic purposes. In child rearing practices during the first year vary from country to country and religion to religion but therapeutic bathing is constant. The amount of bathing that is done is also inconsistent across cultures. Unless contraindicated most infants and children can be bathed in a basin at the bedside or on the bed, or in a standard bath tub located on the ward, which is often conveniently adapted for pediatric use by trained professionals.

Definition

The baby bath is defined as cleaning of baby skin for promoting hygiene, Improving blood circulation, comfort rest and sleep. This procedure can be done at home setting by trained mothers.

A sponge bath is defined as a bath the baby without putting him in a tub. During a sponge bath, a baby on a towel and clean him with a wet washcloth. You should sponge bathe the baby not more than 2 to 3 times each week. A sponge bath should take about 5 to 10 minutes to complete.

Purpose of Baby Bath

- To keep the baby's skin clean
- To refresh the baby
- To stimulate the circulation
- To prevent any skin infection
- To closely observe the body for evidence of any abnormalities and to note infant' growth and development
- To induce sleep.

Contraindications

- Hyperthermia
- Convulsion
- Bronchopneumonia
- Congenital heart disease
- Fresh burns
- Critical illness
- Premature infants.

Assessment of the Skin before Bath

- Temperature
- Pruritis and infection
- Edema around orbit and lower foot
- Texture and turgur of skin
- Moisture of skin
- Lesions and color of skin
- Hirutism of skin
- Erythema and Inflammation
- Rashes over the skin.

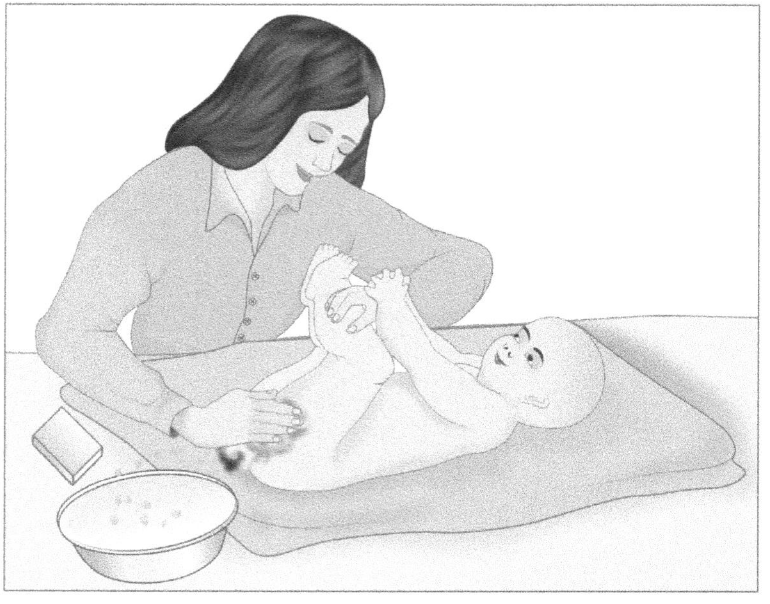

Bathing baby on a pad

Types of Bath

Lap bath	• Lap bathing the baby keeping on the lap. • Here the mother sits on a stool and can sponge and change his dress on her lap itself. So there is no need of having additional stool.
Sponge bath	• Bathing the child in bed. Fill the tub with only 2 or 3 inches of warm water. • Use one hand to support baby's head, then slowly lower him. Using a washcloth or baby bath sponge, wash the face and hair. • The water should feel warm, not hot, on your skin. you have a bath thermometer for measuring water temperature should be 98.6°F to 103.9°F (37°C to 39.9°C).
Hot water tub bath	• Given to reduce muscle tension water temperature 109.4°F. Observe signs and symptoms of dizziness. • A baby bathtub is one used for bathing infants, especially those not yet old enough to sit up on their own. • These can be either a small, stand-alone bath that is filled with water from another source, or a device for supporting the baby that is placed in a standard bathtub.

Equipment

- Clean basin or tub   01
- Baby soap   01
- Sponge or clean wash cloth   01
- Baby shampoo   01
- Warm water   01 bucket
- Clean blanket or bath towel   02
- Clean diaper   01
- Clean clothes   01

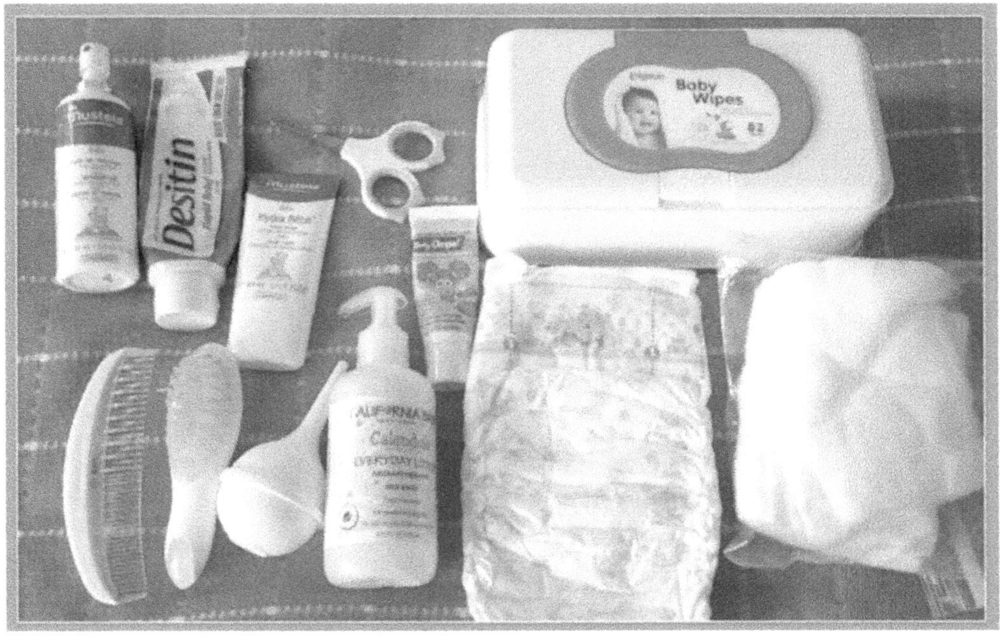

Procedure

- Explain procedure to the mother and encourage her participation.
- Wash your hands.
- Fill the wash basin or baby bathtub with about 3 inches of warm water.
- Test for correct temperature. Do not overfill the tub.
- Arrange all items within reachable place.
- Provide privacy
- Undress baby and place on the pad.
- **Eyes:** Wash baby's eyelids gently with the corner of a soft washcloth and clear water. Start at the inner corner of the eye and wash toward the ears. Use a fresh part of the washcloth for each eye.
- **Face:** Using the washcloth, wash baby's face with clear water. Don't use soap on baby face.
- **Ears:** Wash the outer part of each ear with a washcloth moistened with clear water. Pat ears dry. Do not use cotton swabs inside your baby's ears.
- **Hair and scalp:** Pick up the baby. Support baby head in your hand and his back with your forearm. Rest baby's buttocks on your hip. Holding a baby this way gives him a sense of security. Wet baby's head with clear water. Using a small amount of baby shampoo, make a soapy lather with your hands. Put a small amount of soapy lather on his head, including the "soft spot." Rub gently in a circular motion. Hold a baby's head over the basin to rinse soap off with water using your cupped hand or a wet washcloth. When all the soap is off, pat his head gently with a towel to dry.
- **Body:** Place your baby on the pad. Make a soapy lather with your hands. Start at the neck and lather baby's entire body. Be sure to clean the skin folds, between fingers and toes, and the genital area. (If your baby boy is not circumcised, do not pull back the foreskin on the penis to clean it. This could injure the child's penis). Rinse the soap off with a wet washcloth.
- Wrap the baby in a towel or blanket.
- Finally dress the baby in clean cloth, wrap her in a dry warm blanket.

After the Procedures

- Dry the baby well and dress properly with suitable cloths.
- Do not use powders or oils on baby's body. Babies have their own natural oils, and using oils and powders can decrease the amount of their own oils.
- Brush and comb baby's hair.
- **Nails:** Clean his fingernails and toenails. Carefully clip the nails with baby scissors as needed. If the fingernails are not kept short, the baby may scratch his face.
- Allow a baby to sleep in safe place, while clean the bath area. Put items back on a tray and store it out of the reach of children.

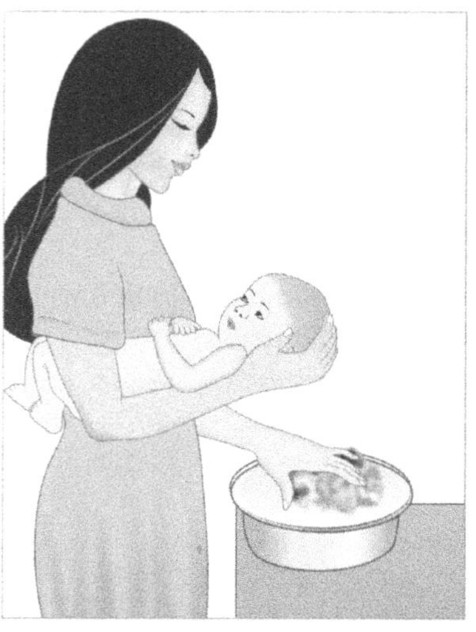

Hold your baby securely

Important Instructions

- Use warm room and warm water
- Bath quickly and gently
- Dry quickly and gently
- Never leave the baby unattended in a bath tub or table
- The infant is given bath after the cord falls and umbilicus is well healed.

Until your baby's umbilical cord stump has healed, sponge baths are the best way to clean your baby. Your baby needs to be bathed only a few times a week—bathing your baby more frequently may dry out her skin

1

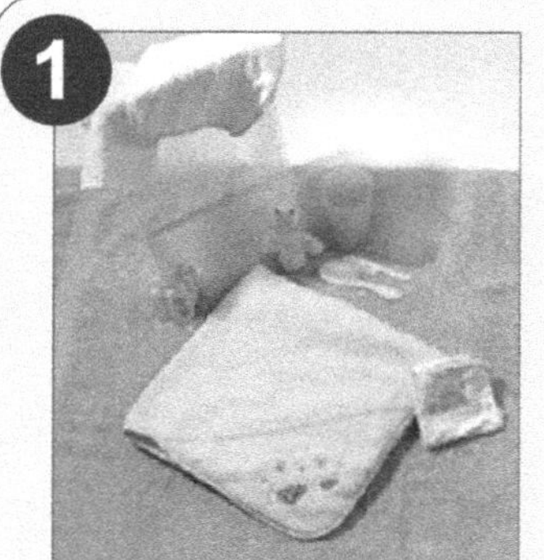

Make sure to bathe your baby in a warm room that doesn't have any drafts. Gather all your supplies, such as a container of warm water, clean washcloths and towels, mild baby soap and shampoo, and diapers and clothes, Lay your baby on a soft, flat surface, and keep one hand on her during the bath, Keep her covered with a towel for warmth, and only expose the area you are cleaning

2

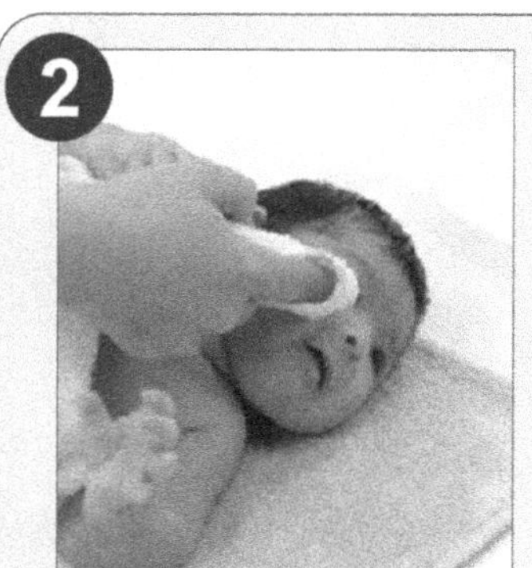

Dip a washcloth in the container, and gently use one corner to wipe your baby's eye from the inner corner to the outer corner. Use a different corner of the washcloth to clean your baby's other eye. Then, finish wiping the rest of your baby's face. Do not use soap when cleaning your baby's eyes and face. You can wash your baby's scalp by applying a pea-size amount of shampoo and using a damp washcloth to rinse it

3

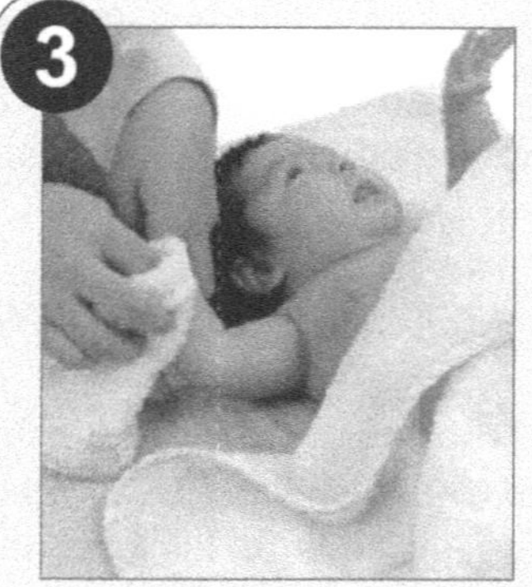

Use a pea-size drop of soap on a washcloth to clean your baby's body. Make sure to clean between the fingers and toes and in skin creases, especially under the arms, behind the ears, and around the neck. Use a clean washcloth to rinse your baby and remove any soap residue, Be gentle around the umbilical cord stump, and make sure the stump doesn't get wet.

4

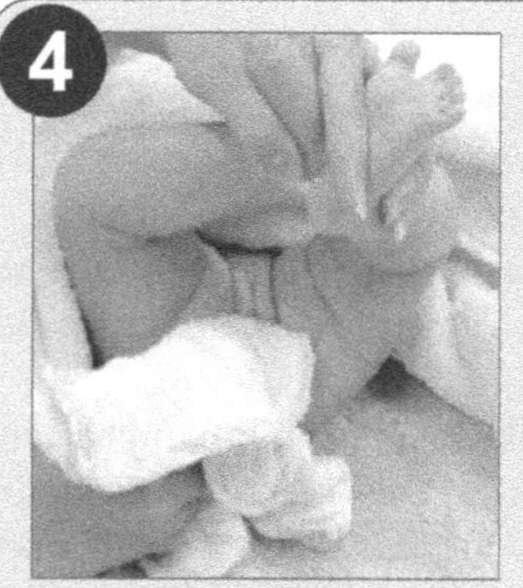

Wipe your baby's genital area with a damp washcloth, making sure to clean in any skin creases. When cleaning a baby girl, wipe from the front to the back. If you are cleaning a baby boy, make sure to lift the testicles and clean underneath them. If the baby is uncircumcised, do not try to pull the foreskin back to clean underneath it.

5

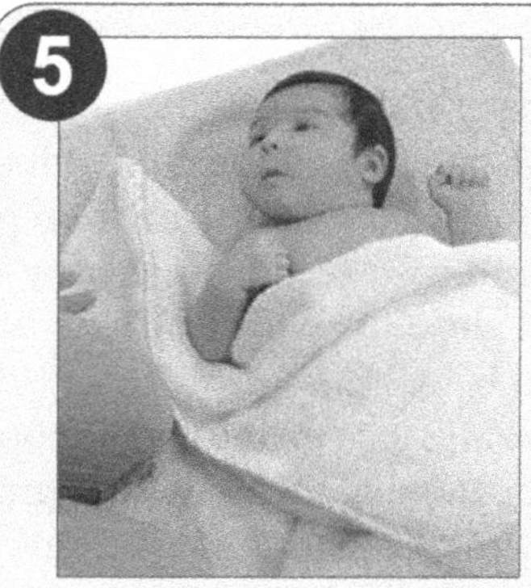

Finish drying your baby by gently using a soft towel—a hooded towel will help keep your baby warm. Use a soft baby brush to comb out your baby's hair, but do not use a hair dryer, Ones she is dry, your baby is ready to be diapered and dressed.

GLASGOW COMA SCORING SCALE

Glasgow Coma Scale for assessment of coma in infants and children			
Category	Score*	Infant and young child criteria	Older child and adult criteria
Eye opening	4 3 2 1	Spontaneous opening To loud noise To pain No response	Spontaneous To verbal stimuli To pain No response
Verbal response	5 4 3 2 1	Smiles, coos, cries to appropriate stimuli Irritable; cries Inappropriate crying Grunts, moans No response	Oriented to time, place, and person; uses appropriate words and phrases Confused Inappropriate words or verbal response Incomprehensible words No response
Motor response	6 5 4 3 2 1	Spontaneous movement Withdraw to touch Withdraws to pain Abnormal flexion (decorticate) Abnormal extension (decerebrate) No response	Obeys commands Localize pain Withdraws to pain Flexion to pain (decorticate) Flexion to pain (decorticate) Extention to pain (decerebrate) No response

*Add the score from each category to get the total. The maximum score is 15, indicating the best level of neurologic functioning. The minimum is 3, indicating total neurologic unresponsiveness.

Score	Eye opening	Verbal response	Motor response
13–15	Mild Injury		
9–12	Moderate Injury		
3–9	Severe Injury		

FEEDING CHILDREN BY KATORI-SPOON AND PALADAI CUP

Definition

The breast milk is the ideal feed for the low birth weight babies. Those unable to feed directly on the breast can be feed expressed breast milk (EBM) by gavage or katori-spoon. Feeding with spoon (or a similar device such as paladai) and katori has been found to be safe in small for gestational age (SGA) infants.

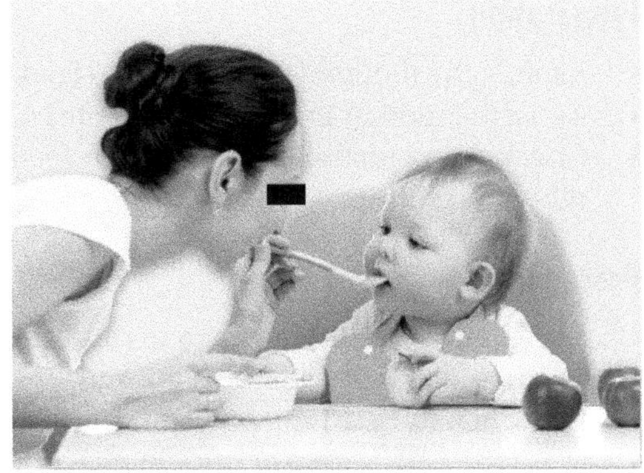

Indications

- Small for gestational age infants.
- Premature babies who have good swallowing reflex but poor sucking reflux.
- Low birth weight baby.

Contraindications

- Extreme LBW babies (<1000 g)
- Absent of sucking reflux
- Congenital anomalies (CL/CP)
- Semiconscious/unconscious level.

Table: Guidelines for the modes of providing fluids and feeding.

Age	Categories of newborn baby		
Birth weight (g)	<1200 g	1200–1800 g	>1800 g
Gestational age (weeks)	<30 weeks	30–34 weeks	>34 weeks
Initial	• Intravenous fluids • Try gavage feeds	Gavage	Breast feeding if unsatisfactory, provide katori-spoon feeds
After 1–3 days	Gavage	Katori-spoon	Breastfeeding
Later (1–3 weeks)	Katori-spoon	Breastfeeding	Breastfeeding
After (4–6 weeks)	Breastfeeding	Breastfeeding	Breastfeeding

Advantages

- This mode of feeding is a bridge between gavage feeding and direct breast-feeding.
- Chances for transmission of infection associated with feeding is less when compare to bottle feeding.
- Best method for stable pre-mature and low birth weight infants.

Disadvantages

- Cannot replace direct breast-feeding advantages.
- Delay in development of sucking reflux.
- Poor bonding between child and mother.
- Oral trauma.
- RDS.

Equipment

Sterile Tray with Sterile Cloth Containing

- Sterile bowl/katori (medium)   : 1
- Bowl teaspoon/paladai   : 1
- Sterile glass/cup for collecting EBM   : 1
- Bib   : 1
- Face towel   : 1
- Ounce glass/measuring cup   : 1

Preparation

- Explain the mother why we need to feed through spoon or paladai.
- Assist the mother in expression of breast milk.
- Check the neonatologist's order for feeding amount, frequency and any other precautions.

Procedure

- Explain the procedure to parents and child.
- Arrange all articles nearby baby unit.
- Perform hand washing procedure.
- Make the baby sitting or upright position.
- Measure the required amount of feed and pour into katori.
- Wear the bib around the child's neck.
- Make the mother to set comfortably and ask the mother to hold baby like cradling.
- The head of the baby should be held at crook of arm of the mother. Ask the mother to support the baby's body with the side of hand.
- Take the milk from the katori with the help of spoon, the spoon should be filled just short of the brim with expressed milk.

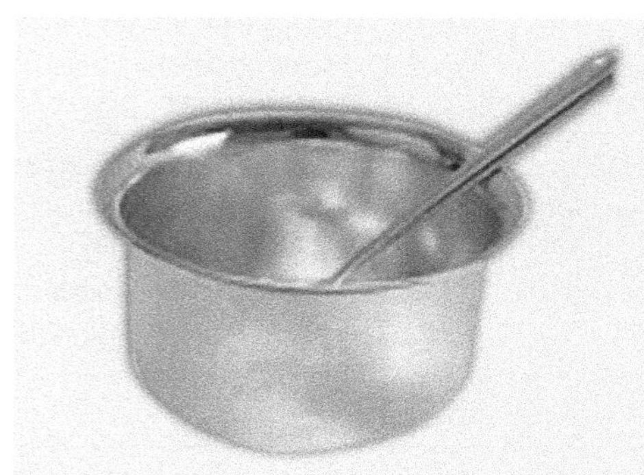

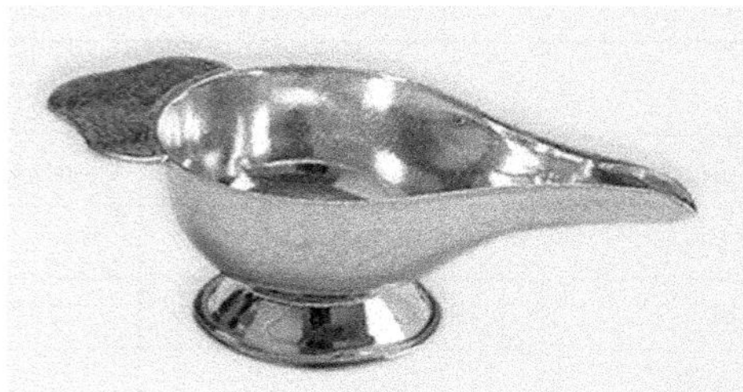

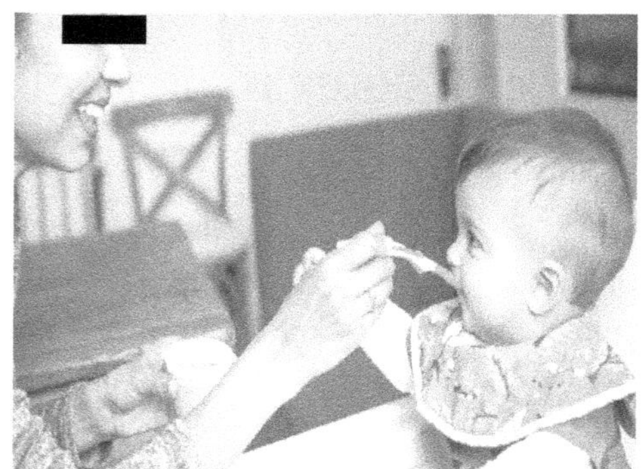

Katori and spoon feeding technique

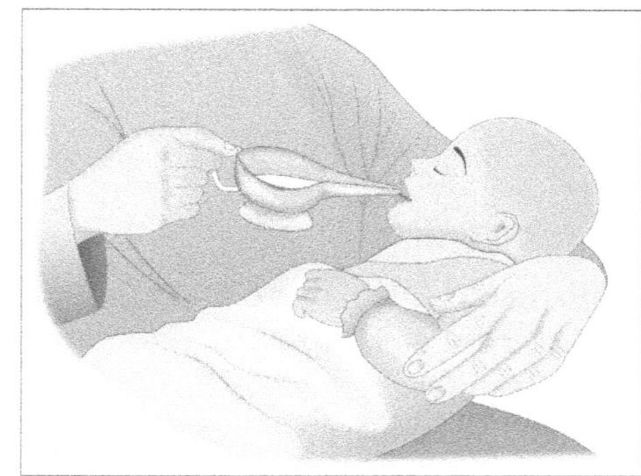

Paladai feeding technique

- Place the spoon or spike of the paladai at the corner of the mouth and milk should be allowed to flow into the infant's mouth slowly, avoiding any spillage.
- The baby would actively swallow the milk.
- This process should be repeated till the required amount has been fed.
- During the procedure, if baby vomit, immediately stop the procedure and report the doctor.
- Maintain Intake and output chart after the procedure.

Post-procedure Care

- Wipe the face of the baby with towel.
- Remove the bib from the neck.
- Burp the child.
- Document the procedure in nurse's record with time, amount of feed, any observation made during feeding.

Nurses Responsibilities

- If the infant does not actively accept and swallow the feed, an attempt should be made to wake the infant with gentle stimulation (tactile stimulation).
- If baby is still sluggish, do not insist in this method. It is better to switch back to gavage feeds till the infant is ready.

FEEDING: NASOGASTRIC, GASTROSTOMY AND JEJUNOSTOMY

Nasogastric/Orogastric Tube Feeding

Introduction

The nutritional needs of the sick and preterm infant must be met in order to promote survival and batter outcome. These needs are different according to the infant's gestation, degree of growth retardation, postnatal age and associated disease.

Bolus feeding has been shown to be more physiological in terms of producing more natural surges in gut hormones. It is usual to start on 2 hourly feeds, but occasionally babies may need hourly feeds. When on full milk feeds the interval between feeds may be increased to 3 and then 4 hourly depending on the individual infant. Continuous feeds are not indicated in babies with gastric tubes in situ.

Definition

Administration of feed directly into the stomach through a tube passed into the stomach through the nose (nasogastric) or mouth (orogastric).

Purpose for Insertion of a Nasogastric Tube

- Decompression of stomach (to remove fluid and gas).
- To prevent or relieve nausea and vomiting after surgery or traumatic events by decompressing the stomach.
- To determine the amount of pressure and motor activity of GI tract (diagnostic studies).
- To give gastric lavage (to irrigate the stomach in case of active bleeding or poisoning).
- To obtain specimen (gastric contents) for laboratory studies.
- To administer medication.
- To give gastric gavage (feed directly).

Purpose of Administration of Nasogastric Tube Feeding

- To provide adequate nourishment to patients who cannot feed themselves.
- To administer medication.
- To provide nourishment to patients who cannot be feed through mouth, e.g. surgery in oral cavity, unconscious or comatosed state.

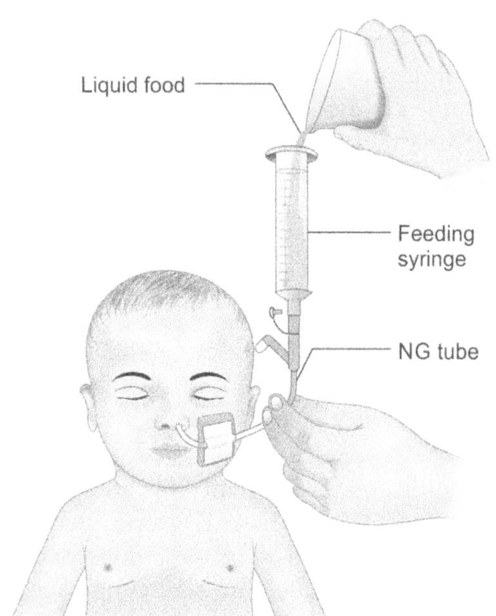

Table: Fluid requirement of neonates (mL/per kg body weight)

Day of newborn baby life	Birth weight	
	> 1500 g	**< 1500 g**
1	60 mL	80 mL
2	75 mL	95 mL
3	90 mL	110 mL
4	105 mL	125 mL
5	120 mL	140 mL
6	135 mL	150 mL
7 onwards	150 mL	150 mL

Note

- On the first day the fluid requirements range from 60 to 80 mL/kg.
- The daily increment in all the groups is around 15 mL per kg till 150 mL/kg is reached.
- Adequacy of therapy is indicated by weight pattern in the expected range.

Indications

- Head and neck injury
- Coma
- Obstruction of esophagus or oropharynx
- Severe anorexia nervosa
- Recurrent episodes of aspiration
- Increased metabolic needs—burns, cancer, etc.
- Poor oral intake or failure to thrive
- Inability to suck
- Respiratory distress.

Contraindications

- Esophageal atresia
- Esophageal fistula
- Esophageal varices.

Articles Need for Procedure

- A sterile tray with tray cloth   : 1
- Sterile gloves   : 1
- Kidney tray with paper bag   : 1
- A bowl with water   : 1
- 5–6 French size polyethylene feeding catheter   : 1 (according to age)
- Water soluble jelly   : 1
- Mackintosh with draw sheet   : 1
- Intake output chart   : 1
- Syringe (10 mL and 20 mL syringe)   : 1 (each one)
- Stethoscope   : 1

Preparation

- Identification cof the right child hand and explaining the procedure to the parents.
- History collection regarding food allergies, time of last feed, bowl sounds.
- Inspect the child's nose and mouth for any deformities that may interfere with the passage of these.
- Select appropriate nasogastric tube according to children age before starting the procedure (Refer below mentioned table).

Table: Typical weights and tube sizes for age

Age	Weight (kg)	NG-tube (Fr)
0–6 months	3.5–7	8–10
1 year	10	10
2 years	12	10
3 years	14	10–12
5 years	18	12
6 years	21	12
8 years	27	14
12 years	varies	14–16

Procedure

- Explain the procedure to parents/child.
- Arrange the articles nearby the baby unit.
- Performing the hand washing technique.
- Wear gloves.
- Position the infant supine with the head slightly elevated and with the neck hyper extended so that nose is pointed upward.
- Assist the order child to sitting position if appropriate (Fowler's position).
- Alternatively have the parents or another person to hold the child to promote comfort and reassurance.
- Place mackintosh and towel across the chest.
- Measure the length of the tube from tip of nose to tip of the ear lobe and to the tip of the xiphoid process and mark with tape.

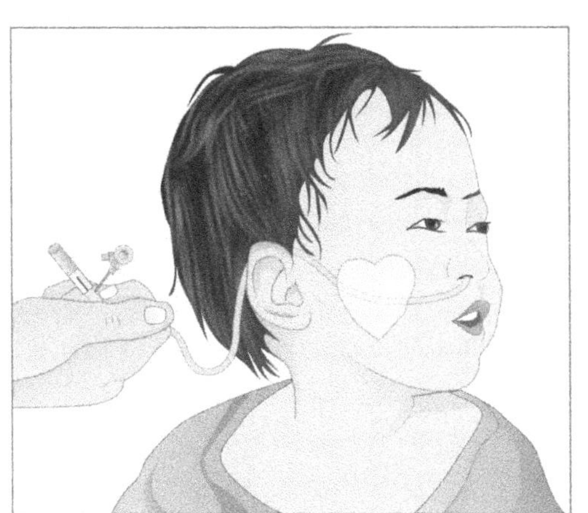
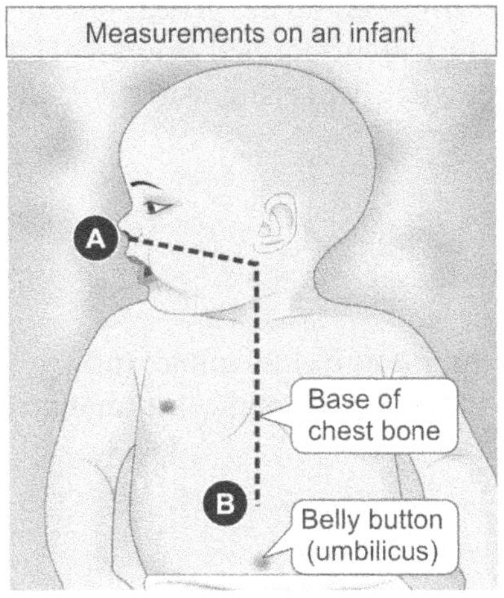

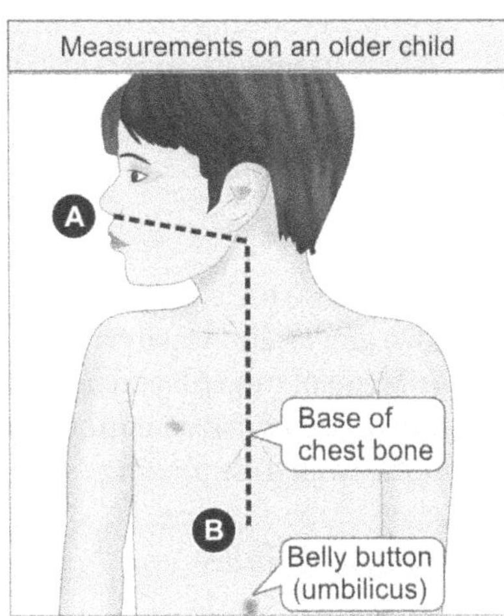

A nasogastric (NG) tube measurement technique

- For orogastric tube insertion, the tube is measured from the lips to the tip of xiphoid process of sternum.
- Cut the adhesive tape of appropriate size and keep ready to fix the tube.
- Lubricate the tip of the tube about 6-8 inches with water soluble lubricant, using gauze piece.
- Insert the tube through the nostril to the back of the throat aiming back.
- Insert the tube gently and very slowly to nostril and give sips of water to older children for drinking, if newborn or infant give bottle nipple to suck when the tube is inserted.
- Flex the patient's head towards the chest after the tube has passed the nasopharynx to reduce the risk of tube entering the trachea.
- Do not force tube when resistance is met or patient starts to gag, cough, choke or become cyanosed, stop advancing tube and pull tube back check for position of tube in back of throat with flash light.
- If there is signs of distress such as gasping, cyanosis, coughing pull back the tube for some length and check if patient distress is relieved, if it is relived develops respiratory distress again, immediately remove the tube because the tube may be in trachea.

- Perform one of the following measures to check for the placement of the tube.
- Aspirated gastric content because aspirated content indicates that the tube is in the stomach then returns ay aspirated contents to the stomach and flush tube with water.
- Place the end of tube in the bowel of water to check for continuous air bubbles indicates that tube is in the respiratory tract.
- If older child ask the speak if she is not able to speak then it means tube is in the trachea.
- Take 2 mL or 5 mL syringe push the air and hear the air entry sound (stethoscope) gargling.
- X-ray may be done.
- Secure tube with tape and avoid pressure on nose. Make sure that mark on the tube is at the nostril.
- Use a piece of tape, split at one end place intact end of tape over bridge of nose. Carefully wrap two ends around tube.
- Secure the tube in check (in neonates). Faster end of tube to gown It reduces friction on nose when patient moves.
- Make patient comfortable in bed and provide oral hygiene every 4–6 hours to promotes comfort and integrity of oral mucous membrane.

Types of Feeding

- **Continuous feeding**- given at a slower rate over long period of time and feeding pump is used to administer the solution at a prescribed rate.
- Bolus feeding—before feeding make sure (twice) the NG tube is in stomach.
    - It may be helpful to have 2 people to do. One person can hold and comfort the child while others can feed.
    - Make sure, the correct amount of formula and warm if to the deserved temperature.
    - Check the tube attach a syringe it the feeding tube.
    - Check the tube placement as above.
    - Clamp the tube attach a syringe to the feeding tube.
    - Pour the formula in the syringe.
    - Unclamp the tube to start flow of formula.
    - During feeding keep the bottom of the syringe no higher than 6 inches above the child stomach.
    - Continue adding formula into the syringe entire the prescribed amount is given.
    - When syringe is empty flush the tube with prescribed amount of lukewarm water and close the tubing.
    - Remove the NG tube. Baby have coughing, wheezing, skin color, difficulty in breathing, can't take, the tube is coming out of the mouth.

Post-Procedure Care

- Discord the waste, clean and replace re-reusable articles.
- Remove gloves and wash hands.
- Record type of tube placed, aspirated returns and child intolerance.
- Measurement of external tube length after insertion and conformation of placement.
- Administering tube feeding.

Nursing Responsibilities

- Proper positioning must be provided according to age group.
- Application of mummy restraints may be necessary to control the child's movements during the insertion.
- Infant hand may be restrained using a necessary soft restrain to prevent grasp of gavage tube and its removal.
- Sterile equipment should be used.
- Feeding amount should be calculated.
- The flow of feeding should be slow. Do not apply pressure.
- Elevate the reservoir of feed 15–20 cm above the child head.
- Weigh the child daily.
- The feeding formula should be at room temperature.
- Taking care to avoid air entry.

Special Considerations

- Insufflations of air into the tube followed by auscultation are no longer considered reliable in determining tube placement from the pleural space into the upper abdomen, thus giving false impression of tube placement.
- Change the tube after 72 hours/according to child condition or according to institution policy.

Gastrostomy Feeding

Definition

Gastrostomy tubes are feeding tubes placed through the abdomen into the stomach. Gastrostomy tubes are used to provide children formula feeding, liquids, and medicines. These tubes are placed by a pediatric surgeon or by a pediatric gastroenterologist.

An enteral feeding is when food is put through a tube directly into the stomach or small intestine. This food is usually a liquid form of protein, carbohydrate and fat. It has all the nutrients, vitamins, and minerals to help a child grow and be as healthy as possible.

A gastrostomy tube is placed in two ways:

1. Surgically insertion
2. Percutaneously insertion.

Surgically Inserted Gastrostomy Tubes

The surgical inserted gastrostomy tube in the operating room under general anesthesia. This operation is done through a small incision (cut) on the abdomen. The surgeon may place a temporary tube, into the gastrostomy opening. A gastrostomy tube is about twelve inches long, and most of the tube extends out of the abdomen.

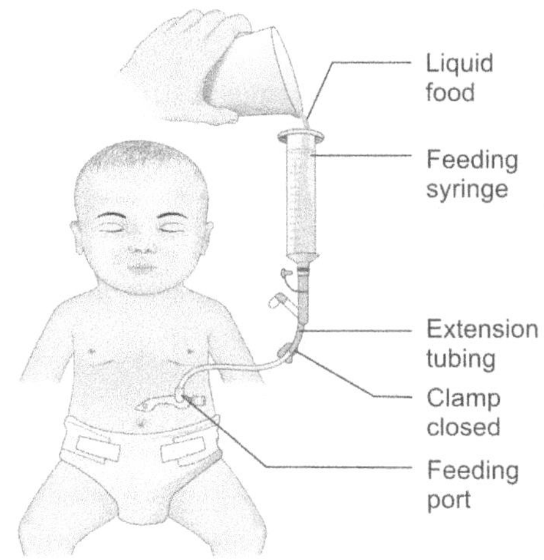

After the gastrostomy tube is placed your child will remain in the hospital for observation and care. An IV (intravenous line) will be placed in the operating room before the procedure and this will be used to give fluids, antibiotics and pain medications while child is recovering. Feedings are usually started the day after the gastronomy is placed.

Percutaneous Endoscopic Gastrostomy (PEG) Tube

- A PEG tube, or percutaneous endoscopic gastrostomy tube, is placed in the operating room by the pediatric surgeon. The PEG tube is inserted using an endoscope.
- The endoscope is a small tube with a light and camera on the end that lets the gastroenterologist see into the esophagus (food tube) and stomach.
- The endoscope allows the doctor to choose the best location in the stomach to place the PEG tube. Once the location is chosen, a small opening is made on the outside of abdomen into the stomach.
- After the opening is made, the top part of the PEG tube is pulled up out of the stomach through this opening.
- The top of the tube rests on the skin and the bottom part of the PEG, which is shaped like bulb, remains inside the stomach. This bulb shape anchors the tube in the stomach and prevents it from coming out.
- After the PEG tube is placed the child will be admitted to the hospital for observation and care. The hospital stay is usually three days.
- Prior to the procedure, an IV (intravenous line) will be placed in the operating room. This will be used to give fluids, antibiotics and pain medication, for one to two days, as your child is recovering. Feedings will be started through the PEG tube within one or two days.
- The PEG tube which is made of silicone, must stay in the stomach for about three months to allow the tract (hole) to heal between the abdomen and the stomach. The tract must be well healed so it is safe for the gastrostomy tube to be changed.

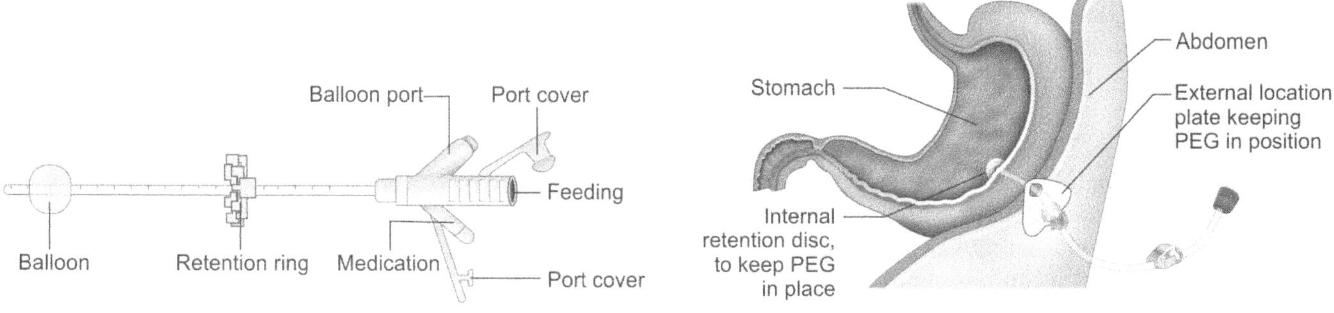

Surgically inserted gastrostomy tubes   Percutaneous endoscopic gastrostomy (PEG) tube

Different types of gastrostomy tubes with insertion methods

Indications

- Congenital abnormalities such as esophageal/choanal atresia or trachea esophageal fistula.
- Conditions which require long term feeding.
- Esophageal injury/dysmotility.
- Child has functioning gastrointestinal tract but is unable to meet his/her total nutritional requirement orally.

Contraindications

- Gross ascites/sever obesity
- Clotting abnormalities
- Gastroparesis
- Esophageal/gastric varices and ulceration
- Complete intestinal obstruction
- Uncontrolled gastroesophageal reflux with a risk of pulmonary aspiration.

Articles Need for Feeding

- Feeding syringe (appropriate to age group) : 1
- Disposable gavage bag with tubing : 1
- IV stand, measuring cup : 1
- Formula, glass of water : 1
- Pair of gloves : 1
- Stethoscope to Auscultate the bowel sound : 1
- Artery forceps : 1

Feeding by Pump

- Feeding set : 1
- Continuous feeding extension set : 1
- Measuring cup with pouring spout : 1
- Formula or blenderized feeding as ordered by your child's doctor : 1
- Glass of water (optional) : 1

Bolus Feeding

- Catheter tip syringe for G-tube : 1
- Feeding extension tube and slip tip syringe : 1
- Measuring cup : 1
- Formula or blenderized feeding : 1
- Glass of water (optional) : 1
- Rubber band : 1
- Clamp for G-tube : 1
- Safety pin : 1

Procedures

- Identification of right child.
- Explain the procedures to parents and get the consent.
- Wash your hands.
- Assess gastrostomy site for skin breakdown, irritation or drainage.
- Place the child in a comfortable position. If possible, place the child in higher chair or at the table during meal time.
- Insert the syringe tip into the feeding tube.
- Flush tubing with 3–5 mL of water to starting the formula feeding.
- Slowly pour the formula into the syringe.
- Unclamp the feeding tube the feeding rate can be controlled by raising or lowering the syringe.
- The feeding should take about the same amount of time as it would take a child drink the formula, about 15–20 minute.
- When all the formula has been given, flush the tubing with water.
- Use formula that is at room temperature. Never microwave formula to bring it to room temperature. Keep opened containers of formula in the refrigerator.
  - This procedure takes about 30 minutes for cold formula to reach room temperature. Measure the amount of formula needed for the feeding 30 minutes before the feeding is due and refrigerate any leftovers promptly.

- – Discard any formula after it has been out of the refrigerator for 4 hours.
  - – Any opened blenderized feeding or commercially prepared formula should be thrown out after it has been in the refrigerator for 24 hours.
- Put two or three drops of formula on your wrist before feeding. The formula should feel warm, not hot or cold.
- Assess the patient for allergies to prevent patient from developing localized or systemic allergic responses.
- Auscultate for bowel sound before feeding because it indicates the presence of peristalsis and obesity of gastrointestinal tract to digest nutrients.
- Verify physician order for formula, rate, and frequency.
- Burp the child after each feeding if appropriate.
- Rinse the feeding tube and record the procedures.

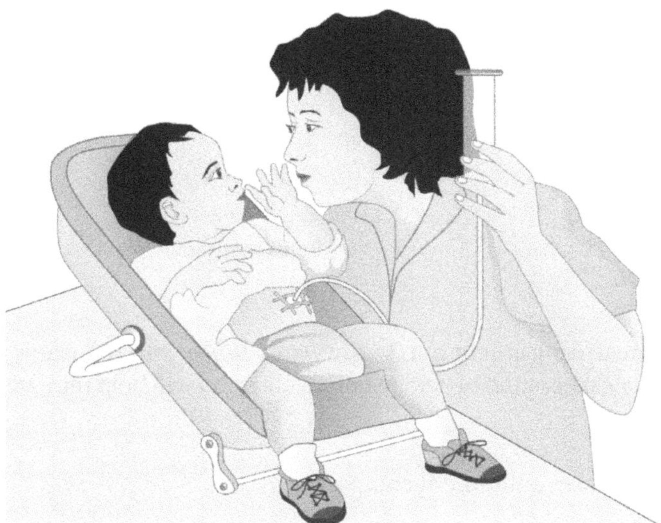

Child upright position

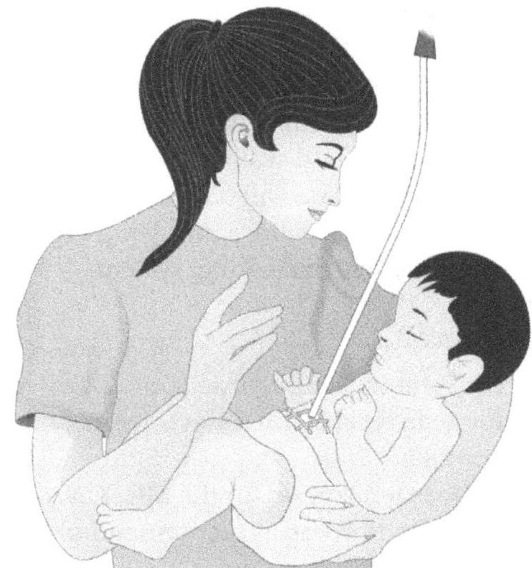

Cuddling position

Gastrostomy feeding position

Pump Feedings

- Close the clamp on the feeding bag. Pour the formula into the bag. Hang the bag high on a hook. Open the clamp and let the formula flow through the tubing until all of the tubing contains formula. Clamp the system. The nurse will show you how to put the tubing through the feeding pump.
- For the G-tube, insert the catheter tip of the feeding tube into the G-tube.
- The child has a skin level device, you will need to attach a feeding extension tube to the feeding system and fill it with formula. After all of the tubing contains formula, clamp the system.
- Next, open the flap of the tube and attach the open end of the feeding extension tube to the device. Open the clamp when you are ready to begin the feeding.
- Set the pump as instructed by the child's nurse and begin the feeding.

Bolus Method

- The child has a skin level device, she will need to attach the extension set to the device and then connect the catheter tip syringe to the extension set. The child has a long G-Tube, connect the catheter tip syringe to the end of the tube.
- Pour the formula into the syringe until it is half full. Filling the syringe full can cause spillage if the child coughs or moves. Next, unclamp the tube or extension tube. Hold the tip of the syringe no higher than your child's shoulders. If the feeding does not start to flow, milk the tube by squeezing it in a downward stroke.

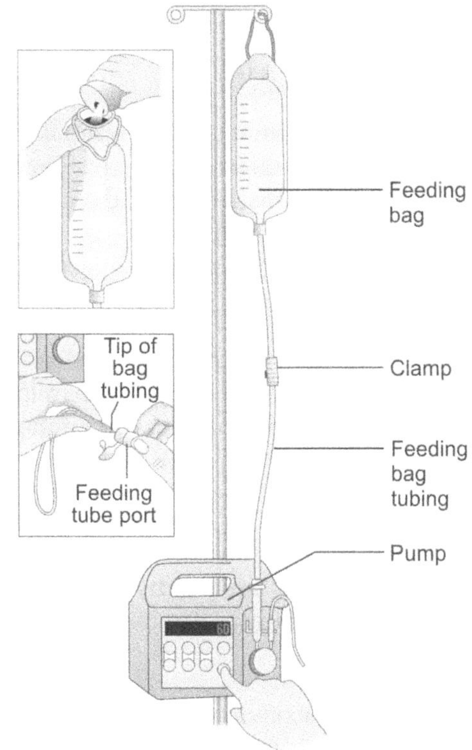

Pump feeding

General Feeding Guidelines

(Both Pump and Bolus Method)

- For a gastrostomy feeding, the child's head must be raised. For an infant, you can hold him in the curve of your arm while feeding (cuddling position). If the child is older, you can feed him in a high chair or any seat as long as his head is raised. The child is fed in these positions, hang the feeding set on a hook in the room.
- The feeding should take the same amount of time as a regular feeding or meal, at least 20–30 minutes. If the child cries during the feeding, stop the feeding until the child is quiet. This can be done by clamping or pinching the tube with your finger and thumb.
- Eating is a social time so make the feeding a happy time for the child. If child needs oral stimulation, follow the instructions given to you by child's occupational therapist or nurse, and the way to grow handout for simulated feedings.
- After the feeding, add water or air to clear the feeding from the tube. The child's nurse will tell you which to use and how much. If the child has a G-tube, close the clamp on the tube and the feeding system and remove the feeding system.

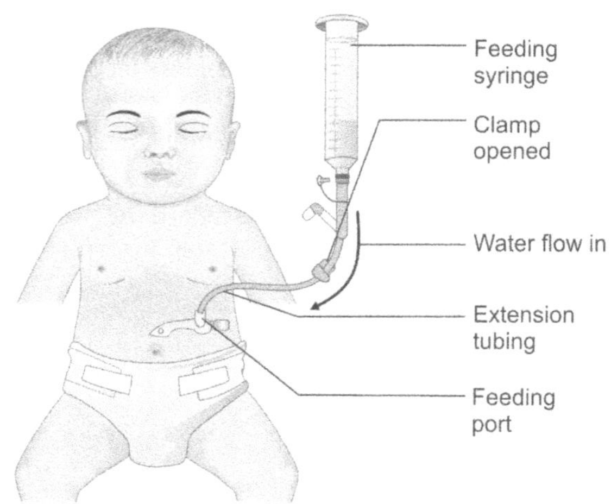

Bolus method

Cleaning the Equipment

- Wash the syringe, feeding extension tube, feeding set and measuring cup in hot, soapy water. Rinse with hot water and dry. If formula is caked on the syringe or tubing, rinsing with a carbonated beverage before cleaning will help remove the dried formula.
- Change the extension set for the Mic-Key, once a week.
- Change the feeding bag as recommended by your home health care equipment company.

Complications

- Large bowl perforation
- Accidental displacement can result in partial closure of stoma
- Infection
- Occlusion.

Nurse's Responsibility

- If the child cannot be fed by mouth, oral stimulation with pacifier can be provided during gastrostomy feeding.
- Encourage oral stimulation by blowing, kissing.
- Disconnect the feeding if the child becomes nauseated shows sign of discomfort abdominal distention, vomiting or difficulty in breathing.
- Remember to flush the feeding tube with water between all feeding and medications.

Care of Feeding Tube

- First 2–3 days the gastrostomy site should be cleaned 2–3 times/day with half strength hydrogen peroxide. After 2–3 days, the site should be cleaned with mild soap and water.
- Take measure to prevent contamination of feed.

Bathing

- Sponging can be given for first 2–3 days to keep the child's new gastrostomy site dry.
- Showering can be given after two days.
- Clean the site and pat dry after showering.
- Swimming is restricted until the stitch is removed.

Venting the Tube

- Place a 60 cc syringe with the plunger remove into the end of the gastrostomy tube. If the tube is clamped open the clamp.
- Hold the syringe above the child stomach for a few minutes. If the gas is present, you can hear the gas bubbles up through the tube or sometimes even see stomach contents backup into the tube and syringe.

- Once the gas is removed allow the formula to flow slowly back into the stomach.
- Make early referral to speech therapist for children requiring long term feeding.

Accidental Tube Expulsion

If tube comes out cover the site with a clean, dry gauze pad or cloth.
- Once the tube is out, hole will begin to close and may close completely in 4–6 hours.
- So the child should be replaced with new gastrostomy tube immediately and should be checked under x-ray for proper placement.
- Balloon devices should be deflated and reinforced weekly to ensure correct amount of fluid remains in the balloon.

Activity Restriction

- Child should not lift anything heavier and should not participate in vigorous activity for two weeks after surgery.
- The school nurse needs instruction filled by the hospital and signed by doctor.

Jejunostomy Feeding

Introduction

Jejunostomy is the surgical creation of an opening (stoma) through the skin at the front of the abdomen and the wall of the jejunum (part of the small intestine). It can be performed either endoscopically, or with open surgery. A jejunostomy may be formed following bowel resection in cases where there is a need to bypassing the distal small bowel and/or colon due to a bowel leak or perforation. Depending on the length of jejunum resected or bypassed the patient may have resultant short bowel syndrome and require parenteral nutrition.

Definition

A jejunostomy tube (J-tube) is a soft, plastic tube placed through the skin of the abdomen into the midsection of the small intestine. The tube delivers food and medicine until the person is healthy enough to eat by mouth.

The Witzel jejunostomy is the most common method of jejunostomy creation. It is an open technique where the jejunosotomy is sited 30 cm distal to the Ligament of Treitz on the antimesenteric border, with the catheter tunneled in a seromuscular groove.

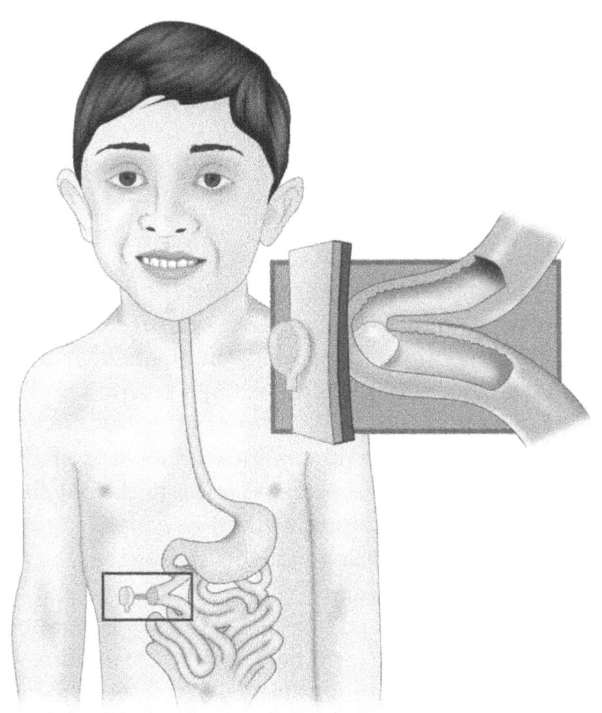

Indication

Jejunal feeding is indicated in child who have a functioning gastrointestinal tract, but who have an absent gag reflex, gastric dysmotility or persistent vomiting resulting in faltering growth.

Articles Need for Feeding

- A clean tray with sterile cloth   : 1
- Mackintosh and towel   : 1
- 10 mL, 20 mL and 50 mL syringe   : 1 in each one
- Feeding tube   : 1
- Bowl with water   : 1
- Stethoscope   : 1
- Ounce class   : 1
- Kidney tray   : 1
- Artery forceps (straight)   : 1
- Adhesive tape with scissors   : 1 in each

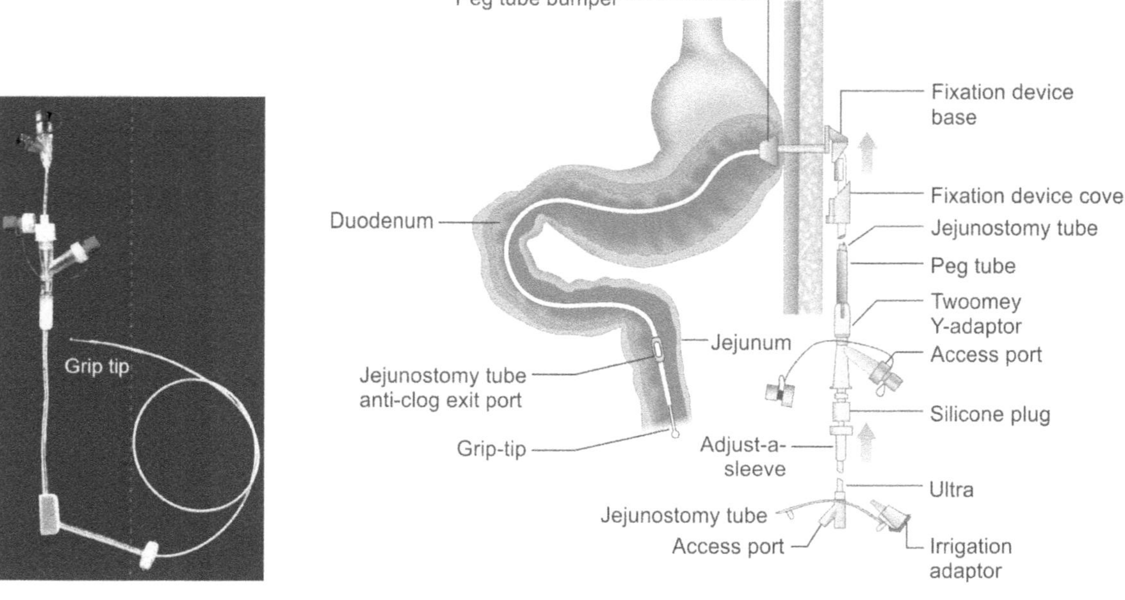

Procedure

- Identification of right child.
- Explain the procedures to parents and get the consent.
- Wash your hands and wear the glove.
- Assess jejunostomy site for skin breakdown, irritation or drainage.
- Place the child in a comfortable position and child should be in semi-Fowler position.
- Insert the syringe tip into the feeding tube.
- Flush tubing with 3–5 mL of water to starting the formula feeding.
- Slowly pour the formula into the syringe.
- Unclamp the feeding tube the feeding rate can be controlled by raising or lowering the syringe.
- The feeding should take about the same amount of time as it would take a child drink the formula, about 15–20 minute.
- When all the formula has been given, flush the tubing with water.
- Use formula that is at room temperature. Never microwave formula to bring it to room temperature. Keep opened containers of formula in the refrigerator.
  - This procedure takes about 30 minutes for cold formula to reach room temperature. Measure the amount of formula needed for the feeding 30 minutes before the feeding is due and refrigerate any leftovers promptly.
  - Discard any formula after it has been out of the refrigerator for 4 hours.
  - Any opened blenderized feeding or commercially prepared formula should be thrown out after it has been in the refrigerator for 24 hours.
- Put two or three drops of formula on your wrist before feeding. The formula should feel warm, not hot or cold.
- Assess the child for allergies to prevent from developing localized or systemic allergic responses.
- Auscultate for bowel sound before feeding because it indicates the presence of peristalsis movements.

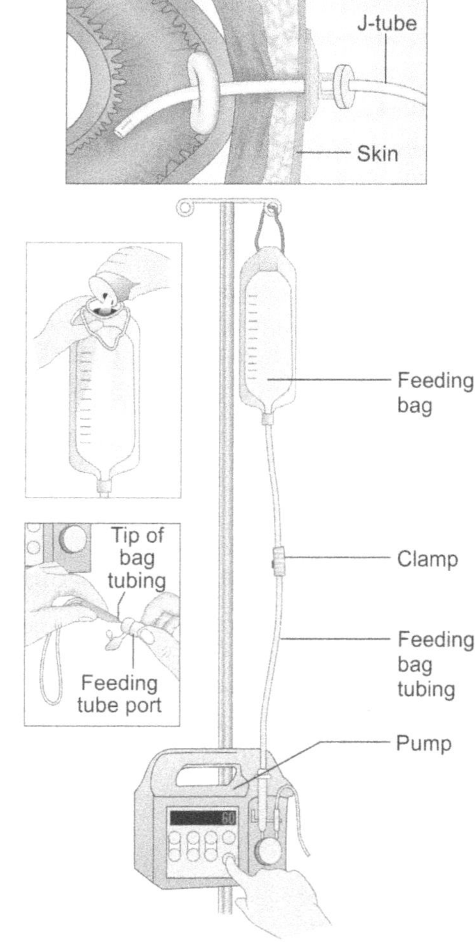

Pump feeding

- Verify physician order for formula, rate, and frequency.
- Rinse the feeding tube and record the procedures.

Nursing Officer Responsibilities

- Proper positioning must be provided according to age group.
- Infant hand may be restrained using a necessary soft restrain to prevent grasp of gavage tube and its removal.
- Sterile equipment should be used.
- Feeding amount should be calculated.
- The flow of feeding should be slow. Do not apply pressure.
- Elevate the reservoir of feed 15–20 cm above the child head.
- Weigh the child daily and maintain the intake output chart.
- The feeding formula should be at room temperature.
- Taking care to avoid air entry.

CARE OF SURGICAL WOUNDS: DRESSING AND SUTURE REMOVAL

Introduction

An incision is a cut through the skin that is made during surgery. It is also called a surgical wound. Some incisions are small, others are long. The size of the incision depends on the kind of surgery child had. Sometimes, an incision breaks open. This may happen along the entire cut or just part of it. Physician decide not to close it again with sutures (stitches).

Definition

A surgical wound defined as a cut or incision in the skin that is usually made by a scalpel during surgery. A surgical wound can also be the result of a drain placed during surgery. Surgical wounds vary greatly in size. They are usually closed with sutures, but are sometimes left open to heal.

Types of Surgical Wounds

Surgical wounds can be classified into one of four categories. These categories depend on how contaminated or clean the wound is, the risk of infection, and where the wound is located on the body.

- **Class I:** These are considered clean wounds. They show no signs of infection or inflammation. They often involve the eye, skin, or vascular system.
- **Class II:** These wounds are considered clean-contaminated. Although the wound may not show signs of infection, it is at an increased risk of becoming infected because of its location. For example, surgical wounds in the gastrointestinal tract may be at a high risk of becoming infected.
- **Class III:** A surgical wound in which an outside object has come into contact with the skin has a high risk of infection and is considered a contaminated wound. For example, a gunshot wound may contaminate the skin around where the surgical repair occurs.
- **Class IV:** This class of wound is considered dirty-contaminated. These include wounds that have been exposed to fecal material.

Risk Factors for Surgical Wound Complication

- Immunocompromised state: Diabetes; autoimmune disease such as rheumatoid arthritis or lupus; cancer; long-term corticosteroid therapy; or any patient receiving chemotherapeutic agents or medications that dampen immune response
- Malnutrition
- Radiation therapy
- Unintentional weight loss
- Obesity
- Longer duration of surgical procedure (greater than two hours)
- Pre-operative sepsis.

Topical Management of Surgical Wounds

- All surgical wounds require a moist environment to support healing. If a dressing change is required within the first 48 hours post-operatively, aseptic technique should be strictly followed.

- Cleansing of surgical incisions is performed for removal of debris, pathogens, and exudate; it should be done with appropriate pressure utilizing a safe agent to avoid cytotoxicity (e.g., normal saline) or mechanical trauma (do not exceed 15 psi).
- Typically, initial surgical dressings are to remain in place for 48–72 hours, and some stay in place for up to seven days.
- Around post-operation day three, the superficial epidermis of a primarily closed incision line may appear "sealed."
- Although the tissue layers are not completely healed and are not able to withstand external forces at this time, the epidermis is the first to resurface, or restratify, to begin to form a barrier to pathogens and contaminants.

Surgical Wound Dressing

Definition

Surgical wound dressing is changing old dressings or applying new dressing, an aseptic technique is used in order to avoid cross infections into a wound. If a wound is already infected, an aseptic technique should be used as it is important that no further infection is introduced. This technique should be used when the patient has a surgical or non-surgical wound.

Equipment

- A clear available work space, such as a stainless-steel trolley
- A sterile dressing/procedure pack
  - One Kocher or Pean forceps
  - One dissecting forceps
  - One pair of surgical scissors or one scalpel to excise necrotic tissue and to cut gauze or sutures
- Access to hand washing sink or alcohol hand wash
- Non-sterile gloves to remove old dressing
- Apron
- Appropriate dressings
- Sterile compresses
  - Non-sterile disposable gloves
  - Adhesive tape and/or crepe or gauze bandage
  - Sterile 0.9% sodium chloride or sterile water
  - Depending on the wound—antiseptic (7.5% povidone iodine scrub solution, 10% povidone iodine dermal solution)
  - Paraffin compresses, analgesics

Removal of an Old Dressing

- Wash hands (ordinary soap) or disinfect them with an alcohol-based hand rub.
- Put on non-sterile gloves and remove the adhesive tape, bandage and superficial compresses.
- Proceed gently with the last compresses. If they stick to the wound, loosen them with 0.9% sodium chloride or sterile water before removal.
- Observe the soiled compresses. If there is significant discharge, a greenish colour or a foul odour, a wound infection is likely.
- Discard the dressing and the non-sterile gloves in the waste container.

Procedure

Technique for Cleaning and Dressing of the Wound

- Explain the procedure to parent and child.
- Wash hands again or disinfect them with an alcohol-based hand rub.
- Open the dressing set or box after checking the date of sterilisation.
- Pick up one of the sterile forceps being careful not to touch anything else.
- Pick up the second forceps with the help of the first one.
- Make a swab by folding a compress in 4 using the forceps.
- Clean sutured wound or clean open wound with red granulation.
- Clean with 0.9% sodium chloride or sterile water to remove any organic residue.
- Work from the cleanest to the dirtiest area (use a clean swab for each stroke).
- Dab dry with a sterile compress.
- Re-cover a sutured wound with sterile compresses or an open wound with paraffin compresses; the dressing should extend a few cm beyond the edges of the wound.
- Keep the dressing in place with adhesive tape or a bandage.

Necrotic or Infected Open Wounds
- A clean with povidone iodine (7.5% scrub solution, 1 part of solution + 4 parts of sterile 0.9% sodium chloride or sterile water).
- Rinse thoroughly then dab dry with a sterile compress; or if not available, sterile 0.9% sodium chloride or sterile water and apply an antiseptic (10% povidone iodine dermal solution).
- Apply sterile vaseline and remove all necrotic tissue at each dressing change until the wound is clean.
- Discard any sharp materials used in an appropriate sharps container and the rest of the waste in a waste container.
- As quickly as possible, soak the instruments in disinfectant.
- Wash hands again or disinfect them with an alcohol-based hand rub.
- The principles remain the same if the dressing is done using instruments or sterile gloves.

Subsequent Dressings
- **Clean, sutured wound:** Remove the initial dressing after 5 days if the wound remains painless and odorless, and if the dressing remains clean.
- The decision to re-cover or to leave the wound uncovered (if it is dry) often depends on the context and local practices.
- **Infected, sutured wound:** Remove one or more sutures and evacuate the pus. Change the dressing at least once daily.
- **Open, dirty wound:** Daily cleaning and dressing change.
- **Open granulating wound:** Change the dressing every 2 to 3 days, except if the granulation is hypertrophic (in this case, apply local corticosteroids).

After the Procedure
- Fold up the dressing/procedure pack and place all contaminated material in a bag designated for clinical waste, making sure all sharps are removed and disposed of in a sharp's container.
- Remove gloves and place in waste bag.
- Wash your hands.
- Clean the trolley with soap and water or disinfectant solution as before.
- Record (document) on the patient's chart your wound assessment, the dressing change and the care you have given.
- Provide the patient with some dressing management education and answer any questions.
- Report any changes to a senior nurse or doctor.

Checklist: Surgical wound dressing	
Safety considerations:	
• Perform hand hygiene. • Check room for additional precautions. • Introduce yourself to patient. • Confirm patient ID using two patient identifiers (e.g., name and date of birth).	• Explain process to patient; offer analgesia, bathroom, etc. • Listen and attend to patient cues. • Ensure patient's privacy and dignity. • Assess ABCCS/suction/oxygen/safety.

Steps	Additional information	
1. Check present dressing with non-sterile gloves.	• Use non-sterile gloves to protect yourself from contamination. • Apply non-sterile gloves	
2. Do the hand wash procedure.	• Hand hygiene prevents spread of microorganisms. • Perform all the 7 steps of hand wash technique	

3. Gather necessary equipment.	• Dressing supplies must be for single patient use only. • Use the smallest size of dressing for the wound. • Gather supplies • Take only the dressing supplies needed for the dressing change to the bedside.
4. Prepare environment, position patient, adjust height of bed, turn on lights.	• Ensure patient's comfort prior to and during the procedure. • Proper lighting allows for good visibility to assess wound.
5. Perform hand hygiene.	• Hand hygiene prevents spread of microorganisms. • Hand hygiene with alcohol-based hand scrub.
6. Arrange sterile gauze pads.	Add sufficient sterile pads: 1. Small size: 4 × 4 cm 2. Medium size: 10 × 10 cm 3. Large size: 10 × 20 cm
7. Add necessary sterile supplies.	Sterile compresses: • Non-sterile disposable gloves • Adhesive tape and/or crepe or gauze bandage • Sterile 0.9% sodium chloride or sterile water • Antiseptic (7.5% povidone iodine scrub solution, 10% povidone iodine dermal solution) • Paraffin compresses, analgesics
8. Pour cleansing solution.	• Pour sterile cleansing solution into sterile tray. • Normal saline or sterile water containers must be used for only one client and must be dated and discarded within at least 24 hours of being opened.
9. Prepare patient and expose dressed wound.	Prepare patient and expose wound

10. Apply non-sterile gloves.	• Use non-sterile gloves to protect yourself from contamination. • Apply non-sterile gloves.	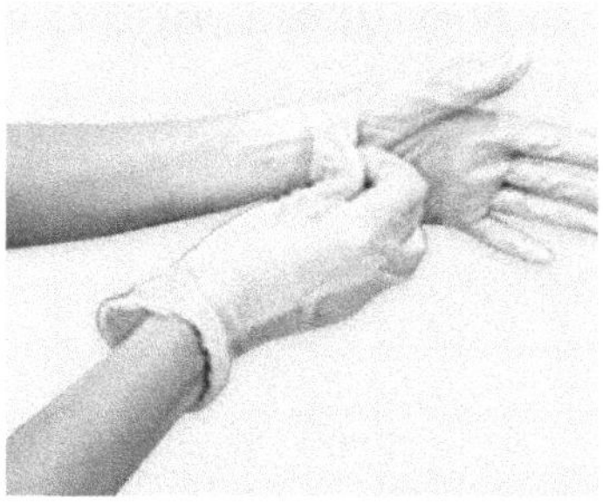
11. Remove outer dressing with non-sterile gloves and discard as per agency policy.	Remove outer dressing with non-sterile gloves.	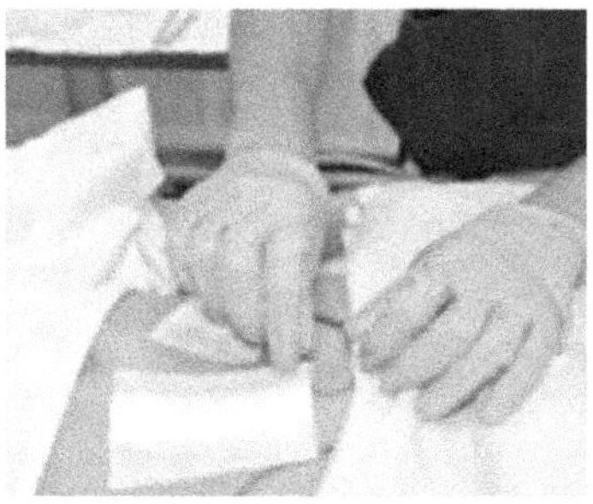
12. Remove inner dressing with transfer forceps, if necessary.	Remove inner dressing with transfer forceps.	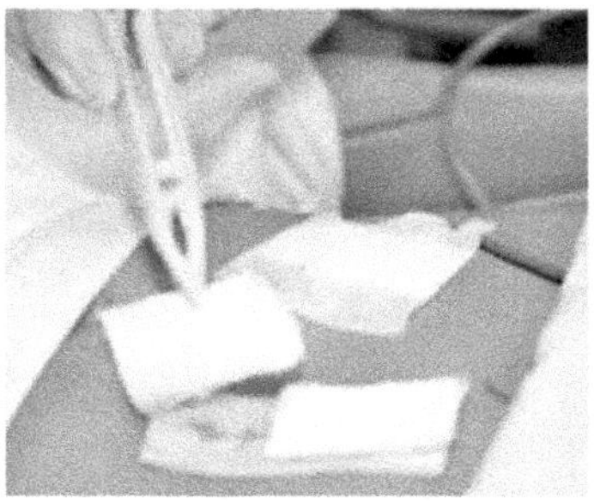
13. Discard transfer forceps and non-sterile gloves according to agency policy.	Discard transfer forceps as per agency policy. Discard gloves.	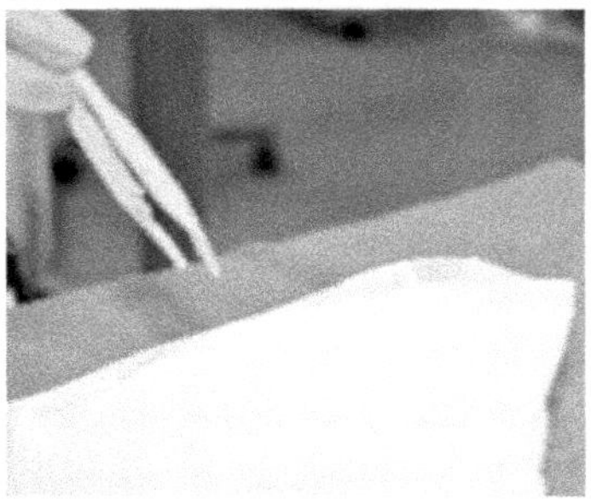 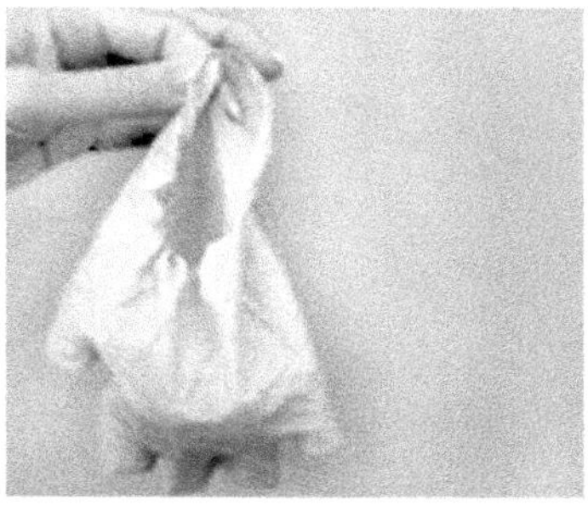
14. Inspect the wound before dressing	Assess the wound condition: 1. Type of wound 2. Color of wound 3. Odor or exudate	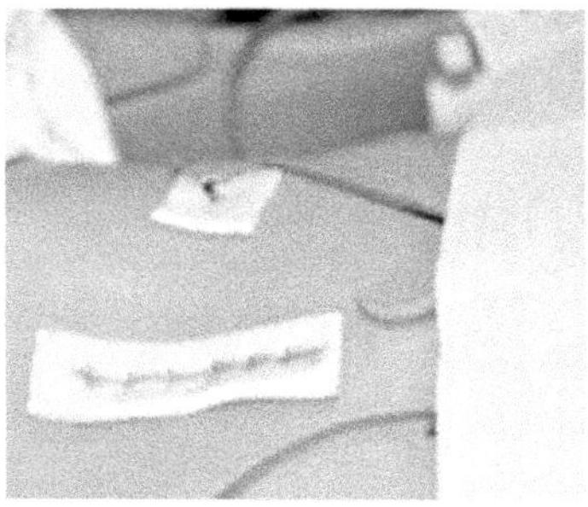

15. Apply non-sterile gloves (optional).	• Use non-sterile gloves to protect yourself from contamination. • Apply non-sterile gloves	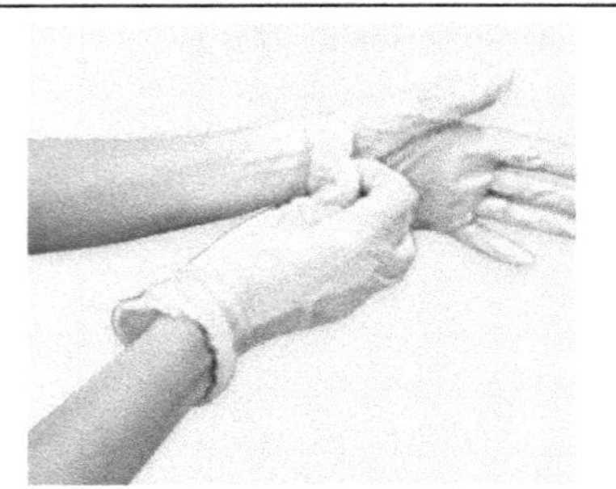
16. Cleanse wound using one 2 x 2 gauze per stroke. Strokes should be: From clean to dirty (incision, then outer edges) From top to bottom	The suture line is considered the "least contaminated" area and is cleansed first. • Using a sterile swab or gauze, clean the suture line by starting at the center and working toward one end.	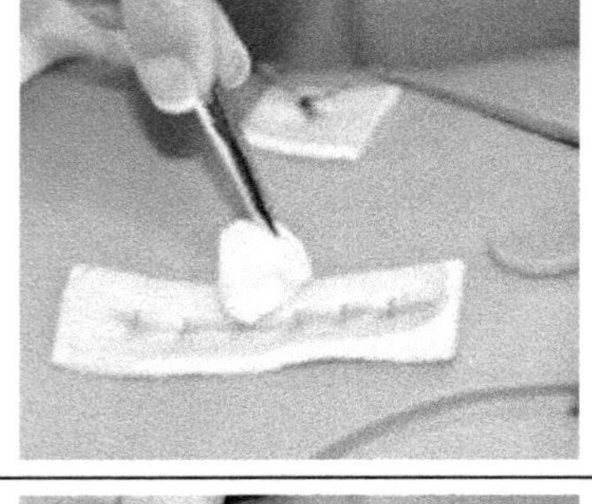
	• With another sterile swab or gauze, start at the center of the incision and work toward the other end.	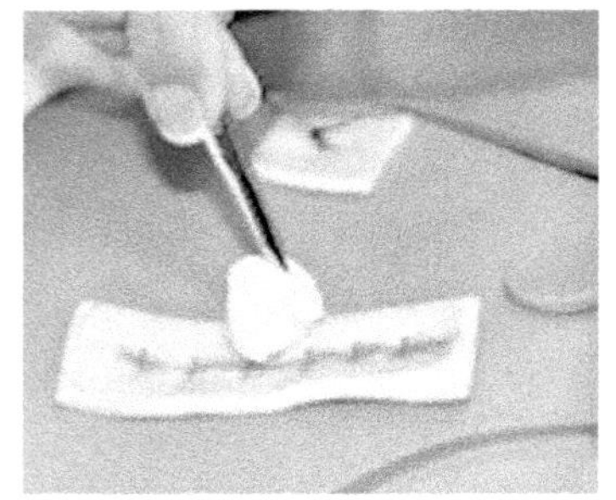
	• All other cleansing involves moving from one end to the other on each side of the incision.	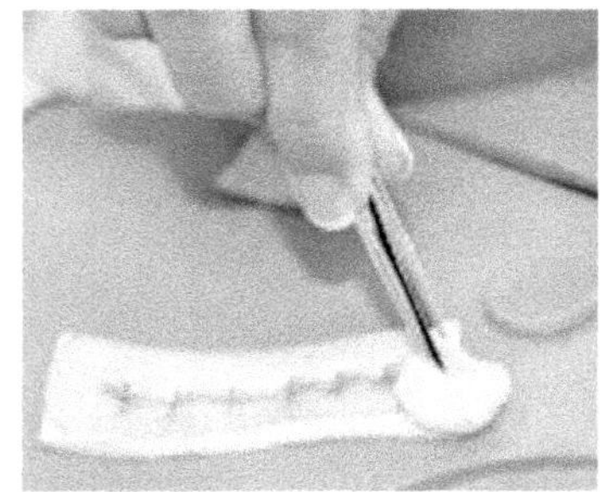
	• Work in straight lines, moving away from the suture line with each successive stroke.	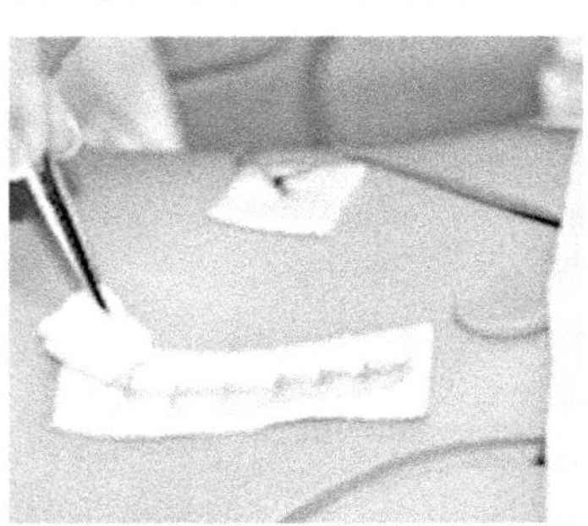
17. Cleanse around drain (if present).	• If a drain is present, clean the drain site using a circular stroke, starting with the area immediately next to the drain. • Using a new swab, cleanse immediately next to the drain and attempt to clean a little further out from the drain. Continue this process with subsequent swabs until the skin surrounding the drain is cleaned. • Cleanse around drain.	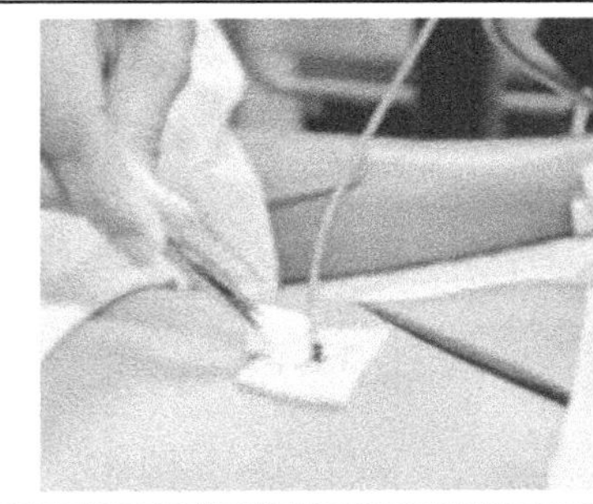

18. Apply inner dressing (4 x 4 gauze) with forceps to incision, then drain site (drain sponges/cut gauze).	• Cover incision.	
	• Cover drain site.	
	• Tape drain tubing to skin.	
19. Discard non-sterile gloves if they were used.	• This step prevents the spread of microorganisms. • Discard gloves.	
20. Apply outer dressing, keeping the inside of the sterile dressing touching the wound.	• This step protects wound from contamination. • Apply outer dressing if required	
21. To complete dressing change: • Assist patient to comfortable position. • Lower patient's bed. • Discard used equipment appropriately. • Perform hand hygiene.	• Taking these step ensures the patient's continued safety. • Hand hygiene with ABHR	

22. Document procedure and findings according to agency policy.	• Record dressing change as per hospital policy. • Document the wound appearance, if the staples are intact, if the incision is well-approximated. • Chart the time, place of wound, size, drainage and amount, type of cleaning solution, and dressing applied. • State how the patient tolerated the procedure. • Report any unusual findings or concerns to the appropriate health care professional.
23. Compare wound to previous wound assessment and determine healing progress, if any.	If there is no movement toward healing, or if there is deterioration, notify the physician or wound care nurse according to agency policy.

Suture Removal

Definition

Sutures are tiny threads, wire, or other material used to sew body tissue and skin together. They may be placed deep in the tissue and/or superficially to close a wound. A variety of suture techniques are used to close a wound, and deciding on a specific technique depends on the location of the wound, thickness of the skin, degree of tensions, and desired cosmetic effect.

Types of Sutures

Sutures are absorbent (dissolvable) or non-absorbent (must be removed). Non-absorbent sutures are usually removed within 7 to 14 days. Suture removal is determined by how well the wound has healed and the extent of the surgery. Sutures must be left in place long enough to establish wound closure with enough strength to support internal tissues and organs.

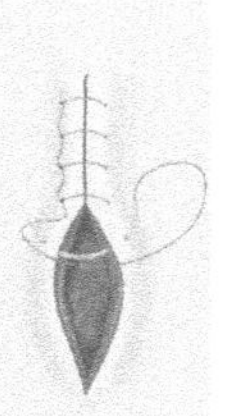

Continuous blanket suture

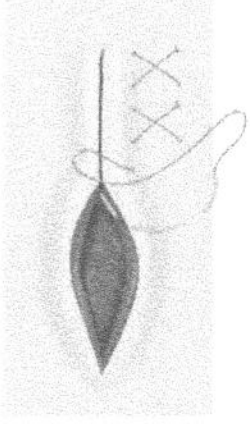

Interrupted cruciate suture

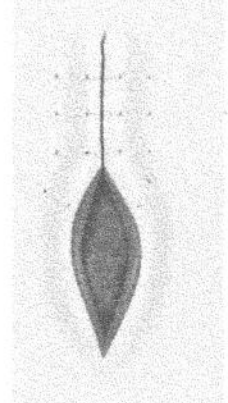

Vertical mattress suture

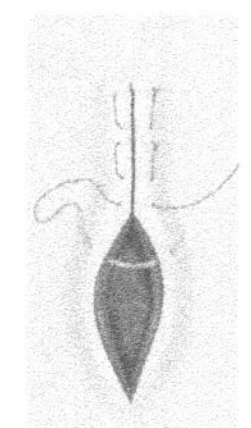

Horizontal mattress suture

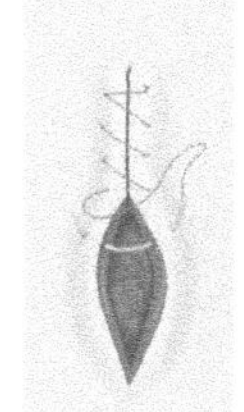

Simple continuous suture

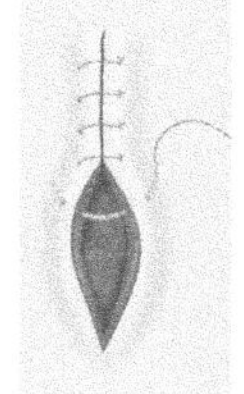

Simple interrupted suture

Types of sutures

Time Duration for Suture Removal

- Abdomen   : 10–12 days
- Back   : 10–12 days
- Chest   : 10–12 days
- Extremity   : 10–14 days
- Hands and feet   : 10–14 days
- Knee and elbow   : 12–14 days
- Scalp   : 10–12 days
- Eyebrow   : 4–5 days
- Eyelid   : 4–5 days
- Face   : 4–5 days
- Lip   : 4–5 days
- Neck   : 5–6 days
- Oral cavity   : 6–8 days
- Pinna (ear)   : 4–6 days

Safety Precautions Considerations

- Perform hand hygiene.
- Check room for additional precautions.
- Introduce yourself to patient.
- Confirm patient ID using two patient identifiers (e.g., name and date of birth).
- Explain process to patient and offer analgesia, bathroom, etc.
- Listen and attend to patient cues.
- Ensure patient's privacy and dignity.
- Complete quick priority assessment (QPA) including safety.
- Assess the patient risk of delayed healing and risk of wound dehiscence.
- Perform a point of care risk assessment for necessary personal protective equipment (PPE).

Equipment List

- Surgical needle   : 1
- Tissue forceps   : 1
- Artery forceps   : 1
- Needle holder   : 1
- Stitch scissors   : 1
- Drapes/gauze pad   : 1
- Antiseptic solution : 1
- Sterile strips   : 1
- Sterile gloves   : 1
- Suture remover kit   : 1

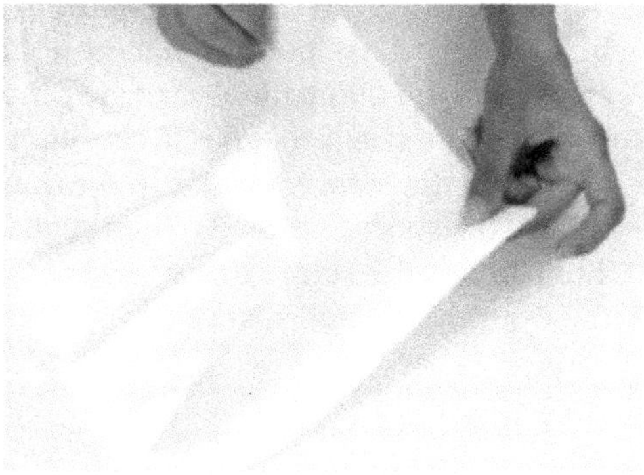
Needed equipment for suturing

Procedures

- Verify the physician's order.
- Explain the procedure to the parents/child and get concerns or obtain their verbal consent to remove the sutures.
- Perform hand hygiene.
- Arranged all the needed equipment's nearby child unit.
- Perform hand hygiene and wear clean gloves to remove the old surgical dressing.
- Observe the wound, if any infection present (excessive redness, warm to the touch, hard, oozing foul looking drainage or a smell) record and report to doctor.
- Doff gloves, perform hand hygiene, and prep supplies
- Open dressing change tray and set-up supplies for procedure
  - The sterile gloves and drape should be at the top of the dressing change tray after you open it carefully grab them and place them down in your work area.
  - Open the sterile drape first (watch the video above to know how to properly open the sterile drape).
  - Then open and **DROP** the suture remover kit supplies and steri-strips onto the sterile drape along with the antiseptic. I prefer to keep them in the tray because there is a chance that once their opened, they will leak onto the drape, which will contaminate the field.

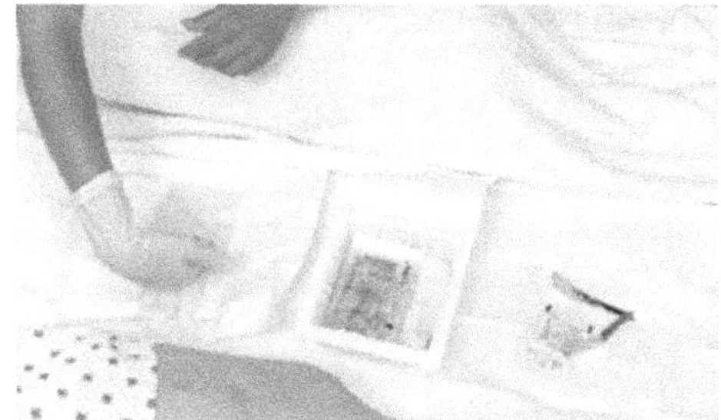
Open the sterile drape first

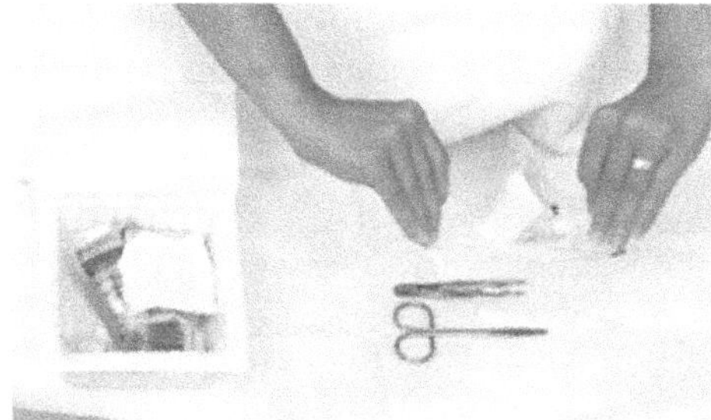
Open and drop the suture remover kit supplies

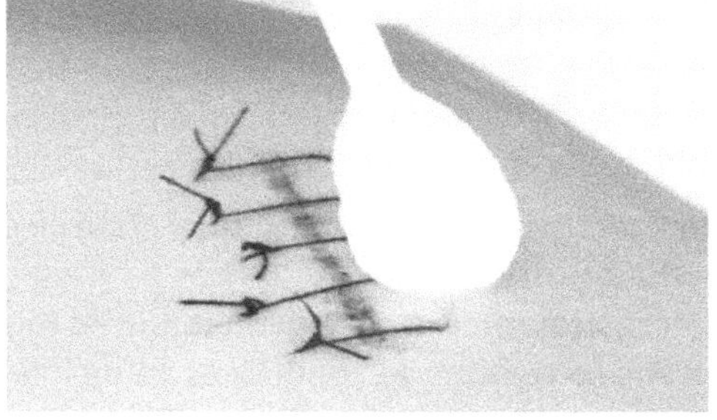
Don the sterile gloves technique

- Open the antiseptic swabs (most have 3 that come in a pack).
- Clean the surgical site with an antiseptic swab and discard.

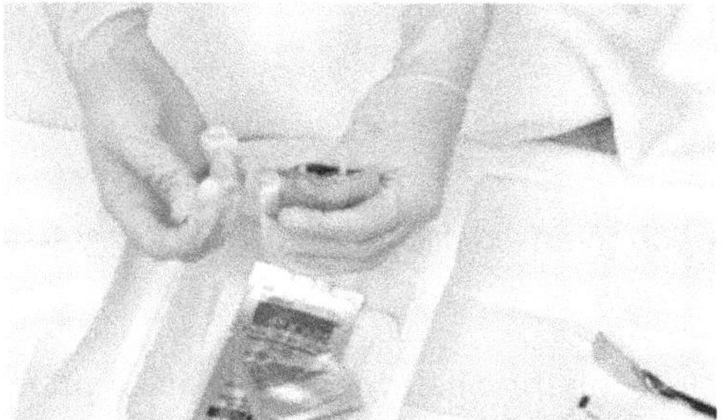
Open the antiseptic swabs

Clean the surgical site

- Let the site completely dry.
- Time to remove the sutures.

First remove every other suture starting with the 2nd suture

A complication of removing surgical sutures is wound dehiscence, this is where the surgical site opens up prematurely before wound healing can occur. By removing every other suture first, this will help decrease this from happening. Before we remove the other sutures, steri-strips will be in place to protect the site.

Start removing the sutures at the 2nd suture thread

- **Important:** When removing simple interrupted sutures DO NOT cut the suture thread that is the longest but cut the suture thread that is closest to the skin near the suture knot (it will be the shortest thread next to the suture knot).
- When you cut the longest suture thread and go to remove it with the tweezers, it will cause the suture thread that has been exposed to the outside environment to pass through the skin (hence the wound) during the removal, which can lead to infection. However, cutting the shortest suture thread will bypass this from happening.
- In addition, when "pulling" out the suture thread via the knot with the tweezers, pull OVER the incision line rather than away from it. Pulling the thread away from the incision line can cause tension and can lead to the incision opening.
- You take the tweezers and lift the knot with your non-dominate hand. Then take the scissors in your dominate hand (gives you the most control with the sharpest item) and cut the thread under the knot where the knot is closest to the skin (hence the shortest thread). Then slightly lift the knot up and pull over the wound.
- Then look at the suture thread and make sure all of it was removed (it not all removed this can alter wound healing and the wound can open again).

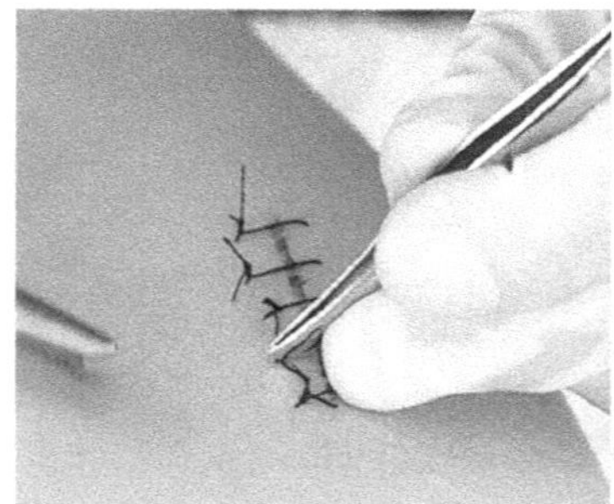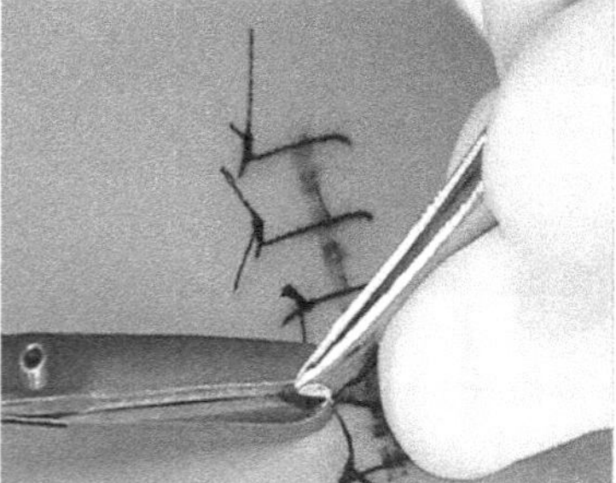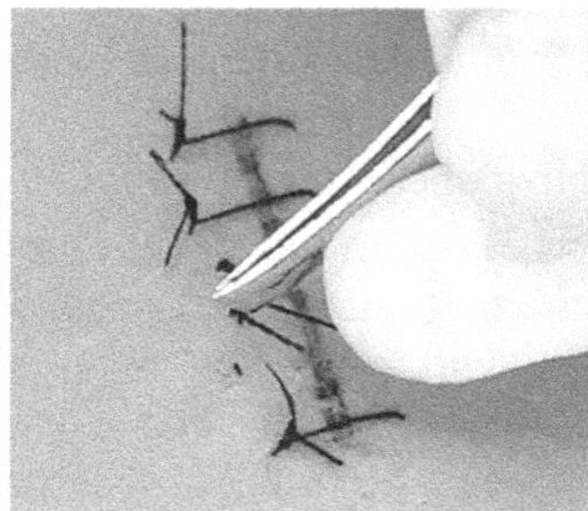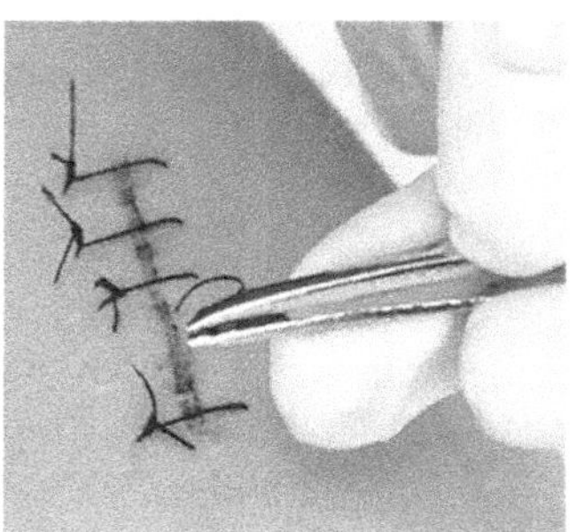

Suture removal technique

- After removing each suture, be sure to place them in a gauze, and don't forget to count them (document it too). This will help prevent the sutures from getting lost and allows you to count them. Should remember this is considered a bio-hazard item and needs to be disposed of properly, according to hospital's protocol.

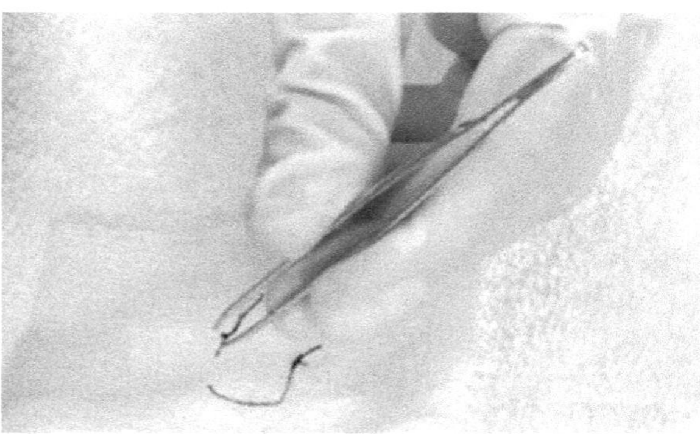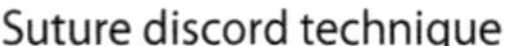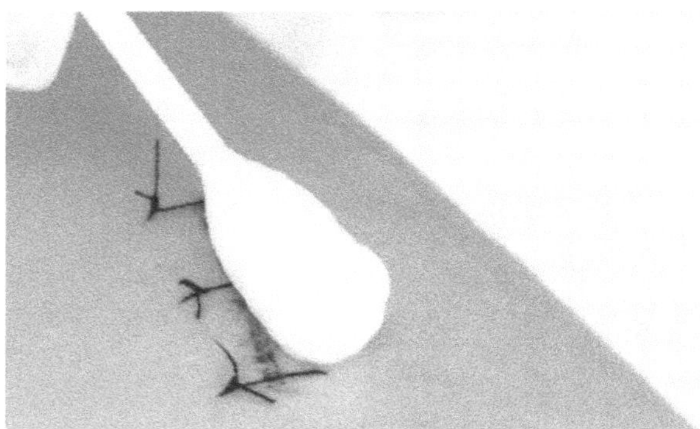

Suture discord technique   Cleaning technique of sutured area

- Continue removing every other suture. Then clean the areas of where you removed the suture with a new antiseptic swab and let the site dry.
- Place steri-strips on the places you removed the sutures.
  - Cut the steri-strips so about ¾ of an inch is on each side of the incision (or whatever the physician prefers or your hospital protocol dictates).
  - In addition, space each strip 1/8 of an inch.

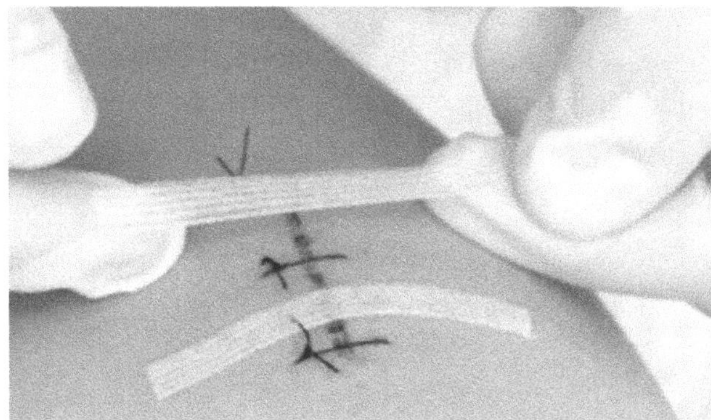

Place steri-strips on the removed sutures area

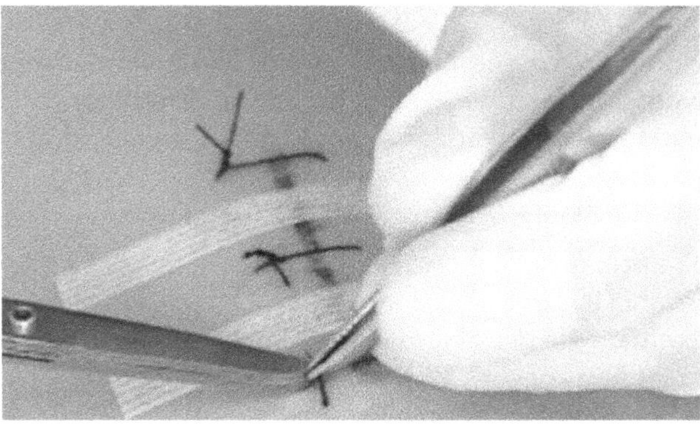

Remove the rest of the sutures

- Remove the rest of the sutures.
- Note (remember) number of sutures you have removed.

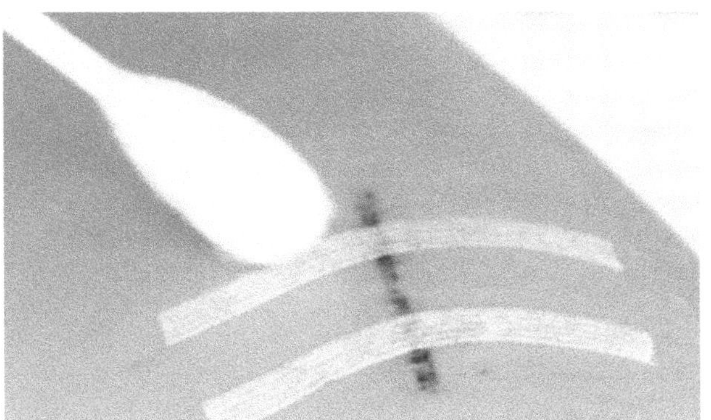

Clean the sites and let them dry

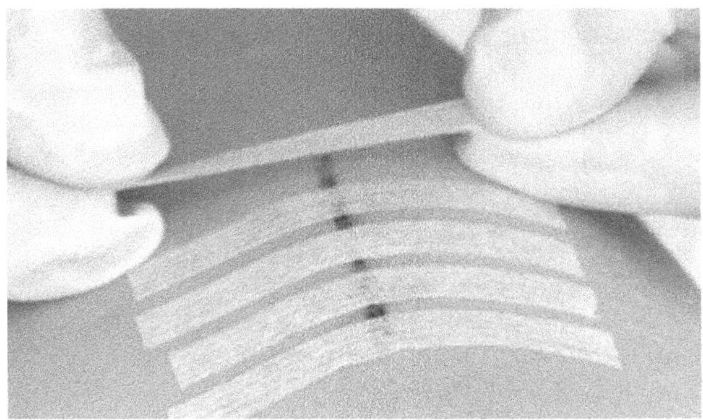

Place steri-strips over the suture removed area

- Clean the sites and let them dry.
- Place steri-strips over the suture removed area.
- **Optional:** Cover the site with a dressing if the site is at risk for friction. Is the site in the groin where the jeans will rub against it. If you place a dressing, EDUCATE the patient how to change it and given them supplies to do so.
- Educate the patient to let the steri-strips fall off naturally (takes about 10 days). Showers are best until the strips fall off.
- Discard the sutures and supplies per hospital protocol.
- Doffing of used gloves
- Perform hand hygiene
- **Documentation:** The number of sutures removed, how the child tolerated the procedure, complications (if available), how the site looked, education provided to the parents and older child.

NUTRITIONAL ASSESSMENT

Introduction

Nutritional status affects every child response to illness. Good nutrition is important for achieving normal growth and development. Nutritional assessment therefore should be an integral part of the care for every pediatric patient. Routine screening measures for abnormalities of growth should be performed on all pediatric patients.

Those patients with chronic illness and those at risk for malnutrition should have detailed nutritional assessments done. Components of a complete nutritional assessment include a medical history, nutritional history including dietary intake, physical examination, anthropometrics (weight, length or stature, head circumference, midarm circumference, and triceps skinfold thickness), pubertal staging, skeletal maturity staging, and biochemical tests of nutritional status.

Definition

Nutritional assessment is the interpretation of anthropometric, biochemical (laboratory), clinical and dietary data to determine whether a person or groups of people are well nourished or malnourished (over-nourished or under-nourished).

Types

- **Nutritional assessment:** Detailed examination of metabolic, nutritional or functional variables by an expert dietician
- **Nutritional screening:** Rapid and simple process conducted by admitting staff or community health care teams-defining patients who are at risk or not at risk of malnutrition.

Nutritional Assessment Goals

- Confirm normal growth and development
- Establish nutritional status
- Evaluate the risk of undernutrition/overweight
- Provide guidelines for nutrition therapy
- Monitor the impact of nutrition therapy

Components of Nutritional Assessment

- Medical history
- Physical examination
- Anthropometric measurements
- Dietary intake and energy requirements
- Body composition
- Biological/biochemical parameters.

Medical and Diet History

Medical history

- Reason for current referral/diagnosis
- Previous illnesses/diagnoses
- Family illnesses/diagnoses (acute or chronic)
- Growth history
- Assess how the client is growing
- Identify growth issues (current and/or previous)
- Calculate body mass index (BMI) and ideal body weight (IBW)

Diet history

- Appetite, composition of typical meals, food preference
- Aversion, food allergy and intolerance

Dietary assessment

- Dietary records
- 24-h recalls
- Food-frequency questionnaire
- Intake observations

Table: Food intake assessment

Causes	Signs and symptoms
Inadequate intake	Lack of food (poverty), incorrect food preparation, abnormalities of sucking, swallowing and deglutition, lack of appetite (anorexia)
Increased loses	Vomiting, diarrhea
Increased metabolic demands	Infection, inflammation, cardiac disorders
Alteration of the nutrients' metabolism	Drugs, hormonal abnormalities
Particular food habits	Vegetarians, vegans

Physical Examination

- Loss of fatty tissue and muscle strength
- Signs of malnutrition or micronutrient deficiency
- Thorough exam of skin, hair, nails, oral cavity, teeth and skeleton.

Assessment features	Manifestations	Possible etiology
General	Underweight, overweight, edema Short stature, apathy, irritability	Caloric/protein malnutrition, caloric excess
Skin and mucous	Pallor, dryness, dermatitis,	Iron, zinc
Membranes	Petechiae, delayed wound heeling	Thiamine, ascorbic acid, essential fatty acid (EFA) deficiency
Subcutaneous tissue	Decreased/increased/edema	Caloric deficit/excess, protein malnutrition
Muscle tissue	Wasting and pain	Caloric/protein malnutrition, thiamine deficiency
Skeleton	Craniotabes, parietal and frontal bossing, epiphyseal, enlargement, pigeon chest, beading of ribs	Calcium, vitamin D deficiency
Hair and nails	Alopecia, thin or sparse, depigmented Friable, koilonychia	Zinc, iron, biotin, vitamin A, K, niacin EFA
Lips and gums	Cheilitis, stomatitis, gingivitis, bleeding	B vitamins, ascorbic acid
Teeth and tongue	Caries, abnormal enamel Smooth, red/pale, painful	Deficiency/excess fluoride Niacin, riboflavin, B12
Eyes	Dryness, keratomalacia Circumcorneal injection Retinitis pigmentosa, photophobia	Vitamin A, riboflavin Vitamin E, zinc

Anthropometric Measurement Tool

Definition

Anthropometric measurement is defined as the study of human body measurements especially on a comparative basis. It is a science which deals with the measurement of the size, weight, and proportions of the human body (Dorland's Medical Dictionary). This procedure will concentrate on non-invasive techniques of determining these parameters.

The term **anthropometric** refers to comparative measurements of the body. Anthropometric measurements are used in nutritional assessments. Those that are used to assess growth and development in infants, children, and adolescents include length, height, weight, weight-for-length, and head circumference (length is used in infants and toddlers, rather than height, because they are unable to stand). Individual measurements are usually compared to reference standards on a growth chart.

Parameters

- Weight measurement
- Height measurement
- Head circumference
- Chest circumference
- Mid-arm circumference
- Abdominal circumference

Weight Measurement Technique

- At birth baby weight is 2.5–3 kg
- Double the birth weight by 5 months = 5–6 kg
- Triple the birth weight by 1 year = 7.5–9 kg

Technique

- Explain the procedures to parents
- Hand wash
- Check the weighing machine reading point, it should be "zero" level before reading the weight
- Remove the baby cloths and place over the weight machine (digital and manual)
- While reading the weight use the play materials for accurate reading
- Take the reading and document.

Height Measurement Technique

- At birth baby height is 50 cm (20 inch)
- Average height is 48–52 cm (18 to 22 inch)

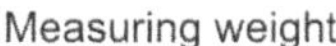

Measuring weight

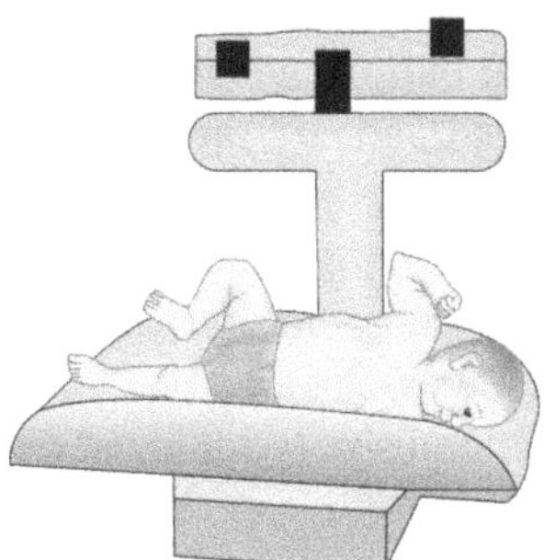

Infant being weighed in a pan scale

Measuring weight

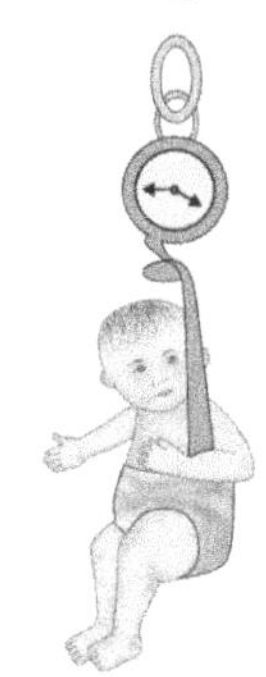

Infant being weighed in a hanging scale

Formula for Pound to Weight Conversion

$$\Rightarrow \frac{\text{Pound}}{2.2\,\text{kg}}$$

Technique

- Explain the procedures to parents
- Hand wash
- Check the infantometer, it should be in working condition
- Place the baby in supine position (digital and manual)
- Ask the child to stand in straight position over the height machine
- Before reading the height observe the child position
- Child head, shoulder, buttocks and heel should touch the measurement board.
- While reading the height use the play materials for accurate reading
- Take the reading and document.

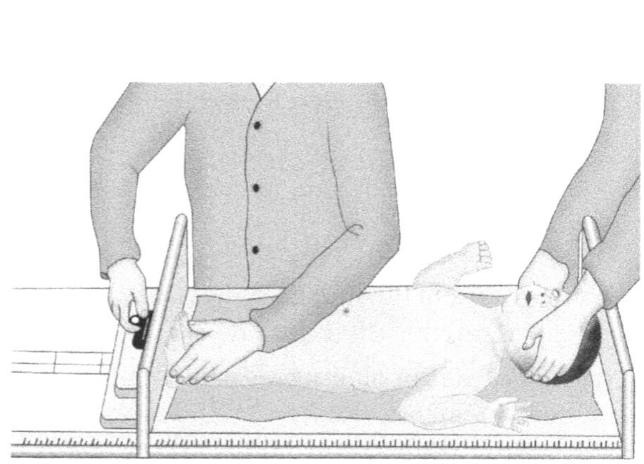 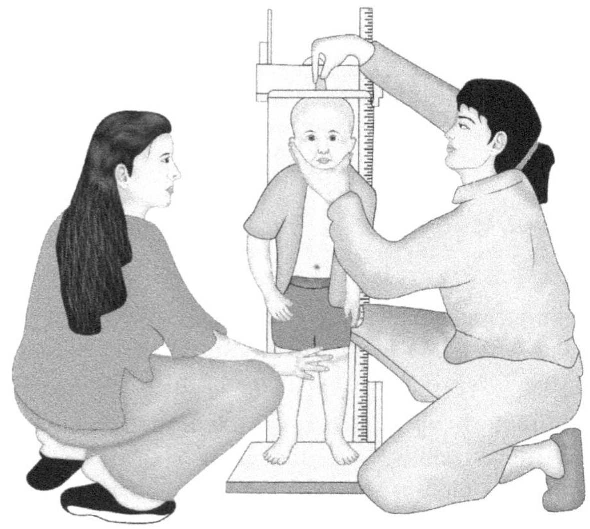

Head Circumference Technique

- At birth baby head circumference is 33–35 cm (13–14 inch)
- Average head circumference is 33–37 cm (13–15 inch)
- The 6 month baby head circumference is 42–44.5 cm (16.5–17.5 inch)
- The 1 year baby head circumference is 45–47.5 cm (17.7–17.7 inch)
- During the 1 year there is 12 cm increased in head circumference
- The 1–5 years of age the child will gain 5 cm
- Adult head size is achieved between 5 and 6 years.

Technique

- Explain the procedures to parents
- Hand wash
- Check the inch tape, it should be working condition
- Place the infant baby in supine position over the bed
- Provide the comfort position to child
- Child head should be measures around the skull
- Hold the measurement tape over the occipital, partial bone (above the earlobe) and four head
- While reading the head circumference use the play materials for accurate reading
- Take the reading and document.

Chest Circumference Measurement Technique

- At birth baby chest circumference is 32–34 cm
- Average chest circumference is 31–33 cm
- At the time of 1 year head and chest will be equal.

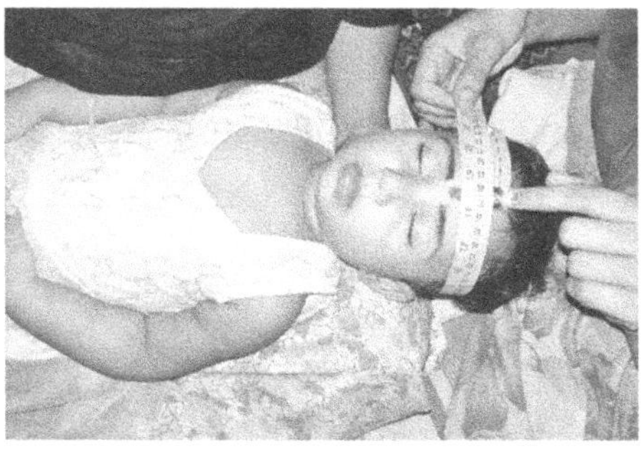 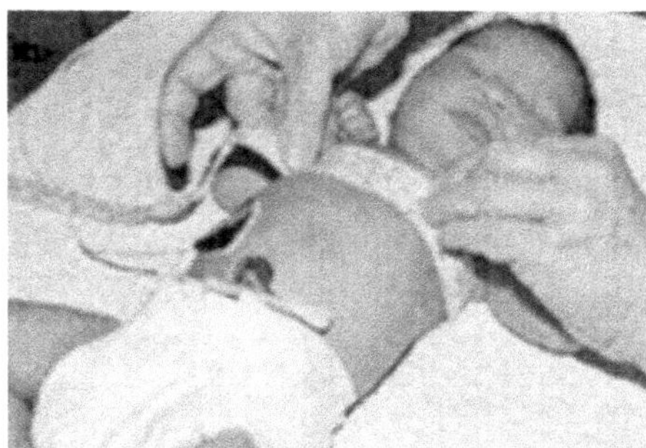 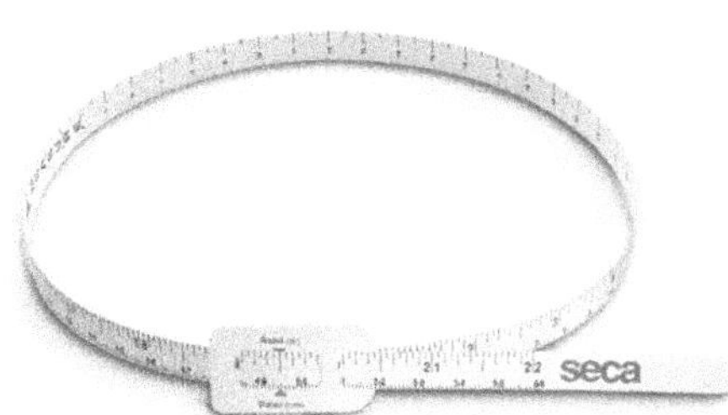

Technique

- Explain the procedures to parents
- Hand wash
- Check the inch tape, it should be working condition
- Place the infant baby in supine position over the bed
- Provide the comfort position to child
- Child chest should be measures around the thoracic cavity
- Hold the measurement tape around chest between the breast nipples
- While reading the chest circumference use the play materials for accurate reading
- Take the reading and document.

Mid-arm Circumference Measurement Technique

- During the 1–5 years of age it remains reasonably static between 15–17 cm among healthy child
- It is conventionally measured over the left upper arm, at the point marked midway between acromion process (shoulder) and olecranon process (elbow) with arm bent at right angle to measure
- To ask the child to site or standing position
- Ask child to hold the hand loose and comfortable
- Reading less than 12.5 cm it indicate severe malnutrition
- Reading between 12.5 and 13.5 cm it is indicate moderate malnutrition.

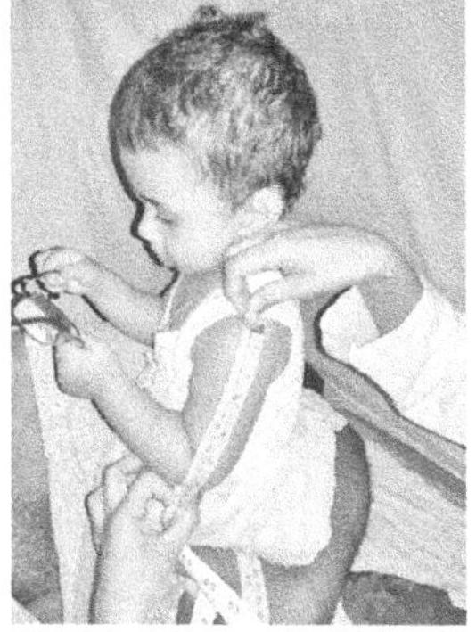 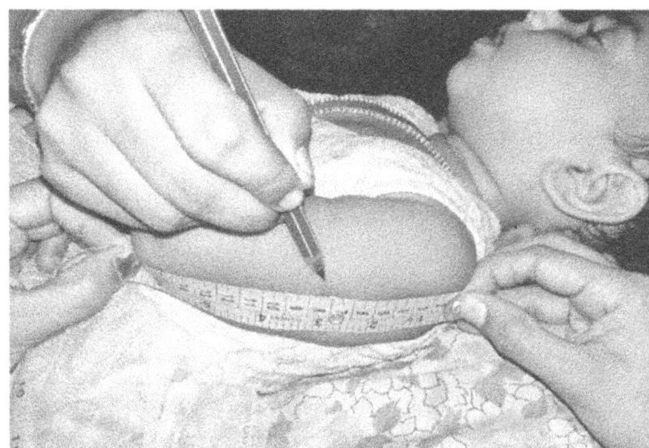 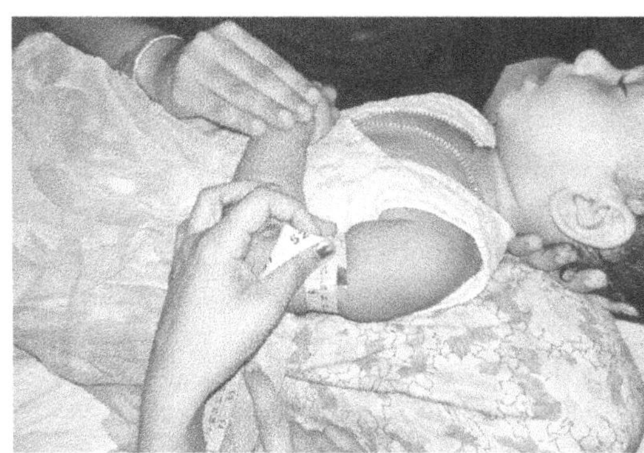

Abdominal Circumference Measurement Technique

- At birth baby abdominal circumference is 32 cm (12.5 inch)
- Average abdominal circumference is 31–33 cm

Technique

- Explain the procedures to parents
- Hand wash
- Check the inch tape, it should be working condition
- Place the infant baby in supine position over the bed
- Provide the comfort position to child
- Child abdomen should be measures around the abdomen cavity
- Hold the measurement tape around abdomen (0.5 cm above the umbilicus)
- While reading the measurement, nurse should use the play materials
- Take the reading and document.

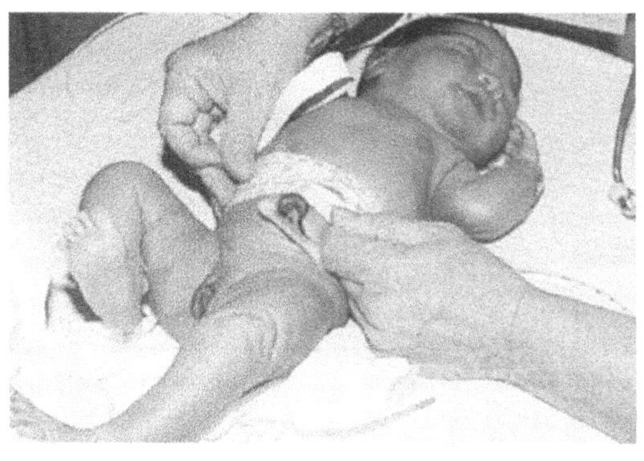

Dietary Intake and Energy Requirements

Daily calorie needs based on age, gender, and activity level

Age (years)	Gender	Sedentary (not active)	Moderately active	Active
2–3	Male or female	1000	1000	1000
4–8	Male Female	1200–1400 1200–1400	1400–1600 1400–1600	1600–2000 1400–1800
9–13	Male Female	1600–2000 1400–1600	1800–2200 1600–2000	2000–2600 1800–2200
14–18	Male Female	2000–2400 1800	2400–2800 2000	2800–3200 2400

Source: US Department of Agriculture and US Department of Health and Human Services. Dietary Guidelines for Americans, 2020, 7th edition. Washington, DC US Government Printing Office, 2010.

Average Daily Intake for a Toddler

Food group	Servings per day	Number of calories per day	One serving equals
Grains	6	250	• Bread—1/4 to 1/2 slide – Cereal, rice, pasta (cooked)—4 tbsps • Cereal (dry)—1/4 cup • Crackers—1 to 2
Vegetables	2–3	75	Vegetables (cooked)—1 tbsp. for each year of age
Fruits	2–3	75	• Fruit (cooked or canned)—1/4 cup • Fruit (fresh)—1/2 piece • Juice—1/4 to 1/2 cup (2–4 oz)
Dairy	2–3	300–450	• Milk—1/2 cup • Cheese—1/2 oz. (1-inch cube) • Yogurt—1/2 cup
Protein (meat, fish, poultry, tofu)	2	200	• 1 oz. (equal to two 1-inch cubes of solid meat or 2 tbsps. of ground meat) • Egg—1/2 any size, yolk and white
Legumes (dried beans, peas, lentils)	2	200	Soaked and cooked—2 tbsps. (1/2 cup)
Peanut butter (smooth only)		95	Spread thin on bread toast or cracker—1 tbsp

Nutritional deficiencies

	Manifestations	Possible etiology
Gastrointestinal	• Diarrhea • Hepatomegaly (fatty liver)	• Zinc • Caloric/protein malnutrition
Cardiovascular	• Cardiomyopathy • Arrhythmia	• Selenium, thiamine • Potasium, calcium, phosphor
Endocrine	• Hypothyroidism, goiter • Glucose intolerance • Hypogonadism	• Iodine • Chromium • Caloric/protein malnutrition
Neurologic	• Peripheral neuropathy • Motor peripheral neuropathy • Vibratory peripheral neuropathy • Sensory peripheral neuropathy • Ataxia • Psychomotor change, confusion	• Thiamine, pyridoxine • Thiamin, B12 • Thiamin, B12 • Thiamin • Vitamin E • Caloric/protein malnutrition
Others	• Altered taste • Parotid enlargement	• Zinc • Caloric/protein malnutrition

Vitamins	Deficiency	Excess
Vitamin A (retinol)	Night blindness, xerophatalmai Follicular keratosis, poor growth	Hepatomegaly, alopecia Headache, high ICP
Vitamin D (cholecalciferol)	Rickets, osteomalacia	Hypercalcemia
Vitamin E (tocopherol)	Hemolygtic anemia	Altered hematopoesis
Vitamin K (menaquinone)	Bleeding bruising	Hemolytic anemia
Vitamin B1 (thiamine)	Beriberi, ataxia, neuritis, cardiomyopathy	None known
Vitamin B2 (riboflavin)	Cheilosis, glossitis, seborrhea	None known
Vitamin B6 (pyridoxine)	Seizures, anemia, hyperirritabilitty	Neuropathy
Pantothenic acid	Infertility, growth delay, vomiting	Diarrhea
Niacin	Pellagra (dermatitis, dementia, diarrhea)	Vasomotor instability, flushing
Folate	Megaloblastic anemia, stomatitis, glossitis, neural tube defect (NTD) in pregnancy	None known
Vitamin B12 (cobalamine)	Megaloblastic anemia, neurologic deterioration, methylmalonic acid (MMA)	None known
Biotin	Dermatitis, vomiting, anorexia, hair loss	None known
Vitamin C (ascorbic acid)	Scurvy (purpura, petechiae, periodonal gingivitis), joint tenderness	Diarrhea, nausea and vomiting, etc.

Body Composition

Dual-energy X-ray Absorptiometry (DXA)

- Used to determine
- Bone mineral content
- Lean tissue mass
- Fat body mass (FBM)

Bio-electrical impedance analysis (BIA)

- Based on conduction of a very week alternating current trough the body which is delivered via two electrodes placed on hand and opposite foot
- BIA is a method for measurement of body water which is used to calculate fat free mass (FFM).

Biological/Biochemical Parameters

Specific Nutrients (as Indicated by History and Examination)

- Immune function
- Total lymphocyte count
- Delayed cutaneous hypersensitivity.

Protein Metabolism

- Nitrogen balance
- Protein turn over studies.

Urinary Elimination of Muscle Metabolites

- Creatinine and 3-methyl histidine (24 hours, correlates with FFM)
- Creatinine-height index (adults).

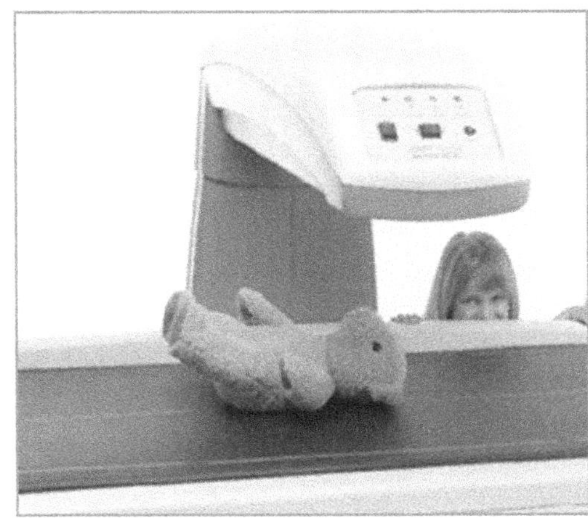

Dual-energy X-ray absorptiometry (DXA)

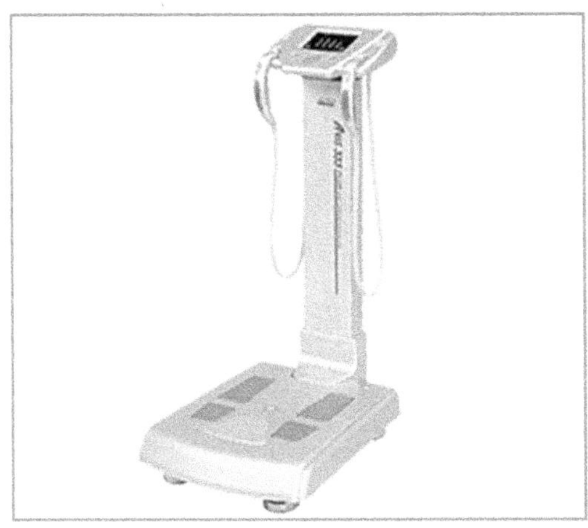

Bio-electrical impedance analysis (BIA)

Plasma protein	Pool size and half-life	Plasma level	Factors of variation
Albumin	Large pool size Half-life: 15–20 days	36–45 g/L	Protein-energy malnutrition Liver failure Protein-losing enteropathy Protracted infectious state
Thyroxin- binding prem-albumin	Small pool size Half-life: 2–3 days	0,32–0,35 g/L	Protein-energy malnutrition Liver disease Hyperthyroidism Inflammatory disease.
Retinol- binding protein	Small pool size Half-life: 12 hours	60+/- mg/L	Protein-energy malnutrition. Inflammatory disease Vitamin A, zinc deficiency. Liver disease (hepatitis, cirrhosis, cancer) Glomerulonephritis and renal tubular defect increase level
Transferrin	Large pool size Half-life: 8 days	2–4 g/L (age dependent)	Glomerulopathy Protein-losing enteropathy Liver failure Protein-energy malnutrition Inflammatory disease Iron deficiency

A Step-by-Step Guide to using STAMP

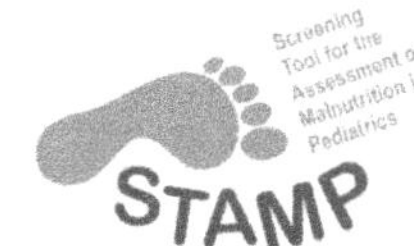

Step 1–Diagnosis			Step 2–Nutritional intake		Step 3–Weight and height	
Does the child have a diagnosis that has any nutritional implications?	Score		What is the child's nutritional intake?	Score	Use a growth chart or the centile quick reference table to determine the child's measurements	Score
			None	3	> 3 centile spaces/ ≥ 3 columns apart (or weight <2nd centile)	3
Definitely	3		Recently decreased/ poor	2		
Possibly	2					
No	0		No change/good	0	> 2 centile spaces/ = 2 columns apart	2
					0 to 1 centile spaces/ columns part	0

Step 4–Overall risk of malnutrition	
Add the scores from steps 1–3 together to calculate the overall risk of malnutrition	Score
High risk	≥ 4
Medium risk	2–3
Low risk	0–1

Step 5–Care plan

Develop a care plan based on the child's overall risk of malnutrition

High risk	Medium risk	Low risk
• Take action • Refer to a dietitian, nutritional support team or consultant • Monitor as per care plan	• Monitor nutritional intake for 3 days • Repeat STAMP screening after 3 days • Amend care plan as required	• Continue routine clinical care • Repeat STAMP screening weekly while child is an in-patient • Amend care plan as required

APPLICATION OF RESTRAINTS

Introduction

Children often undergo potentially painful and frightening medical procedures in hospitals and can experience distress, pain, and anxiety and may express strong and persistent resistance during procedures. Restraint seems to be more frequently used with pre-schoolers during different medical and clinical procedures than with older children and is used to enable safe performance of the medical procedure when the child resists it.

Definition

A special measure are necessary to prevent accidents or injuries from falls. Children may also need restraints to remind them not to pull on tubes or pick at suture lines. Sometimes, enforcing bed rest by applying a child safety device called a restraint is necessary. Small children also should be restrained whenever they are in a high chair, wheelchair, or unattended. However, never substitute the safety device for good observation.

Types of Restraints

- Mummy Restraint
- Jacket Restraint
- Elbow Restraint
- Clove hitch or Extremity Restraint
- Abdominal Restraint
- Mitten or finger Restraint
- Crib with Dome Restraint.

Types of restraints	Image	Purpose
Mummy restraints	A B C D E F	• Mummy restraint is used for the children to restrict the moment of limbs • It is used to the children for examination, procedure and treatment of head, neck and face is required • For example: Like scalp vein puncture, ear examination, and eye irrigation, gastric and gastric lavage
Jacket restraints		• To help of the baby remain flat in bed in a supine position • To prevent of the baby falling from high chair • To prevent of the baby up down on cribs • Chance of strangulation with jacket restraints

Elbow restraints	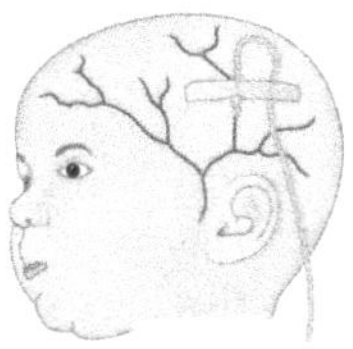 Venipuncture of scalp vein 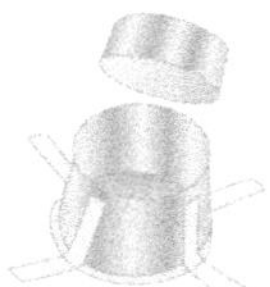 Paper cup taped over venipuncture site for protection. A clear plastic cup may also be used 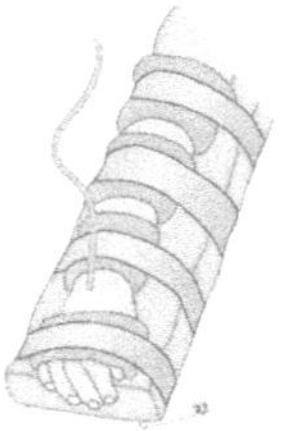 Restraint of arm when hand is site of infusion 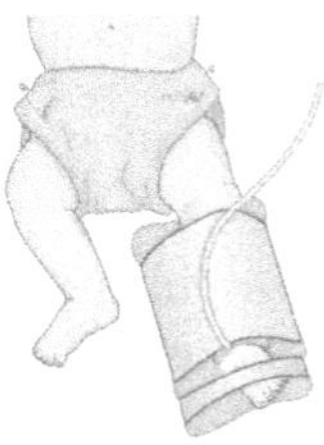 Infant's leg taped to sandbag for immobilization (IV site should be visible)	• To keep of the elbow in extended position so infant cannot reach the face after the surgery of the child's face and head such as cleft palate repair • During in Eczema and skin disorder • When introduce of the scalp vein
Clove hitch or extremity restraints	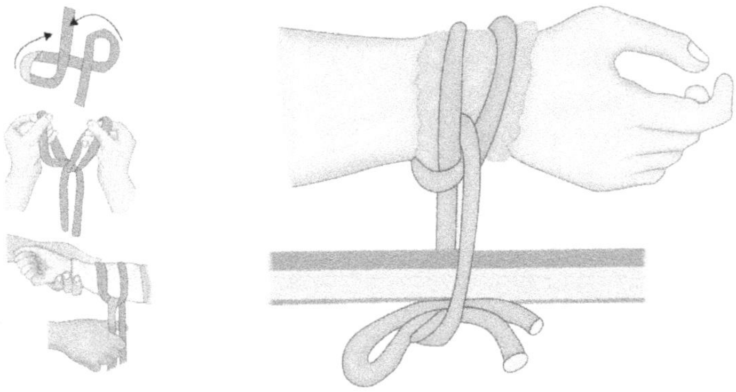	• Clove hitch restraints used to secure an arm or leg; used most often when a child is receiving an intravenous infusion. • The restraint is made of soft cloth formed in a figure eight.
Abdominal restraints	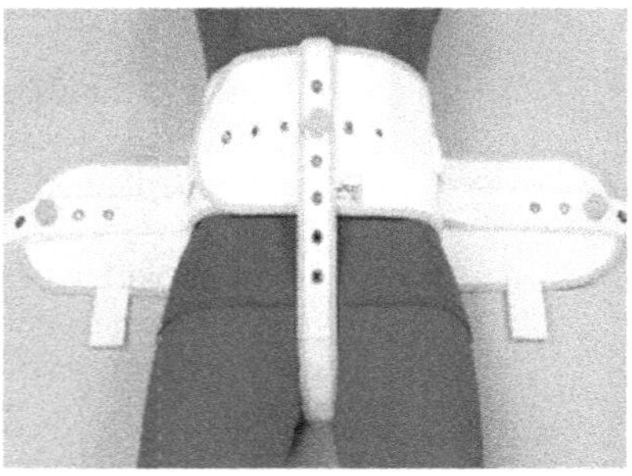 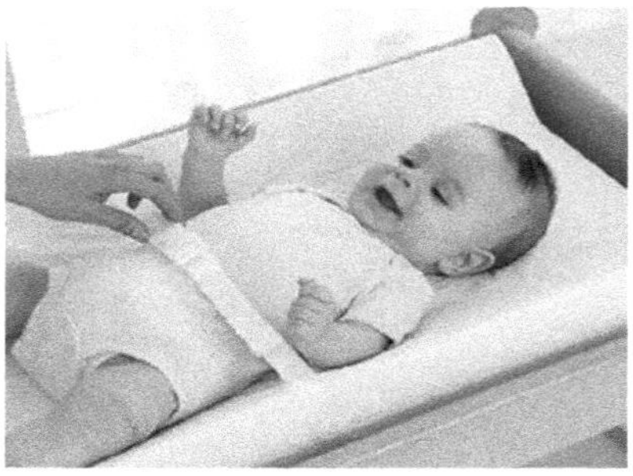	• This holds the infant in supine position on the bed. It must not be applied so securely that respiratory movements of the abdomen are inhibited. • Age group: Infant/toddler/pre-schooler
Mitten or finger	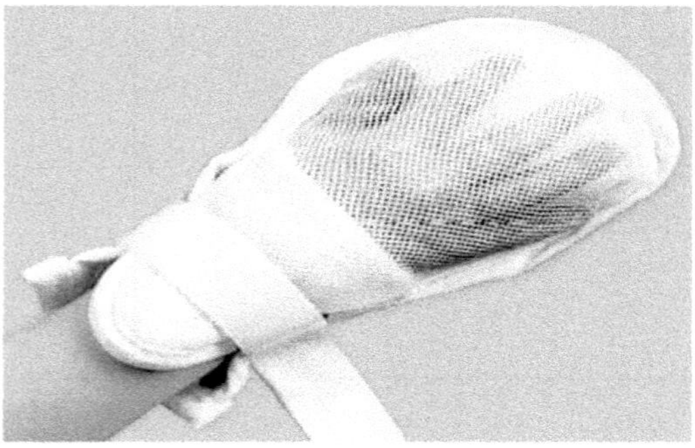	• Mitts are used for infants to prevent self-injury by hands in case of burns, facial injury or operations, eczema of the face or body.
Crib with dome restraint	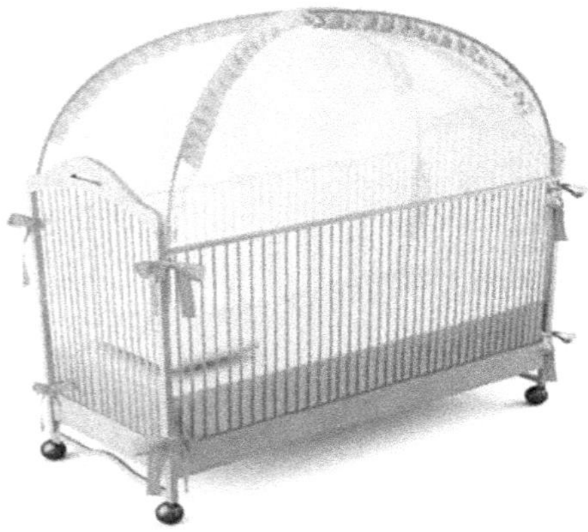	• Restraints designed to totally or partially limit the movement of infants and/or toddlers when they are lying in cribs. • These restraints typically consist of devices that directly restrain the child's movement (e.g., belts, straps) or devices placed on the crib top that limit the child's movement indirectly (e.g., covers, nets). • Crib restraints are used mainly to prevent children from falling out of the crib or climbing the crib rails.

Ethical Considerations

Three important ethical basic principles in health care are:

1. Non-maleficence
2. Beneficence
3. Respect for autonomy

When a painful procedure needs to be performed on a child that resists, it is crucial to weigh off whether applying restraint is in the child's interest. Creating psychological trauma is not in the child's interest; it could actually harm the child. Moreover, knowledge and technology are available for most procedures to make them (more) comfortable for the child. In most non-life-threatening situations, this will not be the case and sufficient time is available to look for an alternative without using restraint.

Complications

Most common restraint complications include:

- Accidental or intentional removal of restraints by children, family, or staff, resulting in possible removal of tubes, intravenous lines, or injury to patient or others
- Injury to restrained extremity (arm or leg)
- Fracture or muscle strains during application with violent patient
- Dislocation or contusion of extremity
- Exposure to blood or body fluid while restraining violent patient (biting, spitting, urinating, etc.)
- Numbness and/or tingling in restrained extremity.

Nursing Care Guidelines

- Assess the client's behavior and the need for restraint and applies as a last resort
- Get written order and obtain consent as per hospital policy
- Must communicates with the client and family members
- Complies with institutional policies and guidelines for restraint
- Explain the client the reason for the restraint and cooperation
- Arrange adequate assistance from competent staff before carrying out the restraint procedure
- Apply the least restrictive, reasonable and appropriate devices
- Arrange the client under restraint in a place for easy, close and regular observation
- Particular attention to his/her safety, comfort, dignity, privacy and physical and mental conditions
- Attend the client's biological and psychosocial needs during restraint at regular intervals
- Reviews the restraint regularly, or according to institutional policies
- Consider the earliest possible discontinuation of restraint
- Explore interventions, practices and alternatives to minimize the use of restraint
- Nurse must maintain his/her competence in the appropriate and effective use of restraint through continuous education
- Document the use of restraint for record and inspection purposes.

ADMINISTRATION OF OXYGEN INHALATION BY DIFFERENT METHODS

Introduction

Administration of oxygen is a process of providing the oxygen to child for the treatment of low concentrations of oxygen in the blood. Children with respiratory dysfunctions are treated with oxygen inhalation to relieve hypoxia. Tissue oxygenation is dependent on optimal or adequate delivery of oxygen to the tissues. Increasing the concentration of inhaled oxygen is an effective method of increasing the partial pressure of oxygen in the blood and correcting hypoxemia.

Definition

Airway management is the highest priority for clinical care. This is because if there is no airway, there can be no breathing, hence no oxygenation of blood and therefore circulation (and hence all the other vital body processes) will soon cease.

Purpose

- To manage the condition of hypoxia
- To maintain the oxygen tension in blood plasma
- To increase the oxy-hemoglobin in red blood cells
- To maintain the ability of cells to carry the normal metabolic function
- To reduce the risk of complications

Indication

Chronic Condition

- Chronic obstructive pulmonary disease (COPD)
- Cystic fibrosis
- Pulmonary fibrosis
- Sarcoidosis.

Acute Conditions

- Medical emergencies requiring high concentrations of oxygen in all cases:
  - Asphyxia and cyanosis
  - Shock and circulatory failure
  - Hemorrhage
  - Sepsis
  - Children who are under anesthesia
  - Major trauma
  - Cardiac arrest and during resuscitation
  - Anaphylaxis
  - Carbon monoxide and cyanide poisonings.
- Medical emergencies which may or may not require oxygen administration
  - Asthma
  - Anemia
  - Pulmonary embolism
  - Transfusion-related acute lung injury (TRALI).

Oxygen Delivery Systems

- Low-flow
- High-flow equipment.

Which provide an uncontrolled or controlled amount of supplemental oxygen to the patient. Selection should be based on preventing and treating hypoxemia and preventing complications of hyper-oxygenation. Factors such as how much oxygen is required, the presence of underlying respiratory disease, age, the environment, the presence of an artificial airway, the need for humidity, a tolerance or a compliance problem, or a need for consistent and accurate oxygen must be considered to select the correct oxygen delivery device.

Low-flow system	Image	High-flow system	Image
Nasal cannula		Venturi system	
Intranasal catheter		Oxy-hood	

Simple mask		Face tent	
Partial rebreathing mask		Oxygen tent	
Non-rebreathing mask		High flow nasal prongs	

Device	Flow rate in liters/minute	Percent FiO$_2$ delivered
Nasal cannula • Indicated for low-flow, low-percentage supplemental oxygen. • Flow rate of 1–6 L/min • Delivers 25–45% oxygen • Patient can eat, drink and talk • Extended use can be very drying; use with a humidifier	1	25%
	2	29%
	3	33%
	4	37%
	5	41%
	6	45%
Simple face mask • Indicated for higher percentage supplemental oxygen • Flow rate of 6–10 L/min • Delivers 35–60% oxygen • Lateral perforations permit exhaled CO$_2$ to escape • Permits humidification	6	35%
	7	41%
	8	47%
	9	53%
	10	60%
Nonrebreather mask • Indicated for high percentage FiO$_2$ • Incorporates use of reservoir bag • Flow rate of 10–15 L/min • Delivers up to 100% oxygen • One-way flaps prevent entrainment of room air during inspiration and retention of exhaled gases (namely CO$_2$) during expiration	10–15	80–100%
	• Both flaps removed results in lower (80–85%) FiO$_2$ • One flaps removed results in higher (85–90%) FiO$_2$ • Both flaps in place results in maximum (95–100%) FiO$_2$	
Venturi mask (venti-mask) • Indicated for precise titration of percentage of oxygen • Flow rate of 4–8 L/min • Delivers 24–60% oxygen • Users either a graduated dial set to desired FiO$_2$ or colored adapters selected to deliver desired FiO$_2$	Blue	24%
	White	28%
	Orange	31%
	Yellow	35%
	Red	40%
	Green	60%

Articles

- Oxygen source—oxygen cylinder/central supply
- Oxygen application device
    - Oxygen face mask
    - Oxygen hood
    - Nasal prongs
    - Nasal catheters
    - Oxygen tent or canopy.
- Humidifier
- Flow meter
- Gauze pieces
- Adhesive tapes
- 'No-smoking' board
- Spanner to remove main valve of oxygen supply
- Bowl with water to check the patency the tube
- Pulse oximetry.

Procedure

- Verify written order for oxygen therapy, including methods of delivery and flow rate.
- Wash hands.
- Explain the procedure to client.
- Assess the client for obstruction of the nasal passages by observing of breathing patterns.
- If using a wall outlet as oxygen source, plug flow meter into outlet by pushing until it snaps into place.
- Adjust the flow rate to the prescribed amount.
- Gently position nasal prongs into client's nares, with curves of prongs pointing toward the floor of the nostrils.
- Loop the cannula tubing over the client's ears; adjust the fit of the tubing by sliding the adjuster upward to hold the cannula in place.
- Assess the client's nares, face, and ears every 4 hours for signs of skin irritation or breakdown and document of findings. At the same time, inspect the nasal prongs for the presence of nasal secretions or crusts.

Complications of Oxygen Administration

- Infection
- Dryness of mucous membrane of respiratory tract
- Combustion (fire)
- Oxygen toxicity
- Atelectasis
- Oxygen induced apnoea
- Asphyxia
- Retrolental fibroplasia.

Role of Nurse in Oxygen Administration

- Review the protocol at your health authority prior to initiating any high-flow oxygen systems, and consult your respiratory therapist.
- In general, nasal prongs and a simple face mask (low-flow oxygen equipment) may be applied by a health care provider. All other oxygen equipment (high-flow systems) must be set up and applied by a respiratory therapist.
- For patients with asthma, nebulizer treatments should use oxygen at a rate greater than 6 L/min. The patient should be changed back to previous oxygen equipment when treatment is complete.
- Oxygenation is reduced in the supine position. Hypoxic patients should be placed in an upright position unless contraindicated (e.g., if they have spinal injuries or loss of consciousness).
- In general, for most patients with COPD, target saturation is 88% to 92%. It is important to recognize COPD patients are at risk for hypercapnic respiratory failure.
- Check the function of the equipment and complete a respiratory assessment at least once each shift for low-flow oxygen and more often for high-flow oxygen.
- In acutely ill patients, oxygen saturation levels may require additional ABGs to regulate and manage oxygen therapy.
- Oxygen saturation levels and delivery equipment should be documented on the patient's chart.

PROCEDURE ON BOWEL WASH

Introduction

A bowel wash performed to decompress the lower intestine and deflate the abdomen by removing gas and stool using small amounts of sodium chloride 0.9% (normal saline).

Definition

A bowel wash is to clean the distal portion of the bowel, decompress the bowel and deflate the abdomen by removing air and feces. Bowel washout facilitates surgery and has been shown to prevent or reduce the risk of postoperative enterocolitis and as such can be used as a mode of temporary management in proven cases of Hirschsprung's until definitive surgery.

Purposes

- To prepare colon for specific surgical or diagnostic procedures
- To dilute and remove toxic agents that may be present n large intestine
- To reduce temperature in hyperpyrexia and heat stroke
- To supply fluid and electrolytes that are absorbed from intestine
- To stimulate peristalsis
- To relieve inflammation
- To keep the individual clean in case of fecal incontinence

Equipment

Rectal Catheter

- Term—14FG or as directed by surgeon
- Preterm—as directed by surgeon
    - A clean big tray and sterile cloth
    - Enema can and tubing
    - Kidney tray
    - Sterile glove
    - Warm water in a basin
    - Bath towel
    - Bedpans or pail for collecting the return flow
    - Irrigating solution
    - Soap, extra rubber sheet, small colon tube, plastic apron, colostomy dressing tray, wash clot
    - The plastic cone-shaped piece at end of the tubing fits snugly against the stoma to run water into the colostomy
    - An irrigation sleeve to carry the irrigation output into the toilet
    - A tail closure clip and a belt for extra irrigation sleeve support (this is optional).

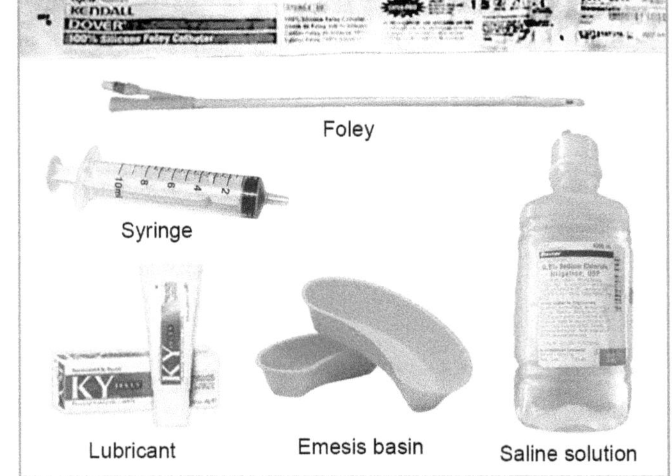

Procedure

- Explain the procedures to parents
- Ensure procedural consent obtained by treating surgical team before commencement
- Consider methods of patient distraction, such as sucrose or distraction.
- Consider second staff member or parent to assist with technique
- Perform hand hygiene
- Position neonate, usually on his/her back with legs in the frog position
- Position older child on their left side
- Swaddling of arms, comfort and play therapy techniques can be used
- Perform hand hygiene
- Select appropriately sized catheter for use

- Warm 0.9% sodium chloride sachets (in a jug of warm tap water) and prime catheter with solution
- Lubricate tip of catheter and gently insert into the rectum
- Length to be determined by surgical instructions
- Instil 0.9% sodium chloride solution in 10–20 mL aliquots (by pushing in with syringe plunger) over 1–2 minutes (there should be no resistance when injecting the normal saline
- Remove syringe and let fluid run into nappy/kidney dish. Procedure may be repeated twice if return is not clear
- If there is 0.9% sodium chloride retention or return volume cannot be determined contact surgeon
- Remove catheter from the rectum and leave the patient clean and dry perform hand hygiene
- Note and record results of rectal washout accurately on fluid balance section of the electronic medical record (EMR) flowsheets
- Sucrose may be administered prior to and throughout the procedure as required
- Do not use excessive force if resistance is felt. Contact medical staff if unsure
- Do not pull back on syringe to aspirate, allow the saline to run out naturally. Sometimes manipulating the catheter in and out a few centimetres gently and massaging the abdomen may encourage fluid returns to be expelled. Do not exceed maximum of 20 mL/kg or total of 250 mL
- After the procedures do the documentation.

After the Procedure

- Time irrigation administered.
- Kind and amount of solution used for the irrigation.
- Dressing applied.
- Condition of the area.
- Results obtained; amount, color, and consistency of the returns.
- Patient's reaction to procedure.

PROCEDURE ON INSERTION OF SUPPOSITORIES

Introduction

Rectal suppositories are solid forms of medication that are inserted into the rectum. It is available in different shapes and sizes, but they are usually narrowed at one end. Rectal suppositories deliver many types of medication. For instance, they may contain glycerin to treat constipation or acetaminophen to treat a fever. Medication from a rectal suppository tends to work quickly. This is because the suppository melts inside the body and is absorbed directly into the bloodstream.

Definition

A suppository is a solid bullet-shaped preparation, which is inserted into the rectum. It is administered when the oral route is not acceptable or when a local effect on the bowel is required.

Types

There are two types of suppositories:

1. A stimulant suppository—stimulates bowel activity, softens stool (for example, glycerine, sodium bicarbonate)
2. A retention suppository—delivers medication (for example, paracetamol).

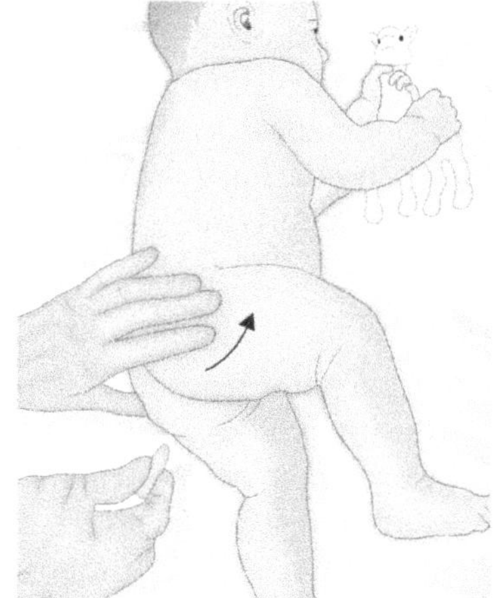

Indications

- Administration of medication
- Oral route contraindicated (nil orally, nausea or vomiting)
- Alternative to an injection (for a very ill child)
- Empty the bowel prior to surgery or endoscopic examination
- Local treatment of hemorrhoids or anal pruritus
- Treatment of constipation (after alternatives of diet or oral laxatives).

Contraindications

- Paralytic ileus
- Colonic obstruction

- Chronic constipation
- Postoperative gastrointestinal or gynaecological surgery
- **Caution:** Children with acute exacerbation of inflammatory bowel disease, diarrhea, rectal trauma, active rectal bleeding or any condition predisposing to rectal injury or abscess
- Suspicion of abuse.

Before the Procedure

- Gather all necessary equipment including—medication, child's chart, prescription sheet, disposable incontinence sheet, tissues, bedpan, toilet or commode (if appropriate); gloves and apron, water-based lubrication gel
- Explain the procedure to the child and family
- Encourage the child to empty their bowels
- Ensure a bedpan, toilet, commode or call bell is easily accessible
- Ensure medication has been stored as per manufacturer's instructions (certain suppositories should be refrigerated)
- Remove all wrapping from suppository and ensure the medication is intact
- To ensure accurate medication dosage—do not cut suppositories
- Place an incontinence pad underneath the buttocks (to prevent soiling of linen and distress to the child).

Administering the Suppository

- Ensure privacy for the child, covering them with a blanket to maintain dignity and prevent embarrassment.
- Wash your hands, put on a disposable apron and gloves to reduce the potential transfer of micro-organisms
- Lie the child on their left side with their knees bent and drawn up towards the abdomen.
- This position allows gravity to assist with the passage of the medication.
- Ask the child to take slow deep breaths to relax the anal sphincter.
- Visualize the peri-anal area, assess for abnormalities.
- Lubricate the apex of the suppository with lubricating gel.
- Insert the suppository apex first into the child's rectum, just past the internal sphincter.
- Gently hold the buttocks for five to 10 minutes, if possible, to reduce pressure on the anal sphincter and also risk of expelling medication.
- Clean away any lubricating jelly to prevent anal irritation and ensure comfort.
- Administer all medications safely as per local nursing policies.

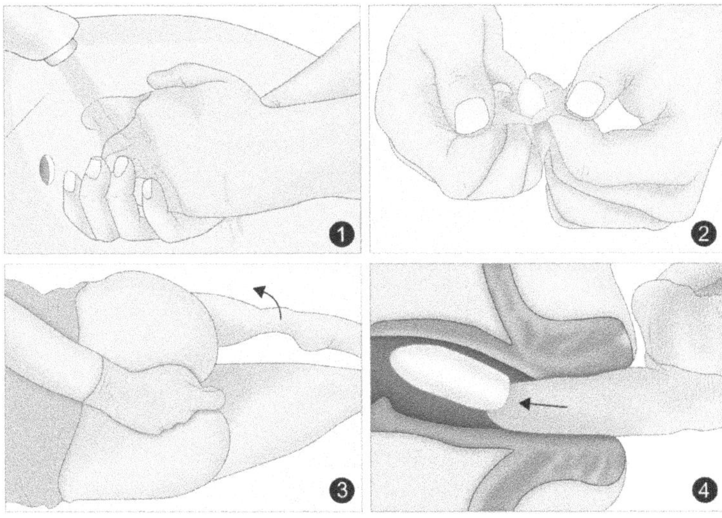

How to insert a suppository

After the Procedure

- Encourage the child to retain the medication for 20 minutes or as long as possible to enhance medication absorption.
- Dispose of equipment appropriately and wash your hands.
- Reassure and praise the child, and ensure they are comfortable.
- Record the medication administration as per local policy, monitor effectiveness of the medication.
- If stool or medication is expelled immediately post-administration, report to medical staff and document within the nursing notes.

Potential Complications

- Anxiety, embarrassment
- Local trauma or discomfort
- Specific adverse effects of individual medication
- Risk of bleeding (children with bleeding disorders).

ENEMA

Introduction

An enema is a technique used to stimulate stool evacuation. It is a liquid treatment most commonly used to help relieve severe constipation. The process helps push waste out of the rectum when child cannot do by own. Other types of enemas are administered to clean out the colon to better detect colon cancer and polyps.

Definition

An enema is defined as a liquid that is introduced into the rectum. It flushes out stool (feces) that has built up (impacted) in the bowel. This process is called disimpaction. Disimpaction helps restore the rectum's normal muscle tone. It can also help your child regain the natural urge to defecate.

Purposes

- To relieve constipation fecal impaction.
- To prevent involuntary escape of fecal matter during surgical procedure and delivery.
- To promote visualization of the intestinal tract during the radiographic or instrumental examination.
- To help establish regular bowel functions during a bowl training program.
- Pre-operative preparation for bowl surgeries.

Indications

- Constipation
- Hyperthermia
- Bowl surgeries
- Examination of intestinal tract.

Contraindications

- Acute renal failure
- Acute myocardial infarction and cardiac problems
- Appendicitis
- Recent surgical procedures involving lower intestinal tract.
- Intestinal obstruction
- Inflammation and infection of abdomen.

Solution Used

- Hypertonic-sodium phosphate
- Hypotonic-Tap water
- Isotonic-physiological saline (one tablespoon salt in 500 mL of tap water
- Others-3–5 mL of concentrated soap solution in 1000 mL of water.

Table: Amount of fluid to be introduced depends upon the size of the child.

Age group	Required amount of fluid
Infants	150–250 mL
Toddler	250–300 mL
Preschooler and school age	300–500 mL
Adolescents	500–750 mL
Adult	750–1000 mL

Catheter size: 10–12 Fr and should be inserted only 2–4 inches into the rectum depending upon the size of the child.

- Infants   : 2.5 cm
- 2–4 years   : 5 cm
- 4–10 years   : 7.5 cm
- > 11 years   : 10 cm
- Temperature of solution   : 105 °F

Equipment Needed

- A clean tray containing with sterile try cloths
- Enema bag or can and tubing with clamp or syringe with rubber tubing
- Lubricant (liquid paraffin)
- Enema solution
- Rectal catheter
- Gauze pieces in bowl
- Pair of gloves
- Bed pan at the edges
- Kidney tray with paper bag
- Lotion thermometer
- Macintosh with draw sheet.

Position of the Child

- Infant and toddler lie on abdomen with knees bent.
- Older children and adolescent left side with right leg flexed toward chest.

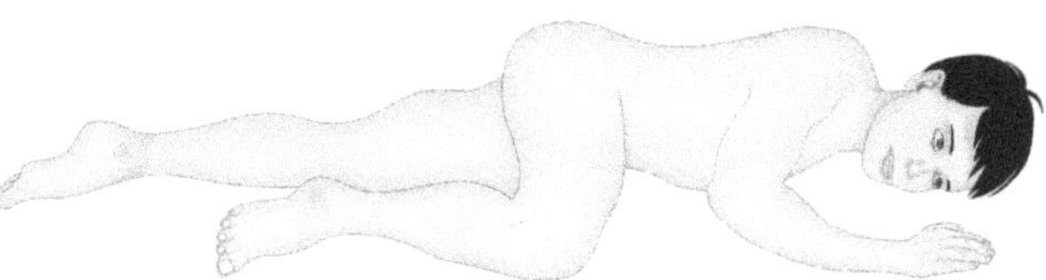

• Left-side position: Lie on left side with knee bent, and arms resting comfortably

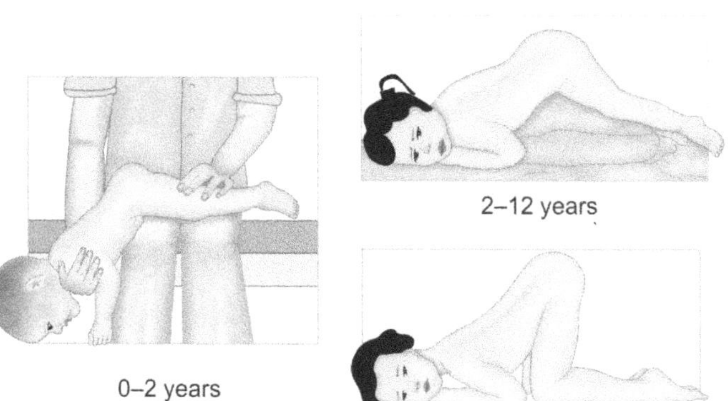

2–12 years

More than 12 years

Position for enemas

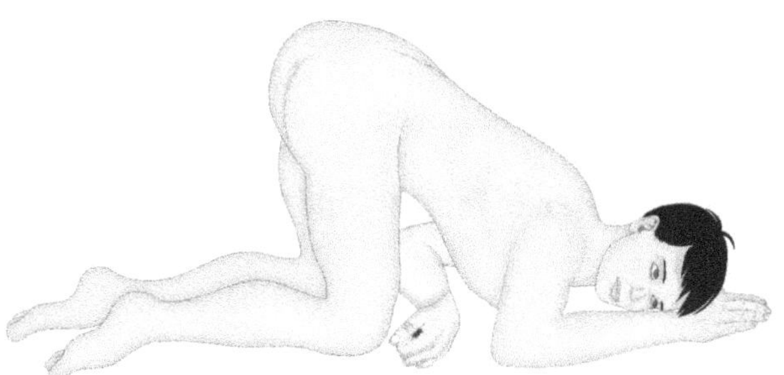

• Knee-chest position: Kneel, then lower head and chest forward until left side of face is resting on surface with left arm folded comfortably

0–2 years

Position for using this enema

Procedure

- Explain the procedures to parents.
- Assess the general status of child—last bowl movement, normal bowl movements, mobility, external sphincter muscles control, abdominal pain and perineal lesion.
- Performa the hand wash procedure and apply gloves.
- Arrange all the articles nearby child unit.
- Provide comfortable positions to child.
- Clamp the enema tubing, remove the cap and apply lubricant to the tip of catheter.
- Insert the tube into the rectum.

- Unclamp the tubing and administer the prescribed volume of enema solution at the rate of about 100 mL per minute.
- Remove the catheter gently and put it in kidney tray.
- Hold the child buttocks together if enema needed to encourage retention of enema for 5–10 minutes.
- Offer bed pan.
- In case of ambulatory and older children assist them to go to toilet.

Nursing Responsibilities

- Praise the child for cooperation.
- Make the child comfort.
- Record the procedure in nurse's record.
- Clean and replace the supplies.
- The Enema Can should not be held more than 18 inches above the child hip. So that the solution may run slowly by against gravity force and maintain proper pressure into the bowl.
- An isotonic solution or physiological saline is used. Tap water alone is not used because of the danger of the fluid shift and overload.
- A cleansing enema can be given 30–40 minutes after the oil retention enema.

URINARY CATHETERIZATION AND DRAINAGE

Definition

A urinary catheterization is defined as a urinary catheter or Foley catheter (hollow tube) is inserted into the bladder to drain or collect urine. The catheter is used as a duct to drain urine from the bladder into an attached bag or container.

There are two main types of urinary catheterization:

1. Indwelling catheterization
2. Clean intermittent catheterization.

Purpose

- Obtain a sterile urine sample
- Obtain accurate measurement of urine output
- Relieve acute or chronic urinary retention
- Evaluate or rule out the presence of obstruction
- Determine amount of residual urine after post void
- Prevent urine contamination of an incision in the perianal region
- Permit urinary drainage in infant with neurogenic bladder/dysfunction/retention.

Anatomy of Male and Female Child Genitalia

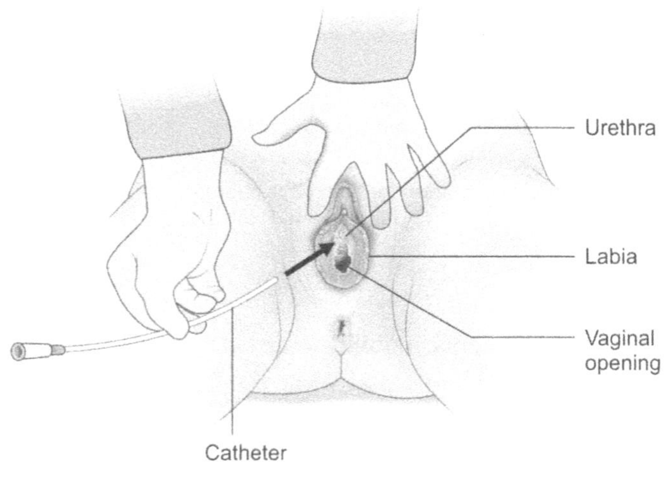

Female child genitalia

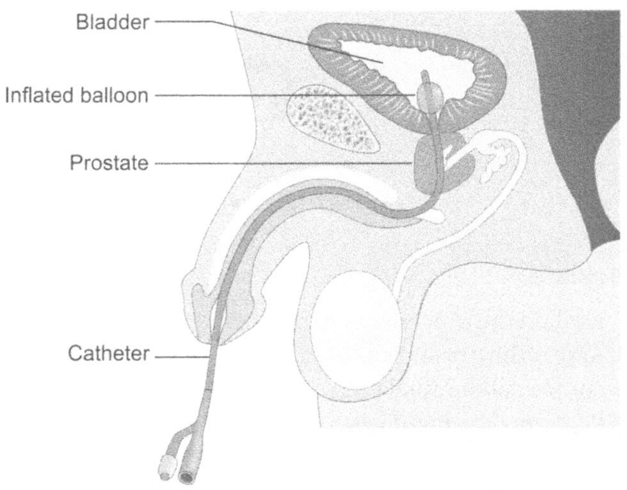

Male child genitalia

Equipment

- Sterile dressing tray
- Kidney tray and bowl-2
- Sterile gloves-1
- 2% chlorhexidine swab sticks (1–3 as needed)
- Sterile gauze
- Two sterile towels
- Two urinary catheter appropriate to size and gestation of the infant (only open one to start)
- Urinary catheter one size smaller than recommended
- Prefilled normal saline syringe if balloon (Foley) catheter is ordered
- Duoderm and Tegaderm to secure catheter if indwelling
- Sterile lubricant
- Sterile water
- Sterile specimen container (s) as required
- Pediatric urine meter or bedside drainage bag if indwelling
- Waterproof tape if indwelling for connection.

Types of Catheter

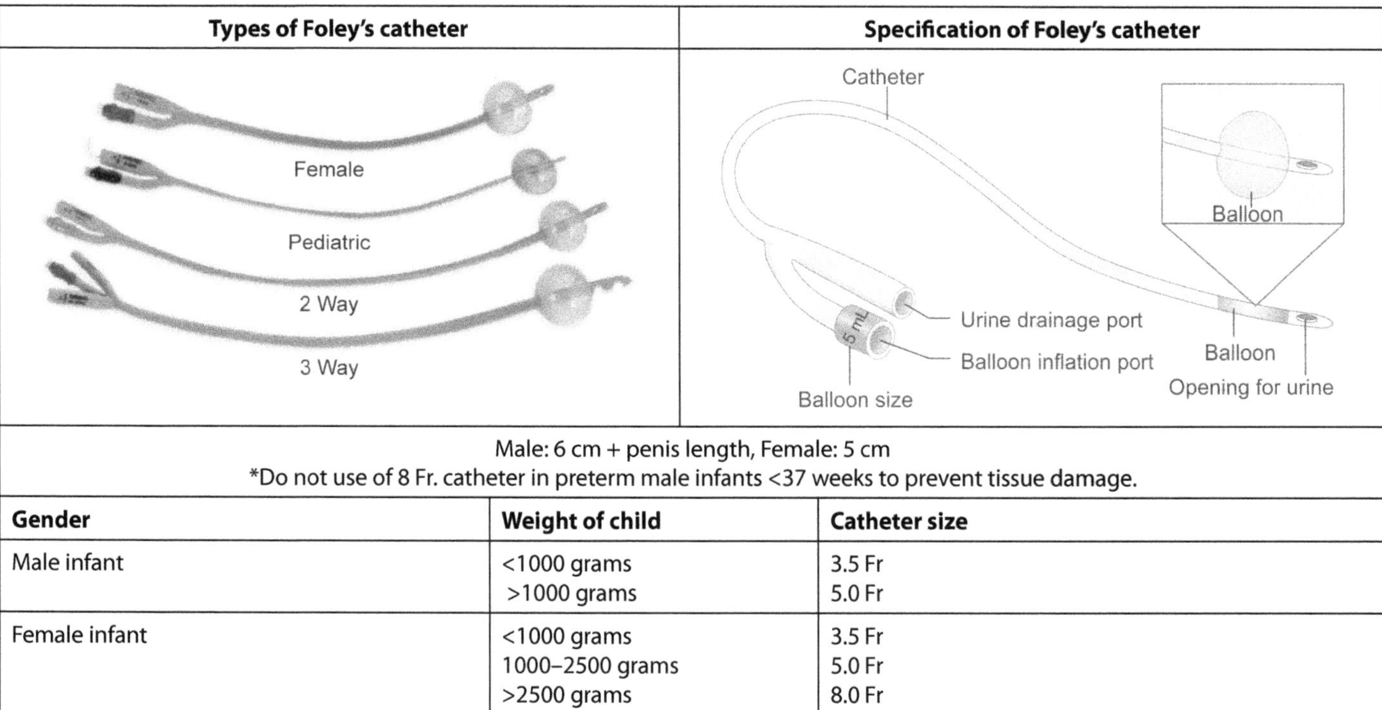

Male: 6 cm + penis length, Female: 5 cm *Do not use of 8 Fr. catheter in preterm male infants <37 weeks to prevent tissue damage.		
Gender	**Weight of child**	**Catheter size**
Male infant	<1000 grams >1000 grams	3.5 Fr 5.0 Fr
Female infant	<1000 grams 1000–2500 grams >2500 grams	3.5 Fr 5.0 Fr 8.0 Fr

Size of Foley's Catheter

Color		Size French	Size Millimeter
	Green	6	2.0
	Blue	8	2.7
	Black	10	3.3
	White	12	4.0
	Green	14	4.7
	Orange	16	5.3
	Red	18	6.0
	Yellow	20	6.7
	Purple	22	7.3
	Blue	24	8.0
	Black	26	8.7

Procedure

Catheterization of Male Infant

Step	Action
1	Use strict aseptic technique
2	Gather equipment. Set-up sterile field. Squeeze a small amount of lubricant on to the sterile field.
3	Place infant supine, with the thighs abducted (frog-like position).
4	Wash hands thoroughly and put on sterile gloves.
5	Stabilise the shaft of the penis with non-dominant hand, perpendicular to the body. This hand is now considered contaminated.
6	Apply gentle pressure at the base of the penis to avoid reflex urination.
7	Clean the penis with antiseptic solution starting at meatus and moving down the shaft of the penis. Allow the antiseptic to dry.
8	Drape sterile guards across the lower abdomen and across the infant's legs.
9	Apply sterile lubricant to catheter tip.
10	Gently insert the catheter into the meatus until urine is seen in the catheter.
11	Slight resistance may be felt as the catheter passes through the external sphincter. Hold the catheter in place with minimal pressure—generally spasm will relax after several minutes allowing easy passage. Never force the catheter.
12	Collect specimen for culture.
13	If the catheter is to remain indwelling, immediately connect the catheter to closed urinary collection system.
14	To prevent dislodgement, tape catheter securely to lower abdomen, rather than the leg to help decrease stricture formation caused by pressure on the posterior urethra. Place duoderm on lower abdomen underneath catheter taping to protect skin.

Catheterization of Female Infant

Step	Action
1	Use strict aseptic technique
2	Gather equipment. Setup sterile field. Squeeze a small amount of lubricant on to the sterile field.
3	Place infant supine, with the thighs abducted (frog-like position).
4	Wash hands thoroughly and put on sterile gloves.
5	With the non-dominant hand separate the labia and using sterile gauze
6	Using the free hand for the rest of the procedure, clean the area around the meatus with antiseptic solution using anterior-to-posterior strokes to prevent drawing faecal material in to the field. Allow the antiseptic to dry.
7	Drape sterile guards across the lower abdomen and across the infant's legs.
8	Apply sterile lubricant to catheter tip.
9	Gently insert catheter until urine is visible in catheter tubing. Do not insert extra tubing.
10	If catheter is accidentally inserted into vagina, leave in place and insert new catheter anterior to the first catheter.
11	Collect specimen for culture.
12	Connect to closed urinary collection system.
13	Secure the catheter by taping to infant's leg, apply duoderm to leg where catheter is to be taped to protect the skin.

Documentation

- Date, time and size of catheter inserted or removed.
- Reason for insertion of catheter.
- Color and consistency of urine.
- Any complications from insertion and notification of physician.
- Record of urine output obtained and lab tests requested.
- For balloon (Foley) catheters:
    - Insertion—include how much fluid was used to inflate the balloon.
    - Removal—include how much fluid was aspirated prior to removal.

CARE OF BABY IN INCUBATOR/RADIANT WARMER

Care of Baby under the Incubator

Introduction

Newborn babies take time to adopt external environment specially if one premature and low birth weight. As they are on risk to develop hypoxia, hypothermia and other many associated adverse conditions, need special care and attention. The term incubation has derived from a latin word 'Incubare' that means "lie on". Incubation is the process of providing an environment to keep them warm and suitable for their development as birds sit on their egg to hatch them.

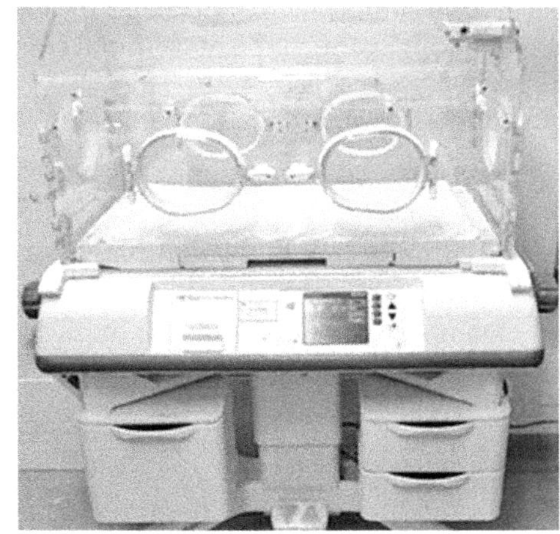

Premature babies or those born with much less weight than normal find it difficult to adjust to the external environment, immediately after being delivered. These infants stand the risk of catching various infections, and hence they need to be isolated and kept in incubators. Incubators provide intensive care to these babies and maintain suitable temperature and environmental conditions for healthy survival.

Indication

- **Premature babies:** Premature babies are weak and underdeveloped. They cannot cope up and sustain the conditions outside the womb, and hence require extra care.
- **Babies with very less weight:** Newborn babies who are underweight are also very weak and susceptible to various diseases. They need a lot of care and vigilance, and thus need to be kept in incubators.
- **Babies suffering from some illness:** Some infants might have infections or ailment that need intensive care and monitoring. Such babies are also kept in incubators for recovery and also to safeguard them from further infections or ailments.

Incubators

- It is an equipment to provide optimal condition of temperature, humidity and oxygen for survival of preterm, low birth weight or high-risk infants.
- It is important to delay or to prevent cold stress that produces additional hazards to the newborn as hypoxia, hypoglycemia and metabolic acidosis.
- Neutral thermal environment is one that permits the infants to maintain normal core temperature, with minimum oxygen consumption and caloric expenditure.
- Consumption of oxygen is minimal at abdominal temperature 36–36.5°C. So when abdominal skin temperature is increased or decreased, oxygen consumption increases.

Types of Incubators for Babies and Infants

- Portable and non-portable
- Open box
- Close type
- Double walled
- Servo controlled

Functions of Incubator

- **Oxygenation:** Providing the required amount of oxygen to the infant via oxygen control valves.
- **Observation:** The baby is kept under observation. The incubator provides detailed measurement of respiration, temperature, brain activity, oxygenation, etc.
- **Isolation and protection:** Placing the baby in an incubator isolates it from external infections, noise, and climate. Incubators provide the required warmth and lessen the exposure of newborns to germs and other external factors.
- **Providing required nutrition:** The baby can be provided with the required nutrition inside an incubator through intravenous catheter or NG tube for fast recovery and development.
- **Medicines:** A baby needs regular medication, which can be easily and effectively provided in incubators.

Other Functions

- Control temperature
- Humidity and oxygen concentration
- It provides high degree of isolation through slight
- It maintains positive pressure by air circulation
- A client probe to the abdominal skin as a guide in controlling the heater output of unit.

Prepare the Incubator

- Pre-warmed to a temperature appropriate to the infant's age, size and condition.
- Use in air mode and must always be switched on with the motor running if in use for a baby.
- Check and record the incubator temperature hourly.
- Position away from draughts or direct sunlight.
- Do not routinely use on the humidity function.

Care of the Baby

Maintaining Temperature

- Pre-warming the incubator up to the desired temperature before placing the infant in it.
- For infant weighing less than 1500 g the incubator pre-warmed to 34–36.1°C.
- For infants weighing more than 1500 g the incubator pre-warmed to 34–35°C.
- When infant removed from incubator should be well wrapped in blanket to conserve heat.

Feeding

- The nurse can feed infant inside the incubator through porthole.
- Lift the baby to semi-sitting position for feeding.
- After the feeding burp the baby then place the baby on prone position or on left side after feeding to facilitate getting out of air and to avoid abdominal distension.

Bathing

- Daily skin care involves using of clean water only. Soiled linen is stripped of from the top slowly slipped down to the bottom.
- It is removed through the porthole at the foot end of the incubator.
- Clean linen is placed inside via the porthole at the head end and should be tucked well under the mattress.
- When infant is removed from incubator, the unit should be cleaned before reuse. All water should be removed from reservoirs.

Nursing Care of Infants in Incubator

Principles	Nursing responsibilities
General use	
Physician order should indicate amount of humidity, liter flow of oxygen and its concentration.	• Observe and record the infant's responses. • Monitor the child reactions like cyanosis, retraction, grunting respiration, or hypothermia. • Give more attention to LBW baby • At least one vacant incubator should be kept ready. • Don't place incubator on direct sunlight or near Radiant warmer.
It is necessary to take body temperature of the infant to determine the amount of external heat required.	• Nurse should record infant temperature every hour until stabilized and then every four hours. • If temperature is elevated or subnormal, the temperature dial of the incubator should be adjusted.
Abrupt changes in the incubator temperature can cause untoward metabolic responses in the newborn that may result in apnea.	• Prewarming to 36.5°–37°C for infants less than 1500 g and to 34°–36.1°C to infants above 1500 g • The normal range of body temperature for a newborn is not always an exact reading of 98.6°F/37°C • Monitor body temperature and respirations
To maintain the atmospheric conditions constant, need not to open during routine care.	• No need of using masks and gowns for caring of infant in incubator. • Use the port holes of the incubator for providing care

Contd...

Contd...

Principles	Nursing responsibilities
Expose the chest for effective observation of respiration	• Infant need not be fully clothed, incubator provides stable atmospheric conditions during routine care.
Oxygen	
Oxygen therapy is more effective when interruptions in the oxygen administration are kept to a minimum.	• When the oxygen supply is not centrally located, the oxygen tank must be changed at intervals to ensure continuous therapy. • When the pressure gauge reading falls below 100 lb, the oxygen technician should be notified.
Low oxygen concentration—hypoxia—cause brain damage.	• The oxygen concentration should be checked every hour
Excessive oxygen concentration damage the optic nerve.	• Incubator care requires organization of nursing care activities to prevent loss of oxygen, warmth and humidity
Weaning	
Should be gradual process to avoid chilling due to the change from incubator temperature to room temperature.	• Dress and wrap the infant and open all the portholes. • After the incubator cooled, the infant may be removed and placed in a regular basinet.
Terminal cleaning	
Stagnant water harbors virulent pathogens. Thorough cleansing of the unit and removal of the water will prevent the spread of infection.	• When infant is removed from incubator, the unit should be cleaned before reuse. All water should be removed from reservoirs. • Alcohol, ether, or acetone should not be used to clean plastic parts

Radiant Warmer

Introduction

Radiant Warmer is a mechanical device which is proving heat and maintains the body normal temperature of the baby. This device helps to maintain the body temperature of the baby and limit the metabolism rate. Heat has a tendency to flow in the heat gradient direction that is from high temperature to low temperature. The heat loss in some newborn babies is rapid such as low birth weight (LBW) baby, preterm baby and hypothermic baby; hence Radiant warmers provide an artificial support to keep the body temperature constant. In certain areas with very cold climate, babies are kept on Radiant Warmer for couple of hours immediately after birth to ensure the baby is stabilized after birth.

Features of Radiant Warmer

Incubator Mode

- Air temperature control
- Baby temperature control
- Integral humidification
- Access doors—two
- Access ports—up to five

Radiant Warmer Mode

- Maximum power—450 W
- Manual control
- Baby temperature control

General Features

- Vertical height adjustment—foot-switch
- Canopy control:
    - Foot-switch (raise only)
    - Finger-switch (raise and lower)
- Mattress rotates—360°
- Electroluminescent control screen
- Radiant warmer have four wheel with locks
- X-ray tray

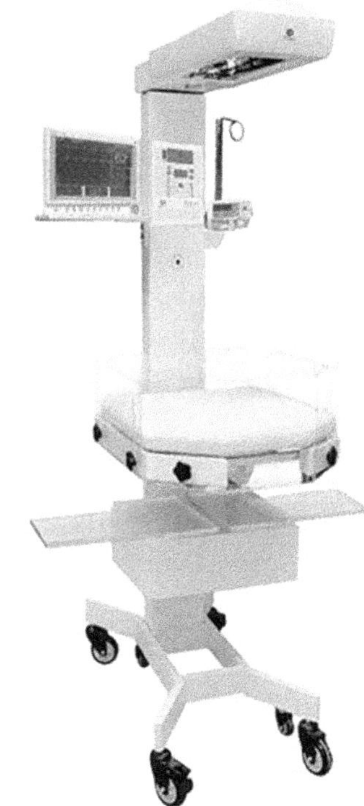

- Sliding storage draw
- Integral scales

Mechanism of Radiant Warmer

Radiant Warmers can be manual or automatic (servo system—heater output is determined automatically based on skin temperature. The skin temperature is set at 36.5°C) depending on the mechanism that the manufacturer employs for temperature control. The heat generated and the temperature of the skin can be individually seen but the basic difference between these two models will be the regulation of temperature. The automatic model increases the heat output in small predetermined steps to reach at the desired temperature of the body. The device may seem simple to handle, but it is always recommended to have a proper training and read the manufacturers guidelines for person handling this equipment. It is necessary to regularly clean and disinfect the instrument.

Servo Mode

- Set temperature at 36.5°C, heater output will adjust automatically to keep baby at set temperature.
- If baby temperature is below the set temperature, the heater
- Output will increase, if baby is at set temperature or higher the heater output will become zero.
- Look for probe displacement when the baby is in servo mode. Check for and ensure proper probe placement every hour.

Manual Mode

- Once connected to mains heater output regulated by knob on front panel.
- The output is displayed as % or bars or bulbs.
- Use maximum (100% output) for rapid warming of bassinet in labour room 10 minutes before delivery.
- Reduce output to 25–75% after 10 minutes depending on ambient temperature.
- If left on with heater output >80% alarm is activated within 15 or 20 minutes later and there after the heater output goes to 40%.
- If alarm is silenced the heater will kept on for another 15–20 minutes as per manufacturers recommendation.
- For low birth weight or sick neonate adjust heater output depending on baby temperature. Never use full (100%) heater output unsupervised.
- Record baby temperature every 2–4 hourly.
- Use this mode only for pre-warming, during resuscitation and initial stabilization.

Indications

- Hypothermic baby
- Low birth weight baby
- Preterm baby
- When an infant reaches 1700 to 1800 grams, has no respiratory distress and only occasional apnea, and has been stable in an incubator operated in the air temperature control mode with air temperature 32°C or less, an attempt can be made to move him to a bassinet.

Role of Nurse in Radiant Warmer

- She should ensure that the temperature of the room is 22°C.
- Place the warmer away from air currents.
- Clean the mattress and platform, and cover the mattress with clean linen sheet.
- The warmer at least 20 minutes prior to pre-warm the linen and mattress so that the baby does not lie on a cold surface initially.
- If baby is in supine position place the skin probe on the right hypochondrium.
- When in prone position, place the probe on the lumbar region of the back. To prevent skin injury.
- Place Tegaderm and fix the probe on it with an adhesive.
- Ensure that the baby's head is covered with cap and feet secured in socks and the baby is clothed or covered unless it is necessary for the baby to be naked.
- Partially undressed for observation or for a procedure.
- Place only one baby under each radiant warmer.
- Turn the baby frequently while under the warmer, if possible.
- Check the temperature of the warmer and of the room every hour, and adjust the temperature setting accordingly. Record the heater output in each shift (every 6 hours). Any sudden increase in heater output is an early indicator of sickness.
- Move the baby to be with the mother as soon as the baby no longer requires

- Frequent procedures and treatment. If in servo mode the heater output is < 20%
- It is safe to shift the baby to mother's side.

Check body temperature in 30 minutes and each hour for 4 hours; if the axillary or rectal temperature drops to below 36.5°C, return infant to incubator, reheat on skin temperature servocontrol as described above, then revert to air temperature control; try again in 2 or 3 days.

Read Temperature on Display

- **High:** If baby temperature is below 36°C.
- **Medium:** If baby temperature is 36–36.5°C.
- **Low:** If baby temperature is 36.5–37.5°C.
- Once the baby's temperature is 36.5–37.5°C, switch on the servo mode/skin mode.

CARE OF A CHILD ON VENTILATOR

Introduction

The Ventilator Care is a multidisciplinary program that provides care to infants with chronic respiratory failure. Many conditions can cause chronic respiratory failure in infants, including interstitial lung diseases and bronchopulmonary dysplasia, the chronic lung disease associated with premature birth. The Ventilator Care was created to improve the complex care that these children require and to make life easier for families.

Definition

Mechanical ventilation refers to the use of life-support technology to perform the work of breathing for patients who are unable to do this on their own.

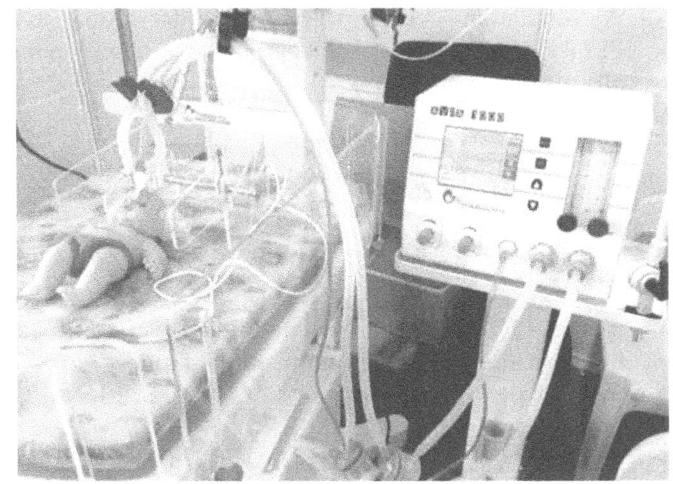

Purpose

- Improved pulmonary gas exchange.
- Relief of respiratory distress (by relieving upper and lower airway obstruction, reducing oxygen consumption, and relieving respiratory fatigue).
- Management of pulmonary mechanisms (by normalizing and maintaining the distribution of lung volume and providing pulmonary toilet).
- Provide airway protection.
- Provide general cardiopulmonary support.

Indications of Mechanical Ventilation

- Respiratory failure–apnea/respiratory arrest, inadequate ventilation, inadequate oxygenation, chronic respiratory insufficiency with failure to thrive (FTT).
- Cardiac insufficiency/shock—eliminates work of breathing and reduces oxygen consumption.
- Neurologic dysfunction—central hypoventilation/frequent apnea, GCS <8, and inability to protect airway.

Initial Ventilator Settings

Initial ventilator settings	Premature neonate	Neonate	Infant/child	Adolescent
Mode	Pressure control mode	Pressure control mode	Volume control with pressure support	Volume control
Rate	40–50	30–40	20–30	12–15
PEEP (cm)	3–6/7	3–6	3–5	3–5
Inspiratory time (cm)	0.3–0.4	0.3–0.4	0.5–0.6	0.7–0.9
PIP	18–22 (if HMD)	18–20	16–18 (in increased ICP); 18–25 (if low compliance)	18–25;35 (in severe ARDS)

(PEEP: positive end expiratory pressure; PIP: peak inspiratory pressure; ICP: intracranial pressure; ARDS: acute respiratory distress syndrome; HMD: hyaline membrane disease)

Choose the Mode

Control every breath if plan for heavy sedation and muscle relaxation. Use synchronised intermittent mandatory ventilation (SIMV) when patient likely to breathe spontaneously. Whenever a breath is supported by the ventilator, regardless of the mode, the limit of the support is determined by:

1. Volume limited—preset tidal volume
2. Pressure limited—preset peak inspiratory pressure (PIP).

- **FiO_2**—start at 100% and quickly wean down to a level < or 60% (to avoid O_2 toxicity) depending on O_2 requirement. 60% may be a starting point.
- **Inspiratory to expiratory (I:E) ratio**—normally set at 1:2–1:3. Higher inspiratory times may be needed to improve oxygenation in difficult situations (inverse ratio ventilation), increasing the risk of air leak. Lower rate and higher expiratory time 1:3–1:4 may be needed in asthma to allow proper expiration due to expiratory obstruction.
- **Trigger sensitivity**—set at 0 to -2. Setting above zero is too sensitive; triggered breath from ventilator will be too frequent while too negative a setting will increase work for patient to trigger a ventilator breath.
- **Volume limited**—Tidal volume—8–10 mL/kg with a goal to get to 6–8 mL/kg. If leak present around endotracheal tube (ETT), set initial tidal volume to 10–12 mL/kg.

Maintenance of Ventilation

- Fine tuning after initiation is based on blood gases and oxygen saturations. Do not make more than 2 alterations at any one time.
- For oxygenation—adjust FiO_2, positive end expiratory pressure (PEEP), inspiratory time, PIP (tidal volume)—increase mean arterial pressure (MAP).
- For ventilation—respiratory rate (RR), tidal volume (in volume limited) and PIP (in pressure limited mode) can be adjusted.
- PEEP is used to prevent alveolar collapse at end of inspiration, to recruit collapsed lung spaces or to stent open floppy airways.

Gas Exchange Related Problems

- Hypoxemia
- Hypercarbia.

Hypoxemia

- Increase FiO_2 and MAP. Need to find a balance as per clinical situation.
- Increase tidal volume if volume limited mode, PEEP, or inspiratory time.
- Increase peak inspiratory pressure (PIP), positive end-expiratory pressure (PEEP)/inspiration (I) time if pressure limited mode.
- If O_2 worse, get CXR to look for air leak, if increasing PEEP decreases saturations, suspect low cardiac output (CO) due to tamponade effect of PEEP (treat by fluids and inotropes) or pneumothorax.
- Other measures—normalize cardiac output (by fluids and inotropes), maintain normal Hb and hematocrit (in neonates), maintain normothermia, deepen sedation/consider neuromuscular block.

Common reasons include:

- Hypoventilation.
- Dead space ventilation (too high a peep, decreased CO, pulmonary vasoconstriction).
- Increased CO_2 production, hyperthermia.
- High carbohydrate diet.
- Shivering inadequate tidal volume delivery (hypoventilation) occurs with ET tube block, malposition, circuit leak, ventilator malfunction.

Hypercarbia

- If volume limited: Increase tidal volume or rate. If asthma—increase expiratory time to >1:3.
- If pressure limited: Increase PIP, decrease positive end expiratory pressure (PEEP), increase rate.
- Decrease dead space (increase cardiac output, decrease PEEP, vasodilator, shorten ET tube).
- Decrease CO_2 production—cool, increase sedation, decrease carbohydrate load.
- Change endotracheal tube if blocked (may be remedied by suction).
- Check proper placement.
- Fix leaks in the circuit, endotracheal tube cuff, humidifier.

Duration of Ventilation

- Duration varies by nature of disease process: Hyaline membrane disease (HMD) may take 3 days to a week, pneumonia 5–7 days, ARDS 10 days to 3 weeks and neurological illness [e.g., Guillain-Barré syndrome (GBS)] from 1 week to few months. Postcardiac surgery ventilation may vary from 24 hours to 7 days or more and postoperative chest or abdominal cases would vary from 24–48 hours.
- Risk of nosocomial infection increases with ventilation >5–7days.

Weaning From Mechanical Ventilation

Weaning begins from the moment ventilation is commenced. When FiO_2 requirement is down to 40%, improvement in secretions and CXRs, improving clinical condition or primary pathology, muscle relaxant drip is stopped and sedation slowly weaned to get patient moving and awake (may take 24 hours or longer if prolonged use).

- Decrease FiO_2 to keep SpO_2>94.
- Decrease synchronized intermittent mandatory ventilation (SIMV) rate to 10 (reduce by 3–4 breaths/min).
- Decrease the PIP to 20 cm of water by reducing 2 cm H_2O each time/tidal volume to no less than 5 mL/kg to prevent atelectasis (usually guided by blood gases).
- Ventilator rate and PIP can be exchanged alternately.
- If at any time patient's oxygen requirement increases greater than 60% or spontaneous ventilation is fast or distressed with accessory muscle use, patient gets agitated or lethargic, hypercarbia on ABGs, pause weaning and increase support level. Patient may not be ready to wean.

Emergency Management

If child fighting ventilator and desaturating immediate measures include: - **"DOPE"**

- **D-Displacement**—check tube placement. When in doubt take ET Tube out and start manual ventilation with 100% O_2 and with bag and mask.
- **O-Obstruction**—is the chest rising. Are breath sounds present and equal? Changes in examination. Atelectasis, treat bronchospasm/tube block/malposition/pneumothorax (consider needle thoracentesis). Examine circulation: Shock or Sepsis.
- **P-Pneumothorax**—check ABG, saturation and CXR for pneumothorax and worsening lung condition.
- **E-Equipment** failure—examine ventilator, ventilator circuit/humidifier/gas source. If no other reason for hypoxemia:- increase sedation/muscle relaxation, put back on the ventilator.

Extubation Procedure

- Keep nil by mouth (NBM) 4 hours before planned extubation.
- Suction endotracheal tube and deflate cuff if using a cuffed tube. Suction the oral cavity and nostrils.
- Suction the NGT before removing to empty the stomach.
- Keep oxygen by face mask ready. Nasal cannula can be taped to the face even before extubation to avoid immediate hypoxia/stress upon extubation.
- Correct size mask and bag with O_2 must be available with a working laryngoscope and correct size ET-Tube.
- Nebulisation with beta stimulant/adrenaline to be ready immediate post extubation.
- Intravenous steroids dexamethasone 0.6 mg/kg IV (maximum dose of 12 mg) stat may be used if indicated by extubation stridor and then continued on prednisone orally at 1 mg/kg 8–12 hourly OR if prolonged intubation or airway edema can give dexamethasone 24 hours prior to planned extubation at 0.15 mg/kg and to be continued for 6–8 doses.
- Intravenous frusemide may be needed to achieve a negative fluid balance as interstitial edema can occur in patients with relative fluid overload or even mild myocardial dysfunction as soon as the positive pressure is taken off from the lower airways and the alveoli during extubation.
- Noninvasive positive pressure ventilation (NIPPV) or a continuous positive airway pressure (CPAP) should also be available to avoid reintubation.
- Do blood gas 20 minutes after extubation; post-extubation CXR not needed routinely but only if clinically indicated by desaturation or increased work of breathing.
- Ideally, ventilator to be on standby at least 24 hours post extubation.
- Anticipate extubation failure in all patients and parents should be made aware earlier on so that there is no disappointment.

Complications of Ventilation

Increased Airway Pressures and Lung Volumes

- Barotrauma (stretch-injury): PIE, pneumothorax, pneumopericardium, pneumoperitoneum, subcutaneous emphysema.
- Decreased cardiac filling and poor perfusion.

- Organ dysfunction-renal, hepatic, and CNS.
- Pulmonary parenchymal damage.
- Adverse effects on gas exchange.
- Increased extravascular lung water.

Endotracheal/Tracheostomy Tube

- Tracheal mucosal swelling, ulceration or damage.
- Sinusitis/middle ear-infection.
- Laryngeal edema, subglottic stenosis.
- Granuloma formation leading to airway obstruction.

Nosocomial Infections

- Ventilator associated pneumonias.
- Sepsis.

Pulmonary Circulation

- Increased pulmonary vascular resistance.
- Compression of alveolar vessels.

Mechanical Operational Problems

- Mechanical ventilator/compressor failure/alarm failure.
- Inadequate humidification.

Nursing Management

Expected outcomes	Activities and interventions	Rationale

Adequate oxygenation ventilation and supported work of breathing	• Assessment of the child receiving mechanical ventilation
	  – *General observations:* Comfort of the child, synchrony between patient and ventilator, chest expansion, color and perfusion and level of consciousness
	  – *Auscultation:* Note symmetry of breath sounds (recall that the thin chest wall of an infant transfer breath sound to opposite side), evaluate quality of breath sounds, note adventitious sounds or absence of breath sounds
	  – Work of breathing
	  – Volume and quality of secretions: Note quantity and characteristics
	  – *Palpation:* Note presence of crepitus, inspiratory crackles, or points of tenderness
	• Provide additional ventilatory support as indicated by signs of hypoxia, hypercarbia and hemodynamic instability (manual breaths and/or adjustment inmechanical ventilation)
	• Continuous pulse oximetry to monitor oxygenation (re-site q2–4 hours to avoid bruns)
	• Consider utilizing ETCO$_2$ monitoring for additional tranding of ventilation therapy
	• Monitor gastric insufflation and remove air from stomach as indicated. Positive pressure ventilation may lead to increased gas flow to stomach.
		• Oxygen consumption is greatly increased with increased work of breathing
		• Ventilator associated pneumonia is a leading cause of nosocomial infection. Changes in the quality of secretions should prompt additional investigations—especially in the presence of a fever.
		• Gastric decompression reduces the risk of aspiration

Correct position and patency of artifical airway	• Verify placement of artifical airway utilizing at least 2 of the below methods:
	  – Chest radiograph
	  – Auscultation of breath sounds across the lung fields
	  – End tidal CO$_2$ monitoring
	  – Verify distance marking on tube
	  – Ensure artificial airway is secure and stabilized in desired position
		• Patient safety
		• Airway verification and securement reduces risk of non-intentional extubation
		• CXR are important to verify ETT or trach position and to evaluate pulmonary process. The decision is determined by the individual needs of the patient

Contd...

Contd...

Expected outcomes	Activities and interventions	Rationale

Adequate airway humidification; mobilization and removal of secretions	• Ensure adequate humidification of ventilation circuit, monitoring temperature of inspired gas (maintain at 35–37°C)
	• Suctioning of the endotracheal or tracheostomy tube should occur when there is evidence of increased airway secretions (coughing, increased PIP, auscultation of upper airway crackles)
	  – Always pre-oxygenate the patient
	  – Suction catheter should be an appropriate size to allow ease of insertion (french size of catheter = 2 × the internal diameter of tube)
	  – Aseptic technique to avoid contamination, consider use inline suction catheters
	  – Insertion distance should be knwon and documented to avoid suctioning below the lip of the artificial airway
	  – Routine instillation of N/S should not be necessary if the humidification is adequate (tenacious secretions may require 0.5–1 mL instillation of N/S, followed by several manual ventilation breaths to disperse instillation prior to suctioning
		• Patient safety
		• Low temperatures may cause secretions to become thick and sticky
		• Body temperature may be altered by high and low temperatures of inspired gas
		• Suctioning clears airway secretions to maintain airway patency.

Maintenance of adequate pH and PaCO$_2$	• Monitor pH and pCO$_2$ through periodic sampling of arterial of capillary blood gases	Arterial and capillary blood sampling are both reliable methods of monitoring pH and pCO$_2$
Hemodynamic stability	• Maintain optimal cardiovascular status of patient, hourly assessment of vital sings and perfusion • Ensure continuous ECG monitoring with alarms limits set to appropriate limits per age • Monitor and optimize perfusion	Increase in intrathoracic pressure that occurs with mechanical ventilation results in a reduciton of venous retrun BP is a late sign of CV decompensation in child. Capillary refill ought to be ≤ 2 seconds.
Maintenance of fluid and electrolyte balances	• Calculation and monitoring of all fluid intake. Fluid restriction may be implemented (usually 80% total fluids orders) to reduce fluid retention that is common with positive • Monitor urine output. Goal should be ≥ 1 mL/kg/hour of urine output • Monitor fluid and electrolyte status through routine evaluation of lab results • Daily weights are very important when can be safely performed • Optimize nutrition through early initiation of feeding via NG or NJ tube	Fluid retention may occur related to underlying disease or non-osmotic ADH release related to positive pressure ventilation. Enteral feeding is the preferred method of nutrition and may be initiated even in the absence of bowel sounds.
Child remains free of nosocomial infection	• Minimize ventilator sources of infection by emptying condensation in tubing • Keep head of bed (HOB) elevated at 30° unless contraindicated • Mobilize patient as able • Consider removal of additional potential sources of hospital acquired infection on a daily basis (central venous line (CVL), Foley catheter)	Ventilator associated pneumonia (VAP) is a cause of mortality in mechanically ventilated children. Elevating the head of bed reduces incidence of aspiration.

Maintenance of skin integrity	• Assess skin integrity every 2–4 hours (attention of bony prominences, areas of nose and mouth in contact with ETT). Assess for
	• Keep skin clean and dry
	• Reposition child every 1–2 hours (including reposition of head) as tolerated
	• Prone positioning every 4–6 hours for all ventilated patients
	• Maintenance of oral hygiene
	  – Brush teeth, gums and tongue at least twice a day
	  – Moisturize lips every 2–4 hours as required
		Repositioning alleviates pressure points and prevents skin breakdown.
		
		Oral care reduces inflammation and plaque (which has been shown to contribute to VAP).

Acceptable level of comfort	• Assess the patient's pain and sedation level q1–4 hours using the Multidisciplinary Assessment of Pain Scale (MAPS) and State Behavioral Scale (SBS) scales (see attached pain and sedation guidelines)
	• Titrate pain and sedation medications as per protocol
	• Provide noninvasive comfort measures
	  – Parental presence
	  – Favorite blanket or toy
	  – Ear plugs to reduce noise
	  – Dim lights
	  – Distraction techniques
		The presence of an artificial airway is uncomfortable.

CONTINUOUS POSITIVE AIRWAY PRESSURE

Definition

CPAP stands for "continuous positive airway pressure." CPAP is a treatment that delivers slightly pressurized air during the breathing cycle. This makes breathing easier for persons with obstructive sleep apnea and other respiratory problems.

Indication

CPAP treatment can be highly effective in treatment of obstructive sleep apnea. For some patients, the improvement in the quality of sleep and quality of life due to CPAP treatment will be noticed after a single night's use. Often, the patient's sleep partner also benefits from markedly improved sleep quality, due to the amelioration of the patient's loud snoring. Given that sleep apnea is a chronic health issue and doesn't go away, ongoing care is needed to maintain CPAP therapy. Based on the study of cognitive behavioral therapy (referenced above), ongoing chronic care management is the best way to help patients continue therapy by educating them on the health risks of sleep apnea and providing motivation and support.

Equipment

- Flow generator (PAP machine) provides the airflow.
- Hose connects the flow generator (sometimes via an in-line humidifier) to the interface.
- Interface (nasal or full face mask, nasal pillows, or less commonly a lip-seal mouthpiece).
- Provides the connection to the user's airway.

Types of CPAP

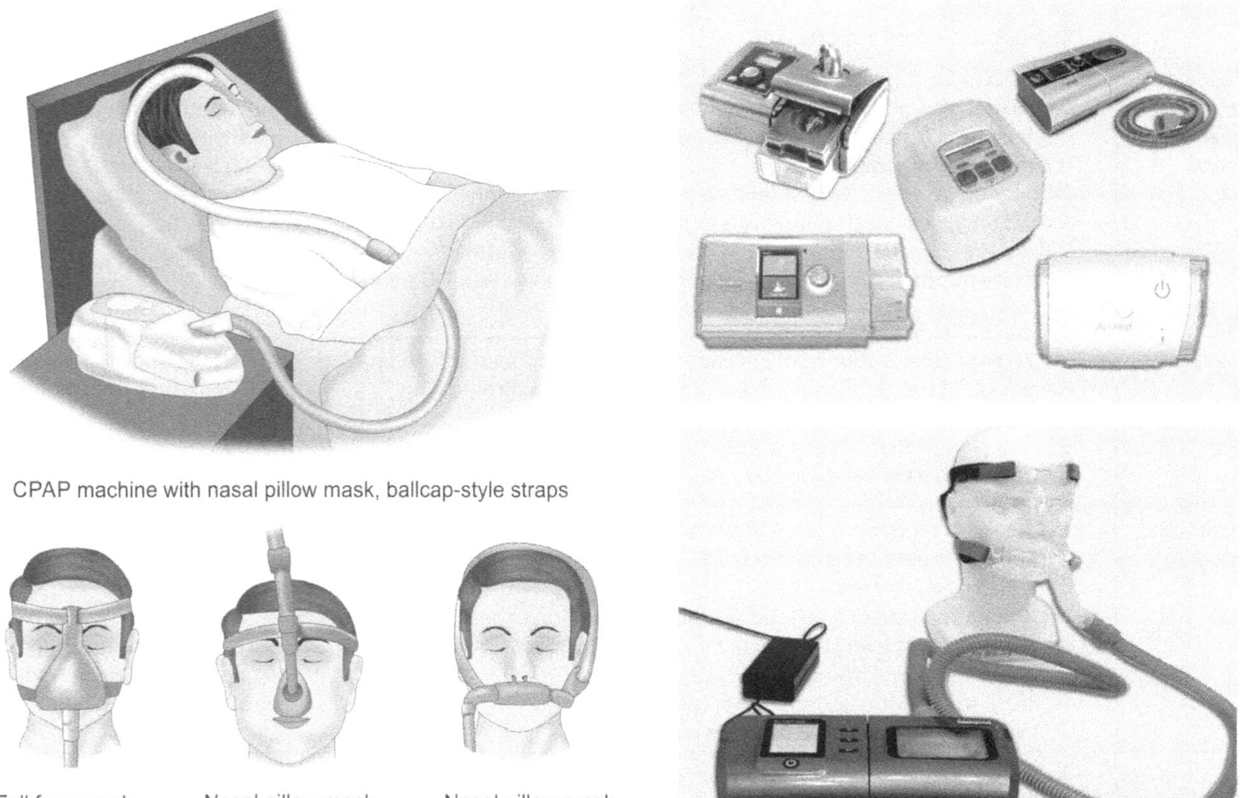

Types of CPAP

Settings and Measurements

- **CPAP:** This is the pressure applied without pause or end to the airway. Generally using flow to generate the pressure.
- **PEEP:** Positive end-expiratory pressure (PEEP) is the pressure in the lungs (alveolar pressure) above atmospheric pressure (the pressure outside of the body) that exists at the end of expiration.

- **Ramp:** This feature is present on many devices and allows the user to reduce the pressure to lowest setting and gradually increase to the set pressure. This allows the user to fall asleep with the pressure at a more comfortable setting.
- **FiO$_2$:** Fractional O$_2$ percentage—that is, the fraction of inspired oxygen that is added to the delivered air.

Mechanism of Action

Continuous Positive Airway Pressure

- A continuous positive airway pressure (CPAP) machine was initially used mainly by patients for the treatment of sleep apnea at home, but now is in widespread use across intensive care units as a form of ventilation.
- Obstructive sleep apnea occurs when the upper airway becomes narrow as the muscles relax naturally during sleep. This reduces oxygen in the blood and causes arousal from sleep.
- The CPAP machine stops this phenomenon by delivering a stream of compressed air via a hose to a nasal pillow, nose mask or full-face mask, splinting the airway (keeping it open under air pressure) so that unobstructed breathing becomes possible, reducing and/or preventing apneas and hypopneas.
- It is important to understand, however, that it is the air pressure, and not the movement of the air, that prevents the apneas. When the machine is turned on, but prior to the mask being placed on the head, a flow of air comes through the mask.
- After the mask is placed on the head, it is sealed to the face and the air stops flowing. At this point, it is only the air pressure that accomplishes the desired result.
- This has the additional benefit of reducing or eliminating the extremely loud snoring that sometimes accompanies sleep apnea.
- The CPAP machine blows air at a prescribed pressure (also called the titrated pressure).
- The necessary pressure is usually determined by a sleep physician after review of a study supervised by a sleep technician during an overnight study (polysomnography) in a sleep laboratory.
- The titrated pressure is the pressure of air at which most (if not all) apneas and hypopneas have been prevented, and it is usually measured in centimeters of water (cm H$_2$O).
- The pressure required by most patients with sleep apnea ranges between 6 and 14 cm H$_2$O. A typical CPAP machine can deliver pressures between 4 and 20 cm H$_2$O. More specialized units can deliver pressures up to 25 or 30 cm H$_2$O.

Disadvantages and Side Effects

Most factors associated with these machines and parts are well known to manufacturers, suppliers, and end-user groups. The Internet has the contacts needed user and manufacturer web sites, local, national and international user groups, with occasional local face-to-face meetings or other forms of user to user interaction. Prospective positive airway pressure (PAP) candidates are often reluctant to use this therapy, since the nose mask and hose to the machine look uncomfortable and clumsy, and the airflow required for some patients can be vigorous. Some patients will develop nasal congestion while others may experience rhinitis or a runny nose. Some patients adjust to the treatment within a few weeks, others struggle for longer periods, and some discontinue treatment entirely.

PAP manufacturers frequently offer different models at different price ranges, and PAP masks have many different sizes and shapes, so that some users need to try several masks before finding a good fit. These different machines may not be comfortable for all users, so proper selection of PAP models may be very important in furthering adherence to therapy. Every few years, advancing technologies may mean the upgrading of your machine and parts.

Nursing Care and Maintenance

- As with all durable medical equipment, proper maintenance is essential for proper functioning, long unit life and patient comfort.
- The care and maintenance required for PAP machines varies with the type and conditions of use, and are typically spelled out in a detailed instruction manual specific to the make and model.
- Most manufacturers recommend that the end user perform daily and weekly maintenance.
- Units must be checked regularly for wear and tear and kept clean. Poorly connected, worn or frayed electrical connections may present a shock or fire hazard; worn hoses and masks may reduce the effectiveness of the unit.
- Most units employ some type of filtration, and the filters must be cleaned or replaced on a regular schedule. Sometimes high efficiency particulate air (HEPA) filters may be purchased or modified for asthma or other allergy clients.
- Hoses and masks accumulate exfoliated skin, particulate matter, and can even develop mold.
- Humidification units must be kept free of mold and algae. Because units use substantial electrical power, housings must be cleaned without immersion.

In cold climates, humidified air may require insulated and or heated air hoses. These may be bought ready-made, or modified from commonly available materials (aluminum foil and bubble-wrap insulation. Noisy machines may be distanced from the sleeper by extension hoses between the machine and the sleeping person.

ADMINISTRATION OF FLUID WITH INFUSION PUMPS

Introduction

An infusion pump draws fluid from a standard bag of intravenous fluid and controls the rate of flow. It provides accurate and continuous therapy. Because it can use any size bag of intravenous fluid, an infusion pump can be used to deliver fluids at either a very slow or very fast infusion rate.

A syringe pump is a different type of infusion delivery device. Instead of drawing fluid from an infusion bag, intravenous medications are drawn into a syringe and installed into the device. Because syringe pumps contain a maximum volume of 50 mL, syringe pumps are used to administer medications that have very small hourly volumes (for example, usually less than 5 mL/h).

An infusion pump infuses fluids, medication or nutrients into a patient's circulatory system. It is generally used intravenously, although subcutaneous, arterial and epidural infusions

Definition

Intravenous infusion pump is defined as an accurate fluid infusion and drug administration is crucial for the optimum management of a critically ill neonate. Controlled intravenous delivery of common medications, such as inotropic agents, vasodilators, aminophylline, insulin, heparin etc. via infusion pump is the preferred mode of therapy in acute care.

Types of Infusion

- Continuous infusion
- Intermittent infusion
- Patient-controlled is infusion on-demand
- Total parenteral nutrition.

Types of Infusion Pump

The two main types of infusion pumps:

1. Syringe pump
2. Large volumetric pump

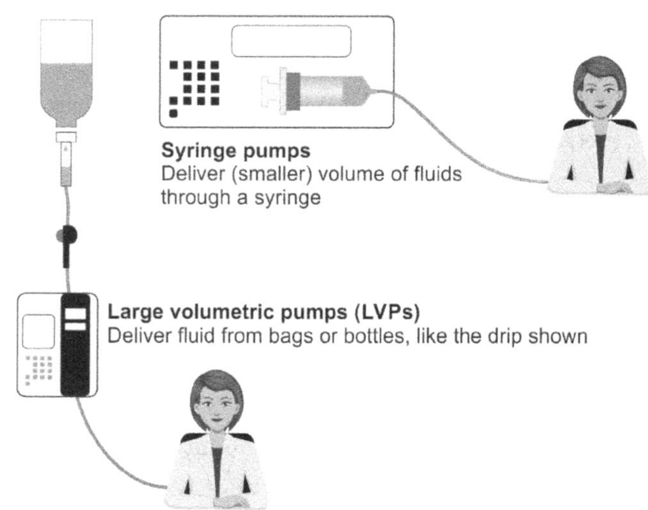

General purpose of volumetric pump	An infusion pump used to accurately deliver intravascular drugs, fluids, whole blood, and blood products to the patient. A linear peristaltic or piston cassette pump insert is utilized to control the prescribed infusion volume.	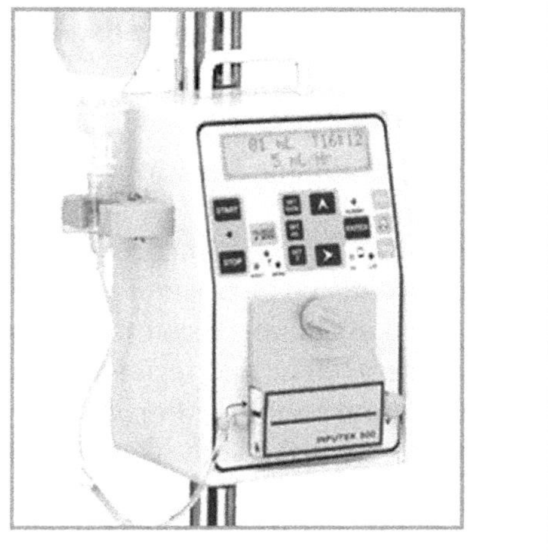

Syringe drivers	The syringe pump utilizes an electronically controlled electric motor to drive a plastic syringe plunger for drug delivery. Accurate syringe size and placement in the pump are imperative.	
Patient-controlled analgesia	An electronic pump that allows the patient to control their own drug delivery by using a hand-held control. It employs predetermined settings with defined limits in respect to frequency and dosage.	
Ambulatory	A portable, battery-powered device. Most devices have minimal alarms; therefore, close attention to administration observations is strongly advised. Portable devices are not recommended for the constant delivery of critical drugs.	

Procedure

- Ensure the machine is plugged correctly into suitable electrical socket, switch on the machine
- Prepare the materials needed and check for expiry date
- Normal saline
- Primary and secondary giving set
- Flush or primary giving set to IV pump
- Set rate, volume
- Connect line to child
- Start infusion
- Check safety—machine, stand and keep line untangled
- Document amount of fluid given for one hour.

Advantages and Disadvantages of Syringe Pumps

Advantages	Disadvantages
• Cheaper than drip rate pumps • Precise control of total volume infused • Suited for small volume • Low cost of disposables • Pressure maintains rate inspite of resistance • Delivery of air impossible • Portable	• Unsuitable for large volume • Comprehensive alarm system not usually provided

PEDIATRIC CARDIOPULMONARY RESUSCITATION (NALS/PLS/PALS)

Introduction

Pediatric Basic Life Support

An infant through adults in cardiac arrest, the Airway, Breathing, and Chest compressions (A-B-C) sequence of basic life support (BLS) has been replaced by a new sequence: Chest compressions, Airway, and Breathing (C-A-B).

In the new C-A-B sequence, "Look, listen, and feel" has been removed from the algorithm, and the guidelines advise that chest compressions should be initiated rapidly to all victims who are responsive and not breathing, without pausing longer than 10 seconds to check for a pulse.

The reason is that studies have shown that both healthcare workers and lay rescuers have difficulty ascertaining if a pulse is present, and compressions administered to a patient with a pulse does no harm.

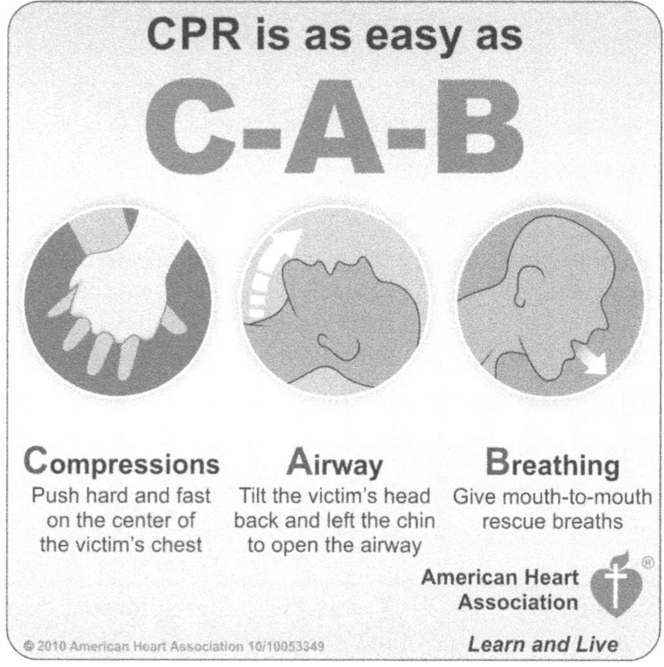

Pediatric Advanced Life Support

- Initial steps in stabilization (provide warmth, position, and clear airway, dry, stimulate, reposition)
- Breathing/ventilation
- Chest compressions
- Administration of drug (epinephrine and/or volume expansion)
- Endotracheal intubation/environment.

Initial Steps

The initial steps of resuscitation are to provide warmth by placing the baby under a radiant heat source, position the head in a "sniffing" position to open the airway, clear the airway with a bulb syringe or suction catheter, and dry the baby and stimulate breathing. Recent studies have examined several aspects of these initial steps. These studies are summarized below.

Approximately 60 seconds ("the Golden Minute") are allotted for completing the initial steps, reevaluating, and beginning ventilation if required. The decision to progress beyond the initial steps is determined by simultaneous assessment of 2 vital characteristics—respirations (apnea, gasping, or labored or unlabored breathing) and heart rate (whether greater than or less than 100 beats per minute). Assessment of heart rate should be done by intermittently auscultating the precordial pulse. When a pulse is detectable, palpation of the umbilical pulse can also provide a rapid estimate of the pulse and is more accurate than palpation at other sites.

Stimulation/Clearing the Airway of Meconium

- Aspiration of meconium before delivery during birth or during resuscitation can cause severe aspiration pneumonia. One obstetrical technique to try to decrease aspiration has been to suction meconium from the infant's airway after delivery of the head (intrapartum suctioning).
- Traditional teaching recommended that meconium-stained infants have endotracheal intubation immediately following birth and that suction be applied to the endotracheal tube as it is withdrawn.
- A vigorous cry infant is defined as one who has strong respiratory efforts, good muscle tone, and a heart rate >100 beats per minute (bpm).
- Endotracheal suctioning for infants who are not vigorous cry should be performed immediately after birth.

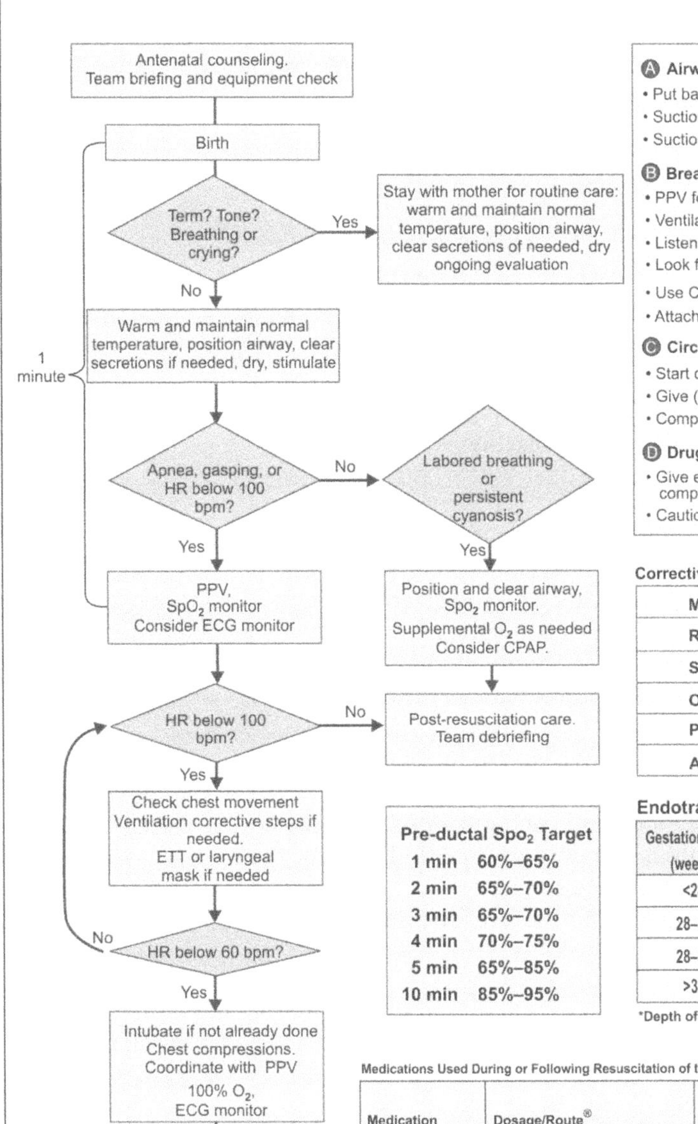

Neonatal Resuscitation Program® - Reference Chart

The most important and effective action in neonatal resuscitaion is ventilation of the baby's lungs.

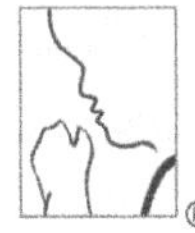

A Airway

- Put baby's head in "shiffing" position
- Suction mouth, then nose
- Suction trachea if meconium-stained and NOT vigorous

B Breathing

- PPV for apnea, gasping, or pulse <100 bpm
- Ventilate at rate of 40–60 breaths/minute
- Listen for rising heart rate, audible breath sounds
- Look for slight chest movement with each breath
- Use CO_2 detector after intubation
- Attach a pulse oximeter

C Circulation

- Start compressions if HR is <60 after 30 seconds of effective PPV
- Give (3 compressions: 1 breath) every 2 seconds
- Compress one-third of the anterior-posterior diameter of the chest

D Drugs

- Give epinephrine if HR is <60 after 45–60 seconds of compressions and ventilation
- Caution: Epinephrine dosage is different for ET and IV routes

Corrective Steps

M	Mask adjustment
R	Reposition airway
S	Suction mouth and nose
O	Open mouth
P	Pressure increase
A	Airway alternative

Pre-ductal Spo₂ Target

1 min	60%–65%
2 min	65%–70%
3 min	65%–70%
4 min	70%–75%
5 min	65%–85%
10 min	85%–95%

Endotracheal Intubation

Gestational Age (weeks)	Height (kg)	ET Tube size (ID, mm)	Depth of insertion® (cm from upper lip)
<28	<1.0	2.5	6–7
28–34	1.0–2.0	3.0	7–8
28–38	2.0–3.0	3.5	8–9
>38	>3.0	3.5–4.0	9–10

*Depth of insertion (cm)=6+ weight (in kg)

Medications Used During or Following Resuscitation of the Newborn

Medication	Dosage/Route®	Concentration	Wt (kg)	Total IV Volume (mL)	Precautions
Epinephrine	IV (UVC preferred route) 0.1–0.3 mL/kg Higher IV doses not recommended Endotracheal 0.5–1 mL/kg	1:10.000	1	0.1–0.3	Give rapidly.
			2	0.2–0.6	Repeat every 3 to 5 minutes
			3	03–0.9	if HR <60 with chest
			4	0.4–1.2	compressions
Volume expanders Isotonic crystalloid (normal saline) or blood	10 mL/kgIV		1	10	Indicated for shock.
			2	20	Give over 5 to 10 minutes.
			3	30	Reassess after each bolus
			4	40	

*Note: Endotracheal dose may not result in effective plasma concentration of drug, so vascular access should be estabilshed as soon as possible. Drugs given endotracheally require higher dosing than when given IV.

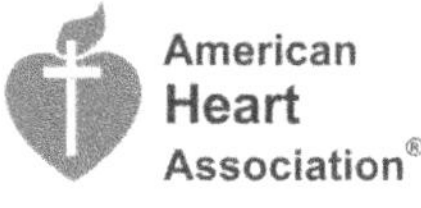

American Heart Association®

life is Why™

American Academy of Pediatrics

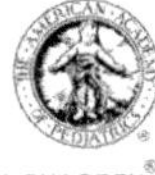

DEDUCATED TO THE HEALTH OF ALL CHILDREN®

(SpO₂: oxygen saturation; PPV: positive pressure ventilation; UVC: ultraviolet C; HR: heart rate; ETT: endotracheal tube)

Temperature Control

- Very low birth weight (<1500 g) preterm babies are likely to become hypothermic despite the use of traditional techniques for decreasing heat loss.
- Placing the child under radiant warmer and temperature must be monitored closely because of the slight but described risk of hyperthermia with this technique.
- Other techniques to maintain temperature during stabilization of the baby in the delivery room (e.g. drying and swaddling, warming pads, increased environmental temperature, placing the baby skin-to-skin with the mother and covering both with a blanket) have been used but they have not been evaluated in controlled trials nor compared with the plastic wrap technique for premature babies.
- All resuscitation procedures, including endotracheal intubation, chest compression, and insertion of lines, can be performed with these temperature-controlling interventions in place.

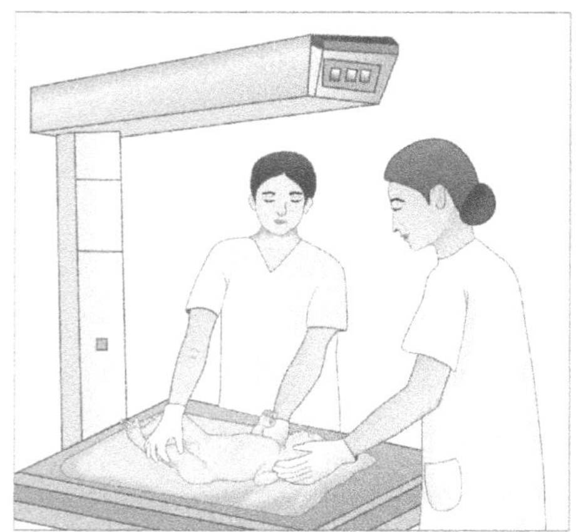

- Infants born to febrile mothers have been reported to have a higher incidence of perinatal respiratory depression, neonatal seizures, and cerebral palsy and increased risk of mortality.

Periodic Evaluation at 30-Second Intervals

- After the immediate post birth assessment and administration of initial steps further resuscitative efforts should be guided by simultaneous assessment of respirations, heart rate, and color.
- After initial respiratory efforts the newly born infant should be able to establish regular respirations that are sufficient to improve color and maintain a heart rate >100 bpm. Gasping and apnea indicate the need for assisted ventilation.
- A newly born infant who is uncompromised will achieve and maintain pink mucous membranes without administration of supplementary oxygen. Evidence obtained with continuous oximetry, however, has shown that neonatal transition is a gradual process.
- Healthy babies born at term may take >10 minutes to achieve a preductal oxygen saturation >95% and nearly 1 hour to achieve postductal saturation >95%.
- Central cyanosis is determined by examining the face, trunk, and mucous membranes.
- Acrocyanosis (blue color of hands and feet alone) is usually a normal finding at birth and is not a reliable indicator of hypoxemia but may indicate other conditions, such as cold stress.
- Pallor or mottling may be a sign of decreased cardiac output, severe anemia, hypovolemia, hypothermia, or acidosis.

Equipment

- Clean big tray with sterile cloth
- Sterile glove and mask—1
- Scissor and adhesive tape—1
- Cotton ball and gauze
- Ambu bag with reservoir (500 mL + 250 mL)—1
- O_2 face mask- 0,1 size—2
- Laryngoscope (0,1 size)—1
- Syringe 1,2,5 and 60 mL—3
- IV cannula (24, 26 Gaze)—2
- NG tube—1
- Umbilical cord clamp—1
- Umbilical catheter—1
- Suction catheter (6, 8 Fr)—1
- ET tube—1
- Inj. Epinephrine—1
- Inj. Adrenalin—1
- Inj. Naloxone—1
- Inj. Sodium bicarbonate—1
- Bowl medium—2
- Tray cloth—1
- Mucous extractor—1
- Shoulder roll—1
- Stethoscope (pediatric)—1

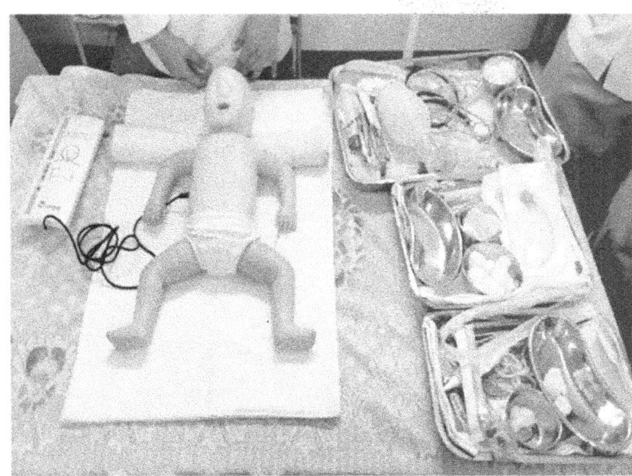 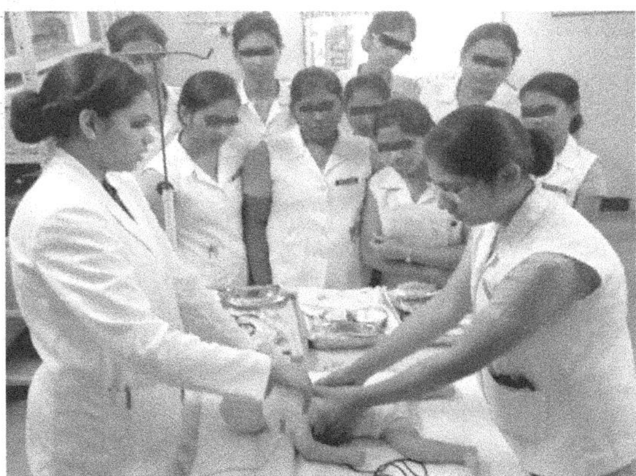

Procedures

A—Airway

- Supplementary oxygen is recommended whenever positive-pressure ventilation is indicated for resuscitation free-flow oxygen should be administered to babies who are breathing but have central cyanosis.
- The standard approach to resuscitation is to use 100% oxygen.
- It is recommended that supplementary oxygen be available to use if there is no appreciable improvement within 90 seconds after birth.
- In situations where supplementary oxygen is not readily available, positive-pressure ventilation should be administered with room air.
- Administration of a variable concentration of oxygen guided by pulse oximetry may improve the ability to achieve normoxia more quickly. Concerns about potential oxidant injury should caution the clinician about the use of excessive oxygen especially in the premature infant.

B—Breathing (Positive-Pressure Ventilation)

If the infant remains apneic or gasping, if the heart rate remains <100 bpm 30 seconds after administering the initial steps, or if the infant continues to have persistent central cyanosis despite administration of supplementary oxygen, start positive-pressure ventilation.

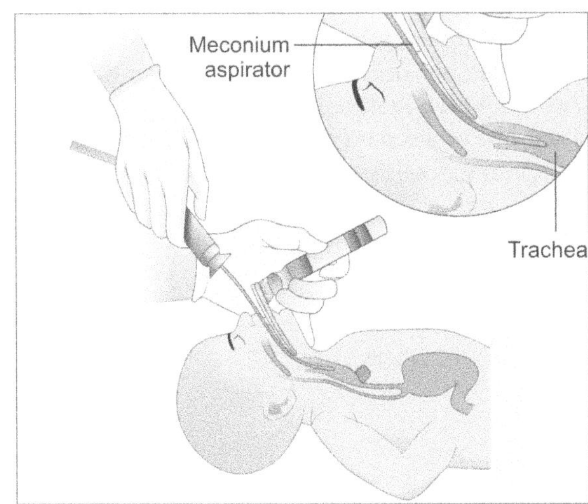

Endotracheal Tube Placement

Endotracheal intubation may be indicated at several points during neonatal resuscitation:

- When tracheal suctioning for meconium is required
- If bag-mask ventilation is ineffective or prolonged
- When chest compressions are performed
- When endotracheal administration of medications is desired special resuscitation circumstances, such as congenital diaphragmatic hernia or extremely low birth weight (<1000 g).

The timing of endotracheal intubation may also depend on the skill and experience of the available providers. After endotracheal intubation and administration of intermittent positive pressure, a prompt increase in heart rate is the best indicator that the tube is in the tracheobronchial tree and providing effective ventilation.

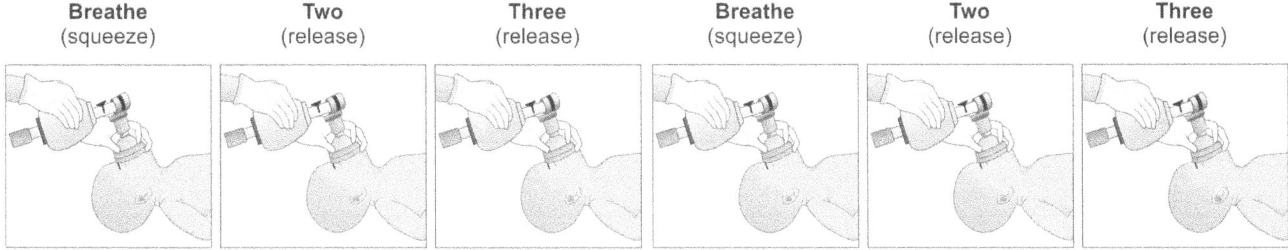

Ambu bag technique

C—Chest Compressions

Chest compressions are indicated for a heart rate that is <60 bpm despite adequate ventilation with supplementary oxygen for 30 seconds. Because ventilation is the most effective action in neonatal resuscitation and because chest compressions are likely to compete with effective ventilation, rescuers should ensure that assisted ventilation is being delivered optimally before starting chest compressions.

Compressions should be delivered on the lower third of the sternum to a depth of approximately one third of the anterior-posterior diameter of the chest.

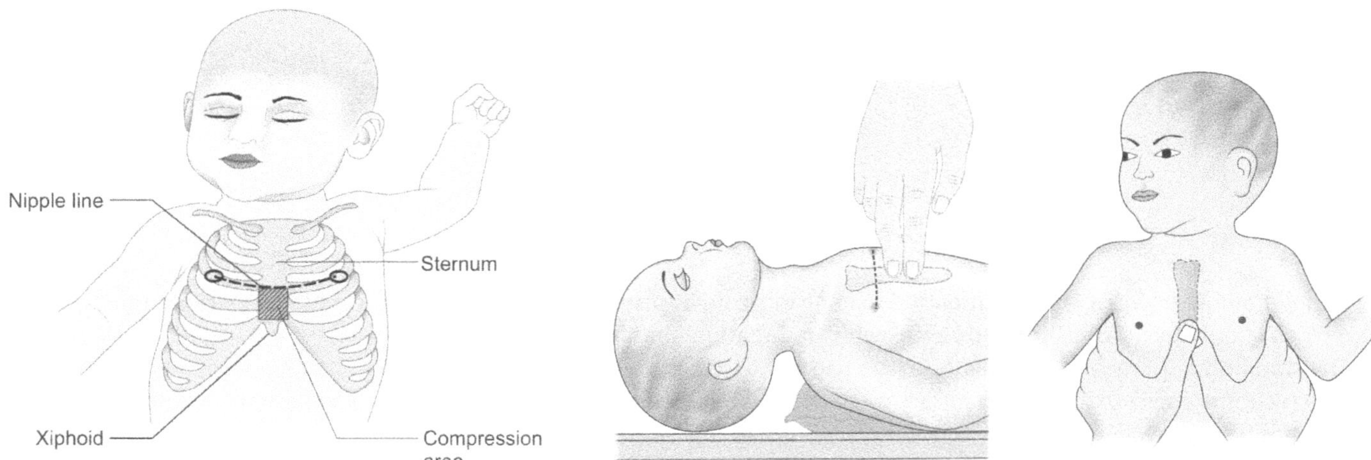

Two techniques have been described: Compression with 2 thumbs with fingers encircling the chest and supporting the back (the 2 thumb–encircling hands technique) or compression with 2 fingers with a second hand supporting the back. Because the 2 thumb–encircling hands technique may generate higher peak systolic and coronary perfusion pressure than the 2-finger technique, the 2 thumb–encircling hands technique is recommended for performing chest compressions in newly born infants. However, the 2-finger technique may be preferable when access to the umbilicus is required during insertion of an umbilical catheter.

There should be a 3:1 ratio of compressions to ventilations with 90 compressions and 30 breaths to achieve approximately 120 events per minute to maximize ventilation at an achievable rate. Thus each event will be allotted approximately 1/2 second, with exhalation occurring during the first compression after each ventilation. Respirations, heart rate, and color should be reassessed about every 30 seconds, and coordinated chest compressions and ventilations should continue until the spontaneous heart rate is ≥ 60 bpm.

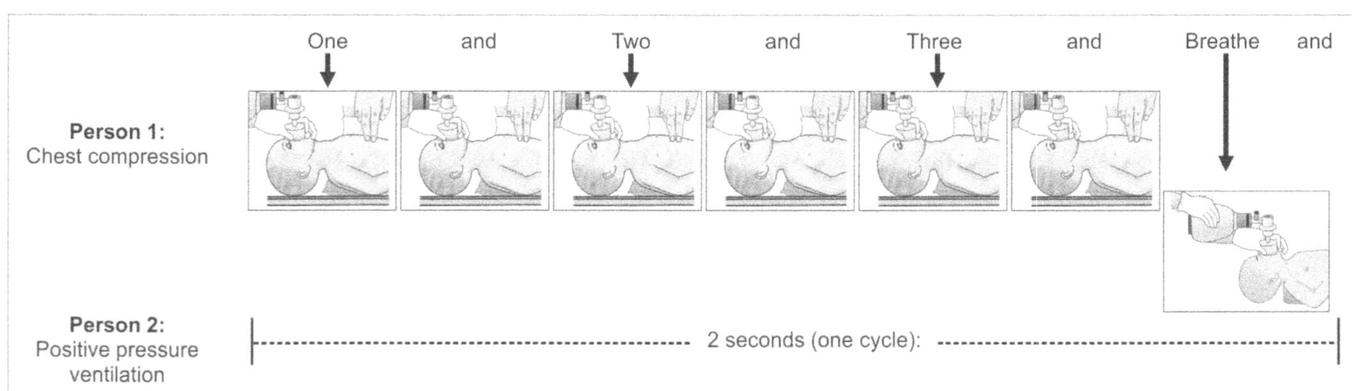

Chest compression coordinating technique

Table: Initiating chest compressions rationale

Features	Newborn	Infant
Rate of compressions	120/minute	at least 100/min
Depth of compressions	0.5–0.75 inches	0.5 to 1 inches
Compression: Ventilation ratio	3:1	5:1
No. of rescuers/staff nurse	2 or more	1 or more
Target heart rate	80/min	60/min

D—Drugs (Medications)

Drugs are rarely indicated in resuscitation of the newly born infant. Bradycardia in the newborn infant is usually the result of inadequate lung inflation or profound hypoxemia, and establishing adequate ventilation is the most important step to correct it. But if the heart rate remains <60 bpm despite adequate ventilation with 100% oxygen and chest compressions, administration of epinephrine or volume expansion or both, may be indicated. Rarely, buffers, a narcotic antagonist, or vasopressors may be useful after resuscitation.

Epinephrine Administration

- The recommended IV dose is 0.01 to 0.03 mg/kg per dose.
- The concentration of epinephrine for either route should be 1:10 000 (0.1 mg/mL).

Volume Expansion

- Consider volume expansion when blood loss is suspected or the infant appears to be in shock (pale skin, poor perfusion, weak pulse) and has not responded adequately to other resuscitative measures.
- An isotonic crystalloid rather than albumin is the solution of choice for volume expansion in the delivery room.
- The recommended dose is 10 mL/kg, which may need to be repeated. When resuscitating premature infants, care should be taken to avoid giving volume expanders too rapidly, because rapid infusions of large volumes have been associated with intraventricular hemorrhage.

Naloxone

- Administration of Naloxone is not recommended as part of initial resuscitative efforts in the delivery room for newborns with respiratory depression. If administration of naloxone is considered, heart rate and color must first be restored by supporting ventilation.
- The preferred route is IV or intramuscular. Given the lack of clinical data in newborns, endotracheal administration of naloxone is not recommended.
- The recommended dose is 0.1 mg/kg, but no studies have examined the efficacy of this dose in newborns. Naloxone may have a shorter half-life than the original maternal opioid; therefore the neonate should be monitored closely for recurrent apnea or hypoventilation, and subsequent doses of Naloxone may be required.

Post-resuscitation Care

- It should be noted that central cyanosis is normally present in the first few minutes after birth. Continuous positive airway pressure may be considered, particularly for preterm infants with laboured respirations or persistent cyanosis; however, if their cardiorespiratory status fails to improve, oxygen, PPV and intubation should be considered.
- As described in the NRP textbook, post resuscitation care includes temperature control, close monitoring of vital signs (e.g. HR, oxygen saturation and blood pressure) and awareness of potential complications and provision of the necessary support.
- It cannot be assumed that a baby who has been successfully resuscitated is healthy and requires only routine care; further stabilization may be necessary as a component of post resuscitation care. For example, the new guidelines provide guidance for the management of newborns considered to be at risk for hypoxic-ischemic encephalopathy.
- Specific recommendations when signs of moderate to severe hypoxic-ischemic encephalopathy are present within 6 hour of age include consideration of therapeutic hypothermia according to an evidence-based protocol, with referral to and follow-up by a regional perinatal center.

Guidelines for Withholding and Discontinuing Resuscitation

Withholding Resuscitation

It is possible to identify conditions associated with high mortality and poor outcome in which withholding resuscitative efforts may be considered reasonable, particularly when there has been the opportunity for parental agreement. A consistent and coordinated approach to individual cases by the obstetric and neonatal teams and the parents is an important goal. No initiation of resuscitation and discontinuation of life-sustaining treatment during or after resuscitation are ethically equivalent, and clinicians should not hesitate to withdraw support when functional survival is highly unlikely.

The following guidelines must be interpreted according to current regional outcomes:

- Low birth weight and congenital anomalies are associated with almost certain early death and when unacceptably high morbidity is likely among the rare survivors, resuscitation is not indicated. Examples may include extreme prematurity

(gestational age <23 weeks or birth weight <400 g), anencephaly, and chromosomal abnormalities incompatible with life, such as trisomy 13.
- In conditions associated with a high rate of survival and acceptable morbidity, resuscitation is nearly always indicated. This will generally include babies with gestational age $\geq$ 25 weeks (unless there is evidence of fetal compromise such as intrauterine infection or hypoxia-ischemia) and those with most congenital malformations.
- In conditions associated with uncertain prognosis in which survival is borderline, the morbidity rate is relatively high, and the anticipated burden to the child is high, parental desires concerning initiation of resuscitation should be supported.

Discontinuing Resuscitative Efforts

- Infants without signs of life (no heart beat and no respiratory effort) after 10 minutes of resuscitation show either a high mortality or severe neurodevelopmental disability.
- After 10 minutes of continuous and adequate resuscitative efforts, discontinuation of resuscitation may be justified if there are no signs of life
- Document the procedures.

ARTERIAL BLOOD GAS ANALYSIS (ABG ANALYSIS)

Definition

Blood gas analysis, also called arterial blood gas (ABG) analysis, is a test which measures the amount of oxygen (O_2) and carbon dioxide (CO_2) in the blood, as well as the acidity (pH) of the blood.
- Drawn from artery-radial, brachial, femoral
- It is an invasive procedure
- Caution must be taken with patient on anticoagulants.

Arterial blood gas analysis is an essential part of diagnosing and managing the patient's oxygenation status, ventilation failure and acid base balance.

Parameters of ABG Analysis

- pH : $[H^+]$
- PCO_2 : Partial pressure CO_2
- PO_2 : Partial pressure O_2
- HCO_3 : Bicarbonate
- BE : Base excess
- SaO_2 : Oxygen saturation

Normal ABG Value

Ideal blood cases			
	pH	pCO_2	pO_2
Preterm	7.28–7.32	3–45	50–80
Term	7.30–7.35	35–45	80–95

Normal values (1 hour age, not ventilated)

Acceptable Arterial Blood Gas

pH	More than 7.2
pCO_2	50–60 mm of Hg
pO_2	50–60 mm of Hg
HCO_3	18–20

Normal ABG values					
	Birth	**1 hour**	**1 day**	**Infant**	**Child**
pH	7.20–7.30	7.30–7.35	7.35–7.40	7.35–7.45	7.35–7.45
pCO_1	45–55	35–40	35–40	35–45	35–45
pO_2	< 60	60–80	70–100	80–100	80–100
HCO_3	20–24	20–24	20–24	22–26	22–26

Purpose of ABG Analysis

- An ABG analysis evaluates how effectively the lungs are delivering oxygen to the blood and how efficiently they are eliminating carbon dioxide from it
- The test also indicates how well the lungs and kidneys are interacting to maintain normal blood pH (acid-base balance)
- Blood gas studies are usually done to assess respiratory disease and other conditions that may affect the lungs, and to manage patients receiving oxygen therapy (respiratory therapy)
- In addition, the acid-base component of the test provides information on kidney function too.
- An ABG is typically requested to determine the pH of the blood and the partial pressures of carbon dioxide ($PaCO_2$) and oxygen (PaO_2) within it.
- It is used to assess the effectiveness of gaseous exchange and ventilation, be it spontaneous or mechanical.
- If the pH becomes deranged, normal cell metabolism is affected.
- The ABG allows patients' metabolic status to be assessed too, giving an indication of how they are coping with their illness.
- It would therefore seem logical to request an ABG on any patient who is or has the potential to become critically ill.
- This includes patients in critical care areas and those on wards who 'trigger' early-warning scoring systems.

Results of ABG Analysis

Respiratory acidosis	Respiratory alkalosis
- Respiratory acidosis is characterized by a **lower pH** and an **increased PCO₂** and is due to respiratory depression (not enough oxygen in and CO_2 out). - This can be caused by many things, including pneumonia, chronic obstructive pulmonary disease (COPD), and over-sedation from narcotics. pH ↓ PCO_2 ↑ **Signs and symptoms** - **Respiratory**: Dyspnea, respiratory distress and/or shallow respiration. - **Nervous**: Headache, restlessness and confusion. If CO_2 level extremely high drowsiness and unresponsiveness may be noted. - **CVS:** Tachycardia and Dysrhythmia.	- Respiratory alkalosis, characterized by a **raised pH** and a **decreased PCO₂**, is due to over ventilation caused by hyperventilating, pain, emotional distress, or certain lung diseases that interfere with oxygen exchange. pH ↑ PCO_2 ↓ **Signs and symptoms** - CNS: Light Headedness, numbness, tingling, confusion, inability to concentrate and blurred vision. - Dysrhythmia and palpitations. - Dry mouth, diaphoresis and tetanic spasms of the arms and legs.
Metabolic acidosis	**Metabolic alkalosis**
Metabolic acidosis is characterized by a lower pH and decreased HCO_3^-; the blood is too acidic on a metabolic/kidney level. Causes include diabetes, shock, and renal failure. pH ↓ HCO_3 ↓ **Signs and symptoms** **CNS:** Headache, confusion and restlessness progressing to lethargy, then stupor or coma. **CVS:** Dysrhythmia. Kussmaul's respirations. Warm, flushed skin as well as nausea and vomiting.	Metabolic alkalosis is characterized by an elevated pH and increased HCO_3^- and is seen in hypokalemia, chronic vomiting (losing acid from the stomach), and sodium bicarbonate overdose. pH ↑ HCO_3 ↑ **Signs and symptoms** **CNS:** Dizziness, lethargy disorientation, seizures and coma. **M/S:** Weakness, muscle twitching, muscle cramps and tetany. Nausea, vomiting and respiratory depression. It is difficult to treat.

Role of Nurse

- After the blood has been taken, the technician or the patient applies pressure to the puncture site for 10–15 minutes to stop the bleeding, and then places a dressing over the puncture.
- The child should rest quietly while applying the pressure to the puncture site. Health care workers will observe the patient for signs of bleeding or circulation problems.

ILLUSTRATED PEDIATRIC PROCEDURE INSTRUMENTS

S. No.	Name of the instruments	Purpose	Image of the instruments
1.	Artery forceps	Artery forceps are primarily use as hemostatic forceps to grasp vessels and allow ligation of those vessels. They vary in size for use on fine, delicate vessels to large vascular pedicles. Artery forceps can also be used to grasp tissues, sutures and other prosthetic materials.	
2.	Dressing forceps	To hold cotton, gauze during dressing procedure	
3.	Cheatle forceps and cheatal jar	• Recognized by their longer length • To take sterile instrument. • It can be used for placing and removing items	
4.	Sponge holding forceps	• Sponge forceps handle sponges, gauzes, or sensitive medical supplies. • Sponge forceps to hold antiseptic cotton swabs and gauge before the surgery.	
5.	Curved mayo scissors	• Both blades are slightly curved and blunt ended tips. • Function: used for cutting deep, heavy, or tough tissue	
6.	Curve Mosquito forceps	• Allow easier placement of ligatures around the forceps • Use in surgery for temporary occlusion of a vessel	

S. No.	Name of the instruments	Purpose	Image of the instruments

7.	Thudichum's nasal speculum	• Function: Used for visualization of external nose.
		   – anterior-inferior part of nasal septum
		   – anterior part of inferior and middle turbinate	

8.	Proctoscope	To examine the anal cavity, Rectum and sigmoid colon	
9.	Crocodile forceps	• To remove foreign body from ear, nose, throat (ENT) procedure.	Closeup of jaws
10.	Tongue holding forceps	• These forceps hold tongue during surgery or to prevent it from falling back so as not to obsutruct breathing	
11.	Trachea dilator	• To keep the tracheostomy open	
12.	Mouth gag	• To open the mouth. • Used during doing mouth toilet at the comatose patient.	
13.	Magill forceps	• To guide a tracheal tube into the larynx or a nasogastric tube into the esophagus under direct vision. • To place pharyngeal packs and remove foreign bodies	Children Adult The handles are specially curved so that operator's hand does not obstruct his view

S. No.	Name of the instruments	Purpose	Image of the instruments
14.	Tuning fork	• Used to dertmine whether a hearing loss is conductive or preceptive • Can be Weber test or Rinne test	
15.	Iris scissors	It small, 3–4 inches long with sharp points, used for ophthalmic surgery, e.g. iridectomy	
16.	Aneurysm needle	Function: To catch small blood vessel and nerve	
17.	Ear syringes	To put irrigation fluid such as normal saline for ears irrigation	
18.	Umbilical cord scissors	Cutting the umbilical cord	
19.	Vulsellum	Used for grasping the cervix (Usually anterior lip of the cervix is grasped)	
20.	Artery forceps	• Straight end→ stay suture • Curved end → hemostal	
21.	Episiotomy scissors	Used in Episiotomy	
22.	Green armytage forceps	Used as a hemostat in caesarean operation	

S. No.	Name of the instruments	Purpose	Image of the instruments
23.	Umbilical cord clamp	Used to clamp the umbilical Cord	
24.	Alli's forceps	• Use to grasp tough structure like Rectus sheath • Use in LSCS, Hysterectomy	
25.	Ayre's spatula	Use in pap smear	
26.	Babcock's forceps	Use to grasp tubular structure like fallopian tube	
27.	Foley's catheter	• Drainage of urine • Induction of labor	
28.	Pinard's fetal stethoscope	Used to auscultate fetal heart	
29.	Needle holder	Used to grasp needle during suture	

COMMON PEDIATRIC HEALTHCARE DEVICES

Ambu Bag

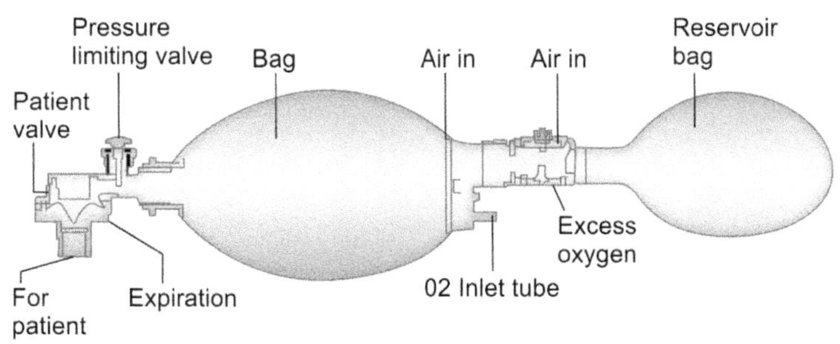

Types of AMBU Bag

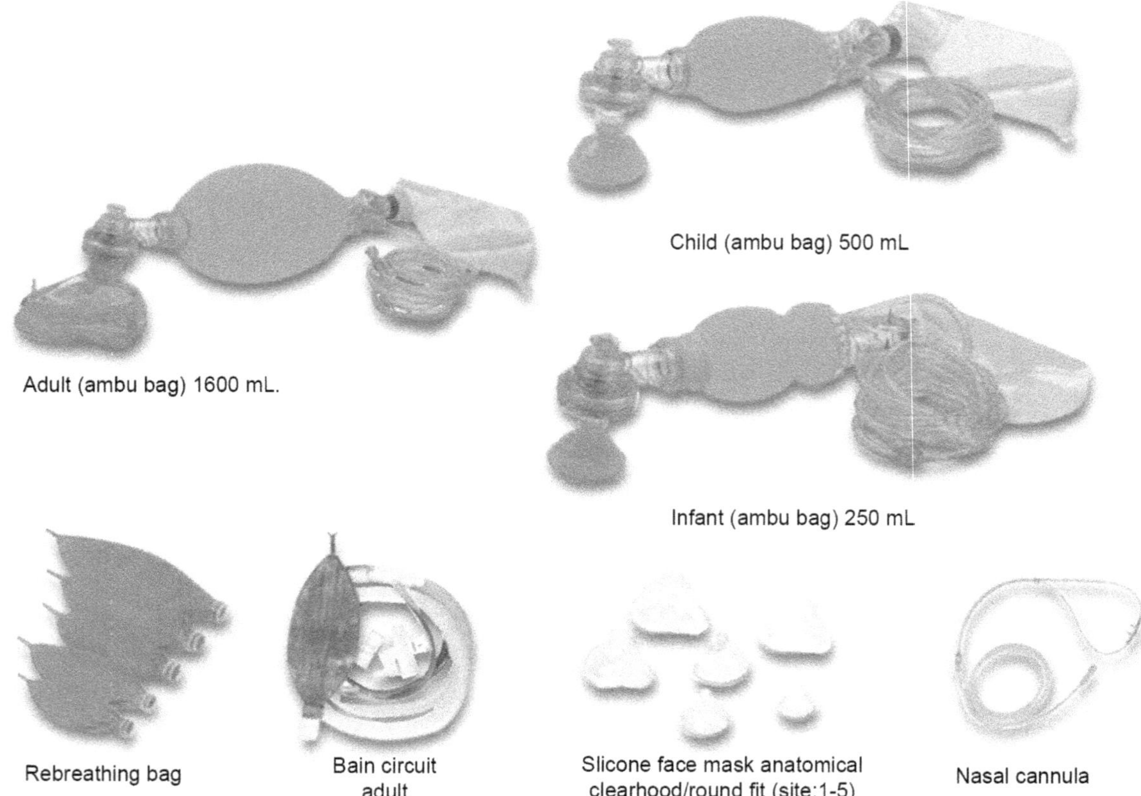

Laryngoscope Sizes

Age	Blade Type and Size
Newborn	Miller 0
1–12 months	Miller 1 or Wis 1.5
12–3 years	Wis 1.5 or Miller 2
3–12 years	Miller 2 or Macintosh 3
12–16 years	Miller 2 or Macintosh 3
> 16 years	Miller 3 or Macintosh 4

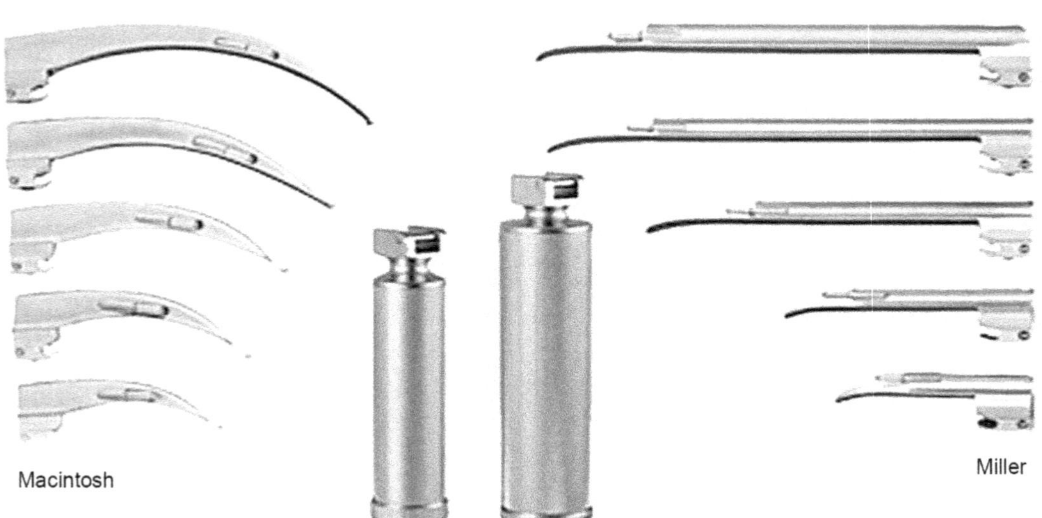

Oral Airway

The American National Standard specifies that the size of oral airways be designated by a no., i.e. the length in cm.

Size	Number	Length (cm)
000	(1)	3.5
00	(2)	4.5
0	(3)	5.5
1	(4)	6.5
2	(5)	7.5
3	(6)	8.5
4	(7)	9.5
5	(8)	10.5

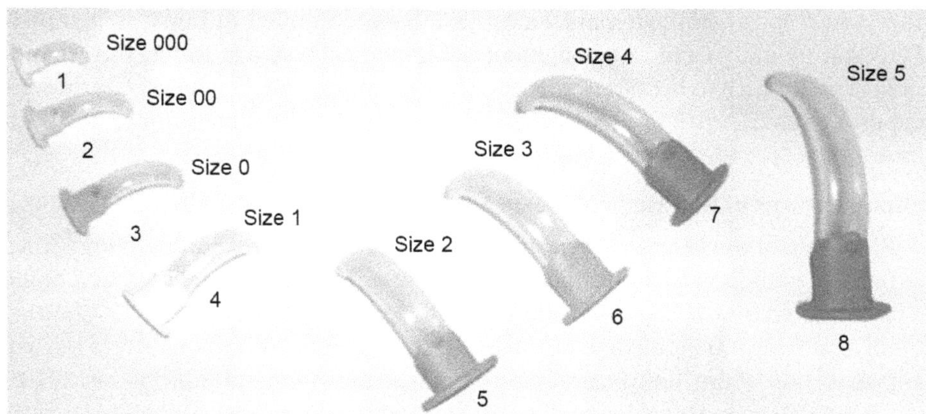

Intravenus Cannula

A cannula is a flexible tube that can be inserted into the body. For medical use, there are 11 different types of cannula. The most commonly used are the intravenous and the nasal cannula.

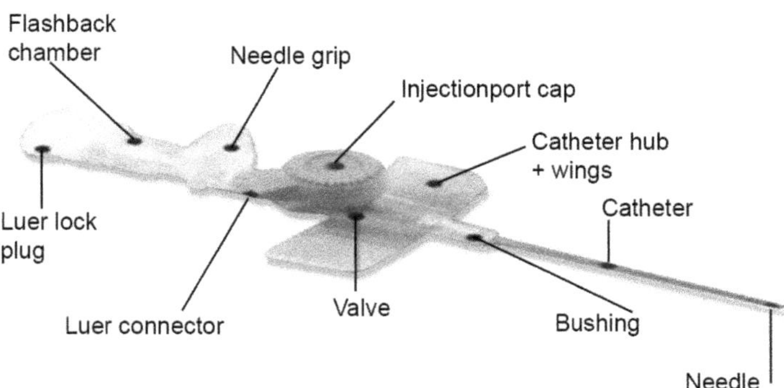

Gauge	Color Code	Ext. Dia. mm	Length mm	Flow Rate mL/min
14 G	Orange	2.1	45	240
16 G	Gray	1.8	45	180
18 G	Green	1.3	32/45	90
20 G	Pink	1.1	32	60
22 G	Blue	0.9	25	36
24 G	Yellow	0.7	19	20
26 G	Violet	0.6	19	13

Infantometer and Baby Weighing Machine

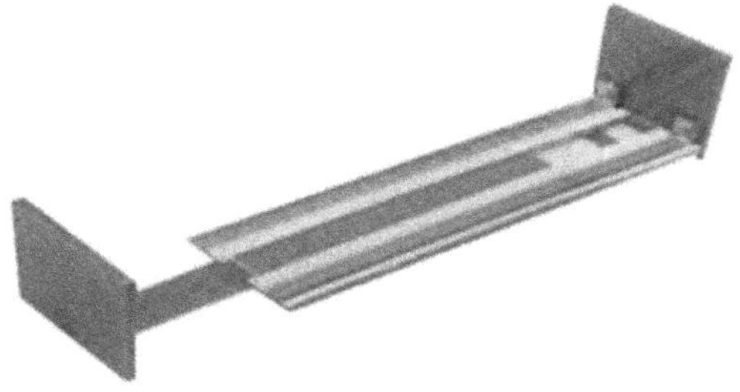

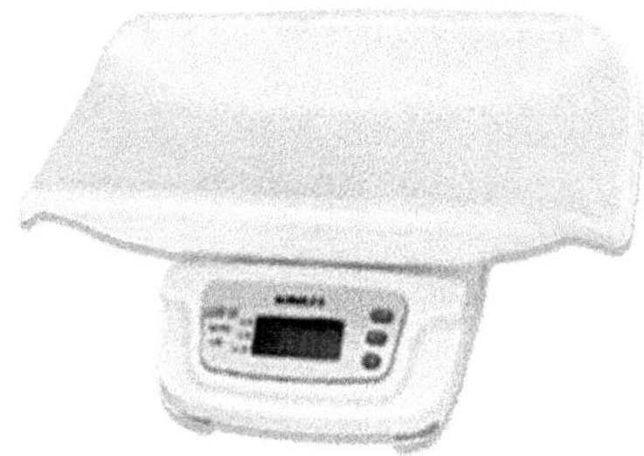

BIO-MEDICAL WASTE MANAGEMENT

Introduction

Bio-Medical Waste Management Rules have been amended to improve compliance and strengthen the implementation of environmentally sound management of biomedical waste in India. The amended rules stipulate that generators of bio-medical waste such as hospitals, nursing homes, clinics, and dispensaries etc will not use chlorinated plastic bags and gloves beyond March 27, 2019 in medical applications to save the environment however the blood bags have been exempted for phase-out, as per the amended BMW rules, 2018.

Salient features of Bio-Medical Waste Management (Amendment) Rules, 2018 are as follows:

- Bio-medical waste generators including hospitals, nursing homes, clinics, dispensaries, veterinary institutions, animal houses, pathological laboratories, blood banks, health care facilities, and clinical establishments will have to phase out chlorinated plastic bags (excluding blood bags) and gloves by March 27, 2019.
- All healthcare facilities shall make available the annual report on its website within a period of two years from the date of publication of the Bio-Medical Waste Management (Amendment) Rules, 2018.
- Operators of common bio-medical waste treatment and disposal facilities shall establish bar coding and global positioning system for handling of bio-medical waste in accordance with guidelines issued by the Central Pollution Control Board by March 27, 2019.
- The State Pollution Control Boards/Pollution Control Committees have to compile, review and analyse the information received and send tis information to the Central Pollution Control Board in a new Form (Form IV A), which seeks detailed information regarding district-wise bio-medical waste generation, information on Health Care Facilities having captive treatment facilities, information on common bio-medical waste treatment and disposal facilities.

Bio-Medical Waste Management Rules

Biomedical wastes categories and their segregation, collection, treatment, processing and disposal options

Category	Type of Waste	Type of Bag or Container to be Used	Treatment and Disposal Options
Yellow	a) Human Anatomical Waste b) Animal Anatomical Waste c) Soiled Waste d) Expired or Discarded Medicines e) Chemical Waste f) Discarded linen, mattresses, beddings contaminated with blood or body fluid, routine mask and gown	Yellow colored non-chlorinated plastic bags or containers	Incineration or Plasma Pyrolysis or deep burial* The discarded medicines shall be either sent back to manufacturer or disposed by incineration
	g) Micro, Bio-t and other clinical lab waste	Autoclave safe plastic bags or containers	
	h) Chemical liquid waste	Separate collection system leading to effluent treatment system	After resource recovery, the chemical liquid waste shall be pre-treated before mixing with other wastewater
Red	Contaminated waste (recyclable)	Red colored nonchlorinated plastic bags or containers	Autoclaving or micro-waving/hydroclaving followed by shredding or mutilation or combination of sterilization and shredding. Treated waste to be sent to recyclers. Plastic waste should not be sent to landfill sites.
White (Translucent)	Waste sharps including metals	Puncture proof, Leak proof, tamper proof containers	Autoclaving or dry heat sterilization followed by shredding or mutilation or encapsulation in metal container or cement concret
Blue	Glassware and metallic body implants	Puncture proof and leak proof boxes or containers with blue colored marking	Disinfection or through autoclaving or microwaving or hydroclaving and then sent for recycling

Source: Bio-Medical Waste Management Rules, 2016 and amended rules 2018

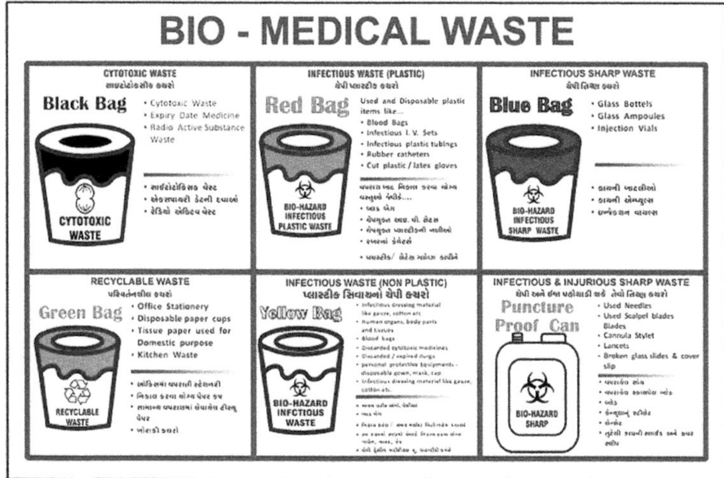

- Every occupier, i.e., a person having administrative control over the institution and the premises generating biomedical waste shall pre-treat the laboratory waste, microbiological waste, blood samples, and blood bags through disinfection or sterilization on-site in the manner as prescribed by the World Health Organization (WHO) or guidelines on safe management of wastes from health care activities and WHO Blue Book 2014 and then sent to the Common bio-medical waste treatment facility for final disposal.

SELECTION OF PLAY MATERIAL

Infants	Adolescents
• Rattles • Soothers • Musical toys • Blanket • Cuddly toys • Board books	• Board games such as monopoly, life, scrabble, risk, trivial pursuit, etc. • CD's • Gift certificates for music stores or department stores such as shoppers drug mart, the bay, sears and body shop • Art supplies such as sketch books, pastels, more advanced craft kits • Word search and crossword puzzle books • Decks of cards • Journals and writing paper • Sports items such as new and packaged sports cards, balls, etc.
Toddlers/preschool	**Other play items**
• Building blocks • 'Little People' sets (fisher price farm, garage, home • Board books, lift the flap books • Dolls • Trucks and cars (durable and sturdy plastic) • Make believe toys such as kitchen utensils, work benches and tools, etc. • Crayons • Construction paper • Magna doodles • Wooden shape puzzles • Interactive toys such as those that light up or make sounds when touched	• DVD's for all ages (toddler to teens) • Bubbles • Character band-aids • Magazine subscriptions (teens, educational such as Chickadee, National Geographic for kids, etc.) • New copies of recent magazines
School age	
• Board games such as guess who, Candy Land, Snakes and Ladders • Decks of playing cards such as Skip-Bo, UNO, Go Fish, Old Maid, etc. • Cuddly toys • Books both early readers and chapter books as well as Look and Find or I Spy books • Markers/crayons/pencil crayons • Crayola model magic • Craft kits and model kits • Small hand held electronic games such as game boy, and Sony PSP • Nintendo, X-box and play station games that are rated "E" for everyone. Please no violent games • Journals • Lego kits • Puzzles under 100 piece	

DEVELOPMENTAL STUDY (GROWTH AND DEVELOPMENTAL ASSESSMENT)

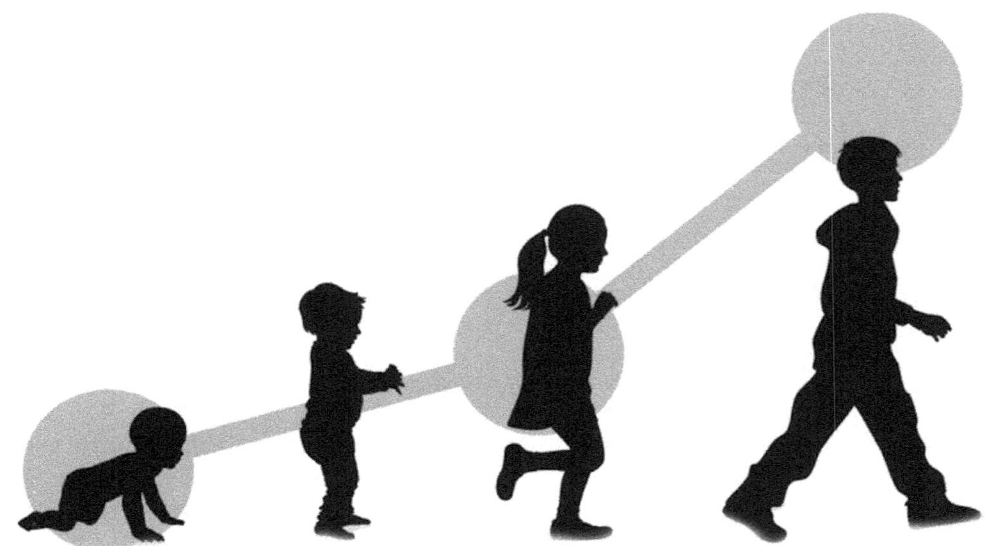

ASSESSMENT OF GROWTH AND DEVELOPMENT

Definition

Definition of Growth

Growth refers to an increase in physical size of the whole or any of its parts and can be measured in inches or centimeters and in pounds or kilograms.

— **Marlow**

Definition of Development

Development refers to a progressive increase in skill and capacity to function. It causes a qualitative change in the child's functioning. Maturation produces an increase in competence, an ability to function at a higher level depending on the child's heredity.

— **Marlow**

Definition of Growth and Development

Growth is the progressive increase in the size of a child or parts of a child. Development is progressive acquisition of various skills (abilities) such as head support, speaking, learning, expressing the feelings and relating with other people. Growth and development go together but at different rates.

Stages of Development

S. No.	Stage	Time period
Prenatal period		
1.	Ovum	0–14 days (after conception)
2.	Embryo	14 days–8 weeks
3.	Fetus	8 weeks–birth (8–40 weeks)
Postnatal period		
1.	Newborn	Birth to 28 days
2.	Infant	1–12 month
3.	Toddler	1–3 years
4.	Preschooler	3–5 years
5.	School-aged child	6–12 years

Contd...

Contd...

S. No.	Stage	Time period
6	Adolescent	13–18 years
	Early Adolescent	13–14 years
	Middle Adolescent	15–16 years
	Late Adolescent	17–18 years

Parameters of Growth and Development Assessment of Child

- Physical/biological development
- Motor development
  - Fine motor development
  - Gross motor development
- Sensory development
- Psychosocial development
- Psychosexual development
- Spiritual development
- Intellectual/cognitive development
- Moral development
- Language development
- Play stimulation

Piaget develops four important stages of cognitive development:

1. Sensorimotor stage (birth to age 2)
2. Preoperational stage (age 2 to 7)
3. Concrete-operational stage (age 7 to 12)
4. Formal-operational stage (age 11 to 12)

Erikson's eight stages consist of the following:

1. Trust vs mistrust (infant)
2. Autonomy vs shame (toddlerhood)
3. Initiative vs guilt (preschooler)
4. Industry vs inferiority (young adolescent)
5. Identity vs role confusion (adolescent)
6. Intimacy vs isolation (young adulthood)
7. Generativity vs stagnation (middle adulthood)
8. Ego integrity vs despair (old age)

Stages of Psychosocial, Psychosexual, Intellectual, and Moral Development

Stage	Age	Tasks	Erikson's psychosocial stages negative counterpart	Freud's psychosexual stages	Significant persons
Infancy	0–12 month	Sense of trust	Mistrust	Oral	Maternal person or substitute
Toddler	1–3 years	Sense of autonomy	Shame and doubt	Anal	Parental persons
Preschooler	3–6 years	Sense of initiative	Guilt	Phallic	Basic family
School going children	6–12 years	Sense of industry	Inferiority	Latency	Neighborhood, school
Early adolescence	Above–12	Sense of identity	Identity diffusion	Puberty	Peer groups and out groups, models of leadership
Late adolescence and young adult	16–18 years	Sense of intimacy and solidarity	Isolation	Geniality	Partners in friendship, sex, competition, cooperation

Principles of Growth and Development

Cephalocaudal direction	Proximodistal direction
The process of **cephalocaudal** direction from **head** down to **tail**. This means that improvement in structure and function come first in the head region, then in the trunk, and last in the leg region.	The process in proximodistal from center or midline to periphery direction. Development proceeds from near to far—outward from central axis of the body toward the extremities.

▮ EVALUATION CRITERIA FOR OVERALL GROWTH AND DEVELOPMENTAL ASSESSMENT

Name of hospital ....Total Marks: 50

Wards:..Duration of posting .... weeks

S. No.	Contents	Score	Marks obtained	Remarks
1.	**Child profile and assessment:**			
	• Identification data	2		
	• Biological assessment/reflexes	4		
	• Motor development	3		
	• Sensory development	2		
	• Psychosocial development	2		
	• Psychosexual development	2		
	• Spiritual development	2		
	• Intellectual development	2		
	• Moral development	2		
	• Language development	2		
	• Play stimulation	2		
	• Impression	2		
2.	**Role of student nurse:**			
	• Set the priority	2		
	• Communication	2		
	• Utilizing the available resources	3		
	• Personal appearance	2		
	• Punctuality	3		
	• Maintain proper dress code	2		
	• Acceptance of criticism	3		
	• Evaluation of the child development	3		
	• Date of submission	2		
	Total	**50**		

Signature of Student   **Incharge Teacher**   **Signature of the HOD**

NEWBORN BABY/NEONATE (BIRTH TO 28 DAYS)

Identification Data

Name of the child   : Baby/Master ....

Chronological age   :

Developmental stage   :

Sex/gender   : Male/Female...

Date of admission   :

IP Number   :

Ward   :

Bed number   :

Diagnosis   :

Name of the surgery   :

Date of the surgery   :

Informant   : Father/Mother/Others ....

Date of assessment   : ....

Address   : ....

                                         : ....

                                         : ....

Physical Assessment Proforma

S. No.	Assessment features	Normal value	Child value	Remarks (achieved/ not achieved)
1.	Anthropometric measurement	Weight: 2.5–3.5 kg Height: 45–50 cm Head circumference: 33–35 cm Chest circumference: 31–33 cm		
2.	Vital signs	Temperature: 36.5–37°C Heart rate: 120/140 beats/minute Respiration: 30–60 breaths/minute Blood pressure: 65/41 mm of Hg		
3.	***Physical Appearance*** Posture	• Flexion of head and extremities, which rest on chest and abdomen		
	Skin	• Bright red, puffy, smooth vernix caseosa, lanugo, edema around eyes, face, legs, hands, feet, scrotum or labia, Mangolian spots		
	Head 1. Anterior fontanel 2. Posterior fontanel	• Diamond shaped 2.5–4 cm • Triangular shaped 0.5–1 cm • Flat, soft and firm fontanels		
	Eyes	• Lids edematous • Color–gray brown • Absence of tears • Presence of red reflex, corneal and papillary reflex and blinking		
	Ears position	• Top of pinna on horizontal line with outer canthus of eye • Pinna flexible cartilage present		

Contd...

Contd...

S. No.	Assessment features	Normal value	Child value	Remarks (achieved/ not achieved)
	Nose	• Nasal potency • Thin and white nasal discharge • Sneezing		
	Mouth and throat	Intact high pitched palate, frenulum of tongue, frenulum of upper lip, suckling reflex, rooting gag and extrusion reflex. Absent or minimal salivation. Vigorous cry		
	Neck	Short thick, surrounded by slais folds, tonic neck reflex		
	Chest	• Anterioposterior and lateral diameters are equal • Xiphoid process evident • Breast enlargement		
	Lungs	Respiration chiefly abdominal, cough reflex present Bilateral equal bronchial sound		
	(a) Heart	Apex-4th to 5th intercostals space, S_2 sharper, S_1 low pitch		
	Abdomen 1. Liver 2. Spleen 3. Kidney 4. Umbilical cord 5. Femoral pulses	Cylindrical in shape Palpable 2–3 cm below right costal margin Tip palpable at end of first week of age Palpable 1–2 cm above umbilicus Bluish white with 2 arteries and one vein Bilaterally Equal		
	Genitalia Female genitalia Male genitalia	• Labia and clitoris edematous • Urethral meats behind clitoris • Vernix caseosa between labia • Urination within 24 hours • Urethral opening at top of glance penis • Palpable Testis at each scrotum • Urination within 24 hours. • Pigmented edematous, pendulous scrotum		
	Rectum Extremities	Spine intact, no opening, masses trunk incurvation, patent and opening passage of meconium within 48 hours. • Ten fingers and toes • Full range of motion • Nail beds pink • Sole usually flat • Symmetry of extremities • Equal muscle tone bilaterally • Equal bilateral brachial pulses		

Impression

Neuromuscular System (Reflexes)

S. No.	Assessment features	Normal value	Child value	Remarks (achieved/ not achieved)
1.	Blinking or corneal reflex	Protection of the eye by rapid eye lid closure when the eyes are exposed to bright light		
2.	Doll's eye reflex	Turn the neonates head slowly to the right or left side, normally eye do not move		
3.	Sneezing and coughing reflex	Foreign substance entering the upper and lower airways, clearing of upper air passages by sneezing and lower air passages by coughing		
4.	Rooting reflex	When the cheek or corner of the mouth is stroked, the infants head should turn towards the stimulus and the mouth should be open		
5.	Sucking reflex	When touching or stroking the lips with the breast, the mouth opens and sucking movement begin.		
6	Swallowing reflex	The passage of food from posterior aspect of the mouth to the stomach		
7.	Gagging reflex	When the posterior pharynx is stimulated with food there is an immediate return of undigested food.		
8.	Extrusion reflex	When substance placed on anterior position of tongue will be expelled out		
9.	Palmer reflex	When the objects are placed in the newborn's palm, the newborn grasps		
10.	Plantar reflex	When object touches the sole of the foot at the base of the toes, toes grasp around very small object		
11.	Dancing or stepping reflex	Hold neonate in a vertical position with the feet touching a flat, firm surface, there will be rapid alternating flexion and extension of legs.		
12.	Babinski reflex	Stroking the lateral aspect of the sole of the foot with a relatively sharp object from the heel up toward the little toe and across the foot toward the big toe, there will be fanning of the toes.		
13.	Tonic neck reflex	Turning the head quickly to one side while the infant is supine, arm and leg on the side the head is turned toward extend. Arm and leg on the opposite side flex.		
14.	Moro reflex	Sudden jarring or change in equilibrium causes sudden extension and abduction of extremities and fanning of fingers with index finger and thumb forming a 'c' shape followed by flexion and adduction of extremities, legs may weakly flex, infant may cry, disappears after age 3–4 months, usually strongest during first 2 months.		
15.	Startle reflex	A sudden loud noise causes abduction of the arms with flexion of elbows, hands remain clenched, disappears by age 4 months.		

Contd...

Contd...

16.	**Perez reflex**	While infant is prone on a firm surface, thumb is pressed along spine from sacrum to neck, infant responds by crying, flexing extremities and elevating pelvis and head lordosis of the spine, as well as defection and urination may occur, disappear by age 4–6 months.		
17.	**Trunk incurvation (gallant) reflex**	Stroking infants back alongside spine causes hips to move toward stimulated side, disappears. By age 4 weeks.		
18.	**Crawl reflex**	When placed on abdomen infant makes crawling movements with arms and legs.		
Impression				

Signature of Student **Incharge Teacher** **Subject Coordinator/HOD**

INFANTS (1 MONTH TO 12 MONTHS)

Identification Data

Name of the Child	: Baby/Master..
Chronological Age	:
Developmental Stage	:
Sex/Gender	: Male/Female..
Date of Admission	:
IP Number	:
Ward	:
Bed Number	:
Diagnosis	:
Name of the Surgery	:
Date of the Surgery	**:**
Informant	: Father/Mother/Others................................
Date of Assessment	: ....
Address	: ....
	: ....
	: ....

Infants (1 Month to 12 Months)

S. No.	Assessment features	Normal value	Child value	Remarks (achieved/not achieved)

1.	Physical/ biological development	**1–6 months**
		Weight:
		• Weight 4.4 ± 0.8 kg: gains above 680 g, a month during first 6 months, or 150 to 210 g a week
		Height:
		• 53±2.5 cm (21 ± 1 in); increases about 2.5 cm (1 in) a month during first 6 months
		Dentition:
		• Full set of 20 temporary teeth.
		Chest circumference:
		• At birth: 35 cm
		• 3 month: 40 cm
		• 6 month: 43 cm
		• 1 year: 45 cm
		Head circumference:
		• Head circumference Increases about 1.5 cm (0.5 in) a month during first 6 months.
		  – Pulse: 130±20 Beats/Minutes
		  – Respirations: 35±10 Breath/Minutes
		  – Blood pressure: 80/50±20/10 mm/Hg		

		Posterior fontanel closed: at 6 to 8 weeks of age ***Expected weight Calculation Formula*** $$\dfrac{Age\ in\ month + 9}{2}$$		

Contd...

Contd...

S. No.	Assessment features	Normal value	Child value	Remarks (achieved/not achieved)
2.	**Motor development**	**2–3 months** • Symmetric posture of head and body. • Head in mid position or side. • Lifts head almost 45 degrees angle. **4–5 months** • Symmetric body postures predominate • Sits with adequate support. • Lifts head and shoulders at a 90° angle **6–8 months** • Sits alone briefly if placed in a favorable leaning position on hard surface. • Holds an arm out back is straight when sitting in high. Chair Pulls to a sitting position. • Bounces actively when held in standing position • Sits alone steadily. • Pulls self into standing position with help **9–12 months** • Raises to a sitting position alone with good coordination. • Pull self to standing position alone while holding on to furniture. • Moves from prone to sitting position. • Makes stepping movements forward when two hands are held. • Stands erect with minimal support and lifts one foot to take a step. • Cruises: walks holding on to furniture. • Stands alone for variable length of time sits down from standing position alone walks in few steps. ***Fine motor*** **1 month** • Holds hands in tight fists. • Can grasp an object placed in the hand (palmer grasp reflex) but drops it immediately. **2–3 months** • Hands may be open • Holds a rattle briefly when placed in the hand. • Hands open or closed loosely. **4–5 months** • Holds hand predominantly open brings hands together in midline sits with adequate support. • Plays with fingers grasps object held near hand. • Attempts to reach objects with hands but overshoots them. • Objects are carried to mouth thumb apposition in grasping occurs between third and fourth months fingers and clutches clothing • Uses thumb in partial opposition to fingers more skillfully • Grasps objects with whole hand, either right or left, holds one object while looking at another **6–8 months** • Grasps with simultaneous flexion of fingers: begins to, use fingers to feed self • Begins to transfer object from one hand to other hand. • Holds own bottle but may prefer for it to be held. • Holds 23 toys at once approaches a toy and grasps it with one hand (ambidextrous) 7 months. • Holds 2 objects while looking at a third persistently reaches for objects beyond range of grasp releases objects from hands voluntarily. • Complete thumb apposition pincer grasp beginning to develop.		

Contd...

Contd...

S. No.	Assessment features	Normal value	Child value	Remarks (achieved/not achieved)
		9–12 months • Bangs two objects together pokes objectives with fingers uses thumb and index finger in early pincer grasp. • Puts nipple in and withdraws it from mouth at will drinks from cup with some spilling (9-12 months), attempts to use a spoon but spills contents • Picks small objects up with index finger and thumb (pincer grasp) releases an object after holding it brings the hands together. • Good pincer grasp picks up small bits of food and transfers them to mouth. Enjoys eating with fingers Attempts to put a small pellet into a narrow-necked bottle but does not succeed. Releases one or more objects inside another object or container		
3.	**Sensory development**	**1–8 months** • Visual acuity, 20/200 **9–12 months** • Visual acuity: 20/100 to 20/50 • Marked interest in very small • Objects Searches for a lost toy with greater persistence.		
4.	**Psychosocial development**	***Trust vs. mistrust*** **1–2 months** • A development of sense of trust. Negative counterpart: mistrust • Totally egocentric • Bonding progresses • A face orientation, smiling, and vocalization are the evidences of attachment between infant and parents. • This is the beginning of social behavior **3–4 months** • Sense of trust • Recognizes and smiles in response to caregiver's (usually the mother's) face. • Stops crying when familiar person seen. • This is the beginning of social behavior. • Shows interest in new stimuli. **5–6 months** • Smiles at self in mirror • Shows displeasure when toy is lost. • Recognizes parents and strangers. • Knows what is liked and disliked **7–8 months** • Sense of trust shows increasing fear of strangers • Responds socially to own name emotional instability • Refuses to play with strangers or even accept toys from them. • Emotional instability still evident dislikes changing clothing and diapers **9–10 months** • Sense of Trust Expresses several beginning recognizable emotions such as anger, sadness, jealousy, anxiety, pleasure, excitement, and affection • Beginning fears about being left alone, as-when put into the crib Dislikes having face washed so covers face with arms and hands. • Shows preference for one toy over another. **11–12 months** • Sense of Trust shows pleasure when a desired act is accomplished. • Becomes frustrated when activities are restricted. • Seeks approval, avoids disapproval		

Contd...

Contd...

S. No.	Assessment features	Normal value	Child value	Remarks (achieved/not achieved)
		• Sense of Trust theoretically achieved. • A sense of mistrust predominates infant's emotion, such as fear, jealousy, anger, can be more clearly interpreted. • Responds to requests for affection such as a kiss or a hug. • Puts arms through sleeves, feet into shoes.		
5.	Psychosexual development	**Oral Stage (0 to 1 year)** • Oral aggressiveness is evidenced by biting and chewing. • Discover genitalia (7 months)		
6.	Spiritual development	**Undifferentiated (0 to 1 year)**		
7.	Intellectual/ cognitive development	***Sensory motor stage (0 to 2 years)*** ***Substage: I (birth to 1 month)*** • Infant uses reflexes to begin to make associations between an act and a sequential response: cannot distinguish self from environment. ***Substage II:*** Primary Circular Reaction (1 to 4 months) • Begins to repeat actions of own body voluntarily (hand to mouth movement permits sucking). ***Substage III:*** Secondary Circular Reaction (4 to 8 months) • Repeats actions that affect an object to get a response (shaking a rattle). • Experiments with old or new responses to produce environmental changes or to reach a goal. ***Substage IV:*** • Coordination of Secondary Schemas **(8 to 12 months)** • Abilities learned earlier are combined and extended to deal with new situations. • Perceptions of space become refined between 8 to 12 months. • Problem solving beginning to develop.		
8.	Moral development	***Pre-conventional morality*** **Stage-0 (0–2 years)** The good is what I like and want.		
9.	Language development	***Receptive language:*** **1–6 months** • Responds to human voices • Alert expression when listening • Direct definite regard soothed by caregiver's, mother, voice • Looks in direction of speaker • Recognizes similar words. **7–12 months** • Recognizes own name responds with gestures to words such as 'come' • Stops activity when own name is spoken verbally • Responds to adult anger • Understand simple commands. ***Expressive language:*** **1–6 months** • Opens and closes mouth as adult speaks • Cry patterns developing, cries when hungry or uncomfortable • Begins to coo		

Contd...

Contd...

S. No.	Assessment features	Normal value	Child value	Remarks (achieved/not achieved)
		• Crying becomes differentiated, varying with the reason for crying, e.g., hunger, sleepiness or pain. Pitch and intensity vary, 'eh,' uh,Coos • Vocalizes several well-defined syllables. **7–12 months** • Vocalizes several well-defined syllables • Vocalizes eagerness vocalizes 'm-m-m' • When crying Imitates simple noises and speech sounds makes polysyllabic vowel sounds vocalizes 'da,' 'ma,' 'ba' Babbling. • Continues syllables: 'da-da' • Cry when scolded • Understands meaning of 'bye-bye' and waves • May speak two or more words besides 'ma-ma' and 'd.t-da' Understands meaning of many more words that an be spoken.		
10.	Play stimulation	**Onlooker play 1–3 months** • Offer a rattle, pull from supine to sitting position Hold or dangle toy in front of infant to encourage eye movement. Change patterns of objects from bright and shiny to dull and dark' for further stimulation. **Solitary play (playpen) 4–7 months** • Place infant when awake where household activities are in progress include infant in family's television viewing and activities. • Continue to encourage playing in water and perhaps 'swimming' in shallow tub or pool. • Gently push infant from a sitting position to improve balance (8 months). **8–12 months** • Continue infant games, including 'pat-a-cake' and "peek-a-boo," with appropriate motions. • Provide opportunities for holding and releasing objects. • Encourage cruising by placing furniture in a circle. Encourage infant to bounce in a standing position by holding the hands for support. • Place infant in a jumper seat to encourage standing and jumping. • Play simple games such as rolling a ball to infant. • Encourage infant to stand alone by gradually decreasing support (furniture or adult's hands). • Encourage infant to walk, eventually holding only one hand.		
Impression:				

Signature of Student **Incharge Teacher** **Subject Coordinator/HOD**

◼ TODDLER (1 TO 3 YEARS)

Identification Data

Name of the Child   : Baby/Master......................................

Chronological Age   :

Developmental Stage   :

Sex/Gender   : Male/Female....................................

Date of Admission   :

IP Number   :

Ward   :

Bed Number   :

Diagnosis   :

Name of the Surgery   :

Date of the Surgery   :

Informant   : Father/Mother/Others........................

Date of Assessment   : ....

Address   : ....

             : ....

             : ....

Toddler

S. No.	Assessment features	Normal value	Child value	Remarks (achieved/ not achieved)
1.	**Physical/ biological development**	**Weight:** Gain about 1.8–2.7 kg per year At 2 years – 12 kg 2½ years – 4 times birth weight **Height:** Increases about 10–12.5 cm per year **Dentition:** Full set of 20 temporary teeth. **Chest circumference:** Exceeds head circumference. **Head circumference:** 49–50 cm. **Pulse:** 110 ± 20 Beats per minutes **Respirations:** 26–28 Breath per minutes **Blood pressure:** 99/64 ± 26/24 mm/Hg ***Expected Weight Calculation Formula*** ***= Age in Year × 2 + 8***		
2.	**Motor development**	**Gross motor:** • Walks sideways and backward • Moves quickly from place to place • Sets self in small chair • Climbs on furniture • Pulls and pushes toy • Kicks large ball without falling • Jumps well in place with both feet off floor. • Rides a walker or pedal car.		

Contd...

Contd...

S. No.	Assessment features	Normal value	Child value	Remarks (achieved/ not achieved)
		Fine motor: • Builds a tower of 6–7 cubes • Scribbles in more controlled way • Imitates a circular and horizontal stroke. • Turns pages of book one at a time • Opens door by turning door knob • Puts block into hole • Eats with spoon, turns spoon in mouth • Plays with food • Drinks well from a small glass held in one hand • Removes most of own clothing.		
3.	**Sensory development**	• Visual acuity: 20/40 • Accommodation well developed • Inserts square object into its appropriate place or hole. • Recalls visual images. • Identifies various shapes.		
4.	**Psychosocial development**	**Sense of autonomy vs doubt/shame** • Separation anxiety • Coping decreased in unfamiliar environment • Begins to imitate parents doing house keeping chores • Autonomous behavior increasing • Begins to have temper tantrums • Bedtime retrials begin • Beginning of possessiveness • Cannot share possessions • Beginning to show early signs of individuality and independence. • Beginning of possessiveness • Cannot share possessions • Beginning to show early signs of individuality and independence.		
5.	**Psychosexual development**	**Anal stage** • Obtains sensuous pleasure from the feeling of a distended bladder and release of faces from rectum. • Pleasure on touching the genitalia.		
6.	**Spiritual development**	**Intuitive projective faith** • Imitates religious behavior such as bowing the head in prayer. • Unable to understand		
7.	**Intellectual/ cognitive development**	**Sensory motor stage** **Substage VI (18–24 months)** • Invention of new means through mental combinations. • Concept of object permanence fully developed. • Can differentiate self from objects. • Short attention span • Begins to think. **Preoperational stage** *Preconceptual phase (2–4 years)* • Preoccupation with symbols in language, dreams fantasy. • Very early understanding of past, present and future. • Increasingly aware of causation while only experiencing the effect. • Symbolic thought begins. • Begins causal thinking.		

Contd...

Contd...

S. No.	Assessment features	Normal value	Child value	Remarks (achieved/ not achieved)
8.	**Moral development**	***Pre-conventional morality*** **Stage-0 (0–2 years)** The good is what I like and want **Stage-1 (2–3 years)** If punished for doing it, it's wrong; if not punished, it must be right.		
9.	**Language development**	**Receptive language:** • Recognizes names of various parts of body. • Responds to familiar, simple commands. • Identifies pictures of familiar objects when named. • Enjoys stores with pictures. • Obeys commands. **Expressive language:** • Says 2–6 words • Names familiar pictures or objects • Vocalizes wants and points to desired object • Shakes head 10 communicate • Use words more than gestures to express desires • Knows about 300 words • Uses pronouns 'I', 'me', 'Mine'. • Asks 'What's that'? • Verbalizes need for drink food and toileting.		
10.	**Play stimulation**	**Parallel play** • Has a favorite toy or transitional object. • Little social interaction with other children. **Motor play** • Large, hollow wooden blocks • Balls • Pulls toys • Low swing with arms and back • Rocking chair • Running and chasing games. **Creative play** • Manipulates play materials such as clay • Finger paints • Sings songs • Brush paints • Record player and cords • Toys to take apart. **Quit play** • Sand toys • Stuffed animals and dolls to drag, sit upon, hug • Enjoys hearing stories illustrated with pictures • Takes favorite toy to bed. **Dramatic play** • Imitates parental actions in play • Enjoys playing with dolls.		

Impression:

Signature of Student	Incharge Teacher	Subject Coordinator/HOD

PRESCHOOLER (3 TO 5 YEARS)

Identification Data

Name of Child	: Baby/Master...
Chronological Age	:
Developmental Stage	:
Sex/Gender	: Male/Female...
Date of Admission	:
IP Number	:
Ward	:
Bed Number	:
Diagnosis	:
Name of the Surgery	:
Date of the Surgery	:
Informant	: Father/Mother/Others ....
Date of Assessment	: ....
Address	: ....
	: ....
	: ....

Preschooler

S. No.	Assessment features	Normal value	Child value	Remarks (achieved/ not achieved)
1.	Biological development	**Weight** • 3 years – 14.5 kgs • 4 years – 16.7 kgs • 5 years – 18.7 kgs **Height** • 3 years – 95 cm • 4 years – 103 cm • 5 years – 110 cm **Mid-arm circumference** • 12.5 to 16 cm **Physical proportions** • Temperature • 37–37.2° C (98.6–99° F) **Pulse** • 105 ± 15 Beats/minute **Respiration** • 25 ± 5 beats/minutes **Blood pressure** • 100/70 ± 20–25 mm/Hg		
2.	Motor developments	*Gross Motor* **3 years** • Rides tricycle, walks on tiptoe, broad jumps. **4 years** • Skips and hops proficiently on one foot. **5 years** • Skips on alternate feet, jumps rope.		

Contd...

Contd...

S. No.	Assessment features	Normal value	Child value	Remarks (achieved/ not achieved)
		Fine Motor **3 years** • Copies a circle puts beads on storing. **4 years** • Copies a square. **5 years** • Copies a triangle crosses vertical lines.		
3.	**Sensory development**	Visual acuity: 20/20		
4.	**Psychosocial development**	**Initiative vs Guilt** **3 years** • Egocentric in though and behavior. • Less dependent on parents but need reassurance and help. • Knows own sex. **4 years** • Egocentric; separate easily from parents. • Physically and verbally aggressive • Sexually arias **5 years** • Independent and trust worthy. • Engages in cooperative play.		
5.	**Psychosexual development**	***Phallic Stage*** • Genitalia are interesting and sensitive area of the body. ***Edipal complex*** *(Male)* ***Electra complex*** *(Female)*		
6.	**Spiritual development**	***Intuitive – projective faith*** • Children imitate the religious gestures and behavior of others.		
7.	**Intellectual (or) cognitive development**	***Preoperational thought:*** **Substage – I:** Preconceptual (2–4 years) • Language acquisition **Substage – II:** Intuitive stage (4–7 years) • Problem solution • Aware of cultural differences.		
8.	**Moral development**	Punishment and obedience orientation. (2–4 years) Native instrumental orientation (4–7 years)		
9.	**Language/ speech development**	***Receptive language*** **3 years** • Can obey two prepositional commands (i.e. on, under). **4 years** • Understands directives (on, under, in back, in front). **5 years** • Understands directives (on, under, in back, in front). ***Expressive Language*** **3 years** • Uses 4 word sentences – asks, why, uses, plurals. Has vocabulary of 800 – 1000 words.		

Contd...

Contd...

S. No.	Assessment features	Normal value	Child value	Remarks (achieved/ not achieved)
		4 years • Uses 3 to 7 word sentences has a vocabulary of 1500 words. **5 years** • Repeats sentence of 12 (or) more syllables. Has a vocabulary of 2100 words.		
10.	**Play stimulation**	• Dramatic play – playing like police officer, storekeeper, teacher (or) nurse. • Cooperative play such as play telephone, music record player, doll house, garden toys, puzzles.		

Impression:

Signature of Student   **Incharge Teacher**   **Subject Coordinator/HOD**

SCHOOL AGE CHILDREN (6–12 YEARS)

Identification Data

Name of the Child	: Baby/Master..
Chronological Age	:
Developmental Stage	:
Sex/Gender	: Male/Female...
Date of Admission	:
IP Number	:
Ward	:
Bed Number	:
Diagnosis	:
Name of the Surgery	:
Date of the Surgery	:
Informant	: Mother/ Father/Other.............................
Date of Assessment	: ....
Address	: ....
	: ....
	: ....

School Age Children (6–12 Years)

S. No.	Assessment features	Normal value	Child value	Remarks (achieved/ not achieved)
1.	**Biological development**	**Weight approximately:** • 18- 39.5 kg. • Gains 3.8 kg yearly. **Height approximately:** • 110–124 cm (43.5–48.5 in). • Gains 1.13 cm yearly. **Pulse:** • 90 ± 15 beats/minute **Respirations:** • 27 ± 3 breath per minute **Blood pressure:** • $100/60 \pm 16/10$ mm/Hg **Dentition:** Starts to lose temporary teeth; acquires first permanent molars, medial incisors, lateral incisors. **Expected Weight Calculation Formula** $$= \frac{\text{Age in year} \times 7-5}{2}$$		
2.	**Motor developments**	***Gross Motor*** **6–8 years** • Rides bicycle without training wheels Runs, jumps, climbs, hops. • Constantly in motion clumsy and awkward coordination improving. **8–10 years** • Performs tricks on bicycle-races • Participate in the sports.		

Contd...

Contd...

S. No.	Assessment features	Normal value	Child value	Remarks (achieved/ not achieved)
		10–12 years • Enjoy in all physical activities. **Fine Motor** **6–8 years** • Knows right from left hand draws a person with 12-16 parts. • Prints the words, lear cursive writing, good eye and hand coordination. **8–10 years** • Use both hands independently. • Draws a Person with 18-20 Parts. • Increase the smoothness and speed in fine motor controls. • Prints fluently and cursive writing. **10–12 years** • Coordination continuous to improve		
3.	**Selfcare development**	**Selfcare** • Feeding skills at 6 years, likes to eat with fingers, stuffs food into mouth, talkative while eating. More interested in eating as beginning of meal • At 7 years, improved table manners, less talking, may bolt food grooming and dressing skills • Self-care managed; has a tendency to dawdle in bathtub, needs to be reminded to wash hands • May need some help with dressing • Wears whatever is selected by parents • Leaves clothes where they are removed can brush and comb hair		
4.	**Sensory development**	Visual acuity: 20/20		
5.	**Psychosocial development**	***Sense of Industry Vs Inferiority*** **6–8 years** • Continues to be egocentric in though bossy, craves attention. • Return of temper tantrums-may use verbal, physical attack. • Uses tensional releases: wiggling, chewing on hair, nose picking. • Wants other children to play. • Jealous of siblings • Fears of getting injury to them self. **8–10 years** • Curious about everything. • Concerned with relationship. • Peer–oriented, Reasonable fear, • Aware of sex role. **10–12 years** • Confident, self control, Respect their Parents. • At the age of 10 yearss they will have a short burst of anger able to control anger. • Hero worship, Fear of darkness. • Know about sexual intercourse.		

Contd...

Contd...

S. No.	Assessment features	Normal value	Child value	Remarks (achieved/not achieved)
6.	**Psychosexual development**	***Latency stage (6-12 years)*** • Sexual impulses are repressed. • Parents are no longer viewed omnipotent. • Privacy becomes more important in later school age child. • Ask questions about reproduction. • Masturbation reduced		
7.	**Spiritual development**	**Mythical-Literal Faith** • Learn specifics about their religion. • Children at this point may drop their religious affiliation or continue to accept the family performance.		
8.	**Intellectual (or) cognitive development**	***Preoperational thought*** **Substage 11 (4-7 years)** • Attention span increasing can describe objects in picture, knows their use language acquisition. **6 years** • Able to understand the abstracts • Child beings to learn to read write and do the arithmetic. **7–11 years (concrete operational stage)** • Thinking, Imagination and language development. **Ordering and seriating:** • Able to arrange things or concrete objects according to the size and relation. **Classification:** • Classify in more complex manner. **Thinking and reasoning:** • They can solve the problems because they can manipulate the symbols. **Time:** • Child can recall the events that happened in the past; they become aware that things exist over a period of time- punctual. • Memory spans increasing. • Ashamed of failure. • Think about vocation. • Preoccupied with right and wrong. ***At 12 years:*** • Ethical sense more realistic than idealistic.		
9.	**Moral development**	***Preconventional Morality*** **Stage 2 (4–7 years)** • Instrumental hedonism and concrete reciprocity. • Children focus on the pleasure motive. • They consider those actions right that meet their own needs or those of action. ***Conventional Morality*** **Stage 3 (7–9 years)** • Orientation to interpersonal relationship of mutuality. "Am I a good person?" **Stage 4 (10–12 years)** • We need law and other maintenance of social order, fixed rules and authority.		

Contd...

Contd...

S. No.	Assessment features	Normal value	Child value	Remarks (achieved/ not achieved)
10.	Language, speech development	**Receptive language** **6–8 years** • Follow the series of three commends response. **8–10 years** • Follow the suggestion better than commends. **10–12 years** • Follow the suggestion better than request, is obedient. **Expressive language** **6–8 years** • Can repeat 10 to 12 words vocabulary of 2500 words. • Number combination up to 10 develops sense of humor. **8–10 yearss** • Begins to use shorter and more compact sentence. **10–12 years** • Oral vocabulary 7200 words • Reading vocabulary 50000 words • Use number beyond 100 with meaning.		
11.	Play stimulation	**Competitive play/team play** **6–8 years** • Like rough and tumble play • Loves active play. • Prefers group play. • Doll play, table game, bicycle, puppets, puzzles etc. **8–10 years** • Prefers companionship. • Likes to complete. • Continues to require super vision in play. • Enjoy the Dramatic play — playing like police officer, storekeeper, teacher (or) nurse. **10–12 years** • Enjoy large musical activity and outdoor activity. like bicycle, reading, collecting, construction activities. **12 years** **Enjoys** • Parties (with supervision) • Athletic sports • Talking on telephone. • Reading loves stories • Solitary play • Sex differences notices in play.		

Impression:

Signature of Student	Incharge Teacher	Subject Coordinator/HOD

ADOLESCENTS (13–18 YEARS)

Identification Data

Name of the Child : Baby/Master.......................................

Chronological Age :

Developmental Stage :

Sex/Gender : Male/Female..

Date of Admission :

IP Number :

Ward :

Bed Number :

Diagnosis :

Name of the Surgery :

Date of the Surgery :

Informant : Mother/Father/Other...........................

Date of Assessment : ....

Address : ....

: ....

: ....

Adolescents (12–18 Years)

S. No.	Assessment features	Normal value	Child value	Remarks (achieved/ not achieved)
1.	Physical/ biological development	**Weight** **Early adolescence (12–13 years)** • Male: 38–60 kgs • Female: 40–60 kgs **Middle adolescence (14–16 years)** • Male: 50–60 kgs • Female: 42–64 kgs **Late adolescence (17–21 years)** • Male: 56–80 kgs • Female: 48–72 kgs **Height** **Early adolescence (12–13 years)** • Male: 154–172 cms • Female: 153–167 cms **Middle adolescence (14–16 years)** • Male: 164–180 cms • Female: 155–169 cms **Late adolescence (17–21 years)** • Male: 163–182 cms • Female: 156–170 cms • Temperature: 36.5–37°C • Heart rate: 60–80 beats/min • Respiration: 14–20 breaths/min • Blood pressure: 124/74 = 17/16 mm of Hg.		

Contd...

Contd...

S. No.	Assessment features	Normal value	Child value	Remarks (achieved/ not achieved)
		Secondary sexual development **Boys** • Broadening of shoulders from the age of 13 years. • Increase in size of breast • Increase in size of genitalia • Growth of pubic, axillary chest and face hair. • Deepening of voice. • Production of spermatozoa. **Girls** • Broadening of hips • Developing of breast • Increase in size of genitalia • Growth of pubic, axillaries hair. • Attending menarche. • Menstrual cycle regular • Change in vaginal secretion • Remaining in permanent in teeth eruptions. • Expected Weight Calculation Formula $$= \frac{\text{Age in Year} \times 7 - 5}{2}$$		
2.	**Motor developments**	• Refine gross and fine motor skills • Clumsiness occurs due to rapid physical growth motor function comparable to adult. • Eye-hand coordination at adult level possesses manual dexterity. • Can do the craft works.		
4.	**Sensory development**	Visual acuity: 20/20		
5.	**Psycho-social development (Erick and Erickson)**	*Early Adolescent (12–13 years)* **Identity Vs Role confusion** "who am I?" *Middle Adolescent (14–16 years)* **Intimacy Versus Isolation** *Late Adolescent (17–21 years)* **Integrity Versus despair** • Shows mood swings and extremes of behavior experiences sense of loss as begins to separate from parents • Peer relationship of greatest importance. • Daydreams over heroes Continues same–sex friendships • Heterosexual relationship and interests common • Verbally attacks parents beliefs and values		
6.	**Psycho-sexual development**	***Genital stage*** (12-18 years) • The secondary sexual character will develop. • Masturbation occurs • Heterosexual genital Expression but is denied it. • Sexual tension during this period.		
7.	**Spiritual development**	***Synthetic–conventional faith*** • Personal and social value evolved to support their Identity. • Explore religious affiliation.		
8.	**Intellectual (or) cognitive development**	***Formal operational thought*** (11 years – Adulthood) • Generates hypotheses • Uses the scientific method for problem–solving • Expresses concern for education vs. vocational choice		

Contd...

Contd...

S. No.	Assessment features	Normal value	Child value	Remarks (achieved/ not achieved)
9.	**Moral development**	***Post conventional stage*** Stage 5 (13 + years) • 'The individual conforms to maintain other's respect' • Orientation toward decisions of conscience 'Universal ethical principles'		
10.	**Language, speech development**	• Fluent in spoken language • Uses slang within and outside peer group • Uses distinct meanings for words • Oral vocabulary 72,000 words • Reading vocabulary 50,000 words • Continuous to learn new concept.		
11.	**Play stimulation**	• Recreational activities • Chooses activities according to individual interests • Parties, conversation • Interest in world affairs • Expressive arts, hobbies crafts • Social drinking • Engages in organized competitive sports.		
Impression				

Signature of Student　　　　　　　　　　**Incharge Teacher**　　　　　　　　　　**Subject Coordinator/HOD**

NURSING CARE PLAN

MEDICAL CARE PLAN

Pediatric Nursing Care Plan

Definition

The nursing process is a series of organized steps designed for nurses to provide excellent client and family care. Learn the five phases, including assessing, diagnosing, planning, implementing, and evaluating.

Purpose of Nursing Process in Child Care

The nursing process provides an organizing framework for meeting the individual needs of the child and family.

- The nursing process provides an organized, systematic method of problem-solving (while still allowing for creative solutions) that may minimize dangerous errors or omissions in care giving and avoid time-consuming repetition in care and documentation.
- The use of the nursing process promotes the active involvement of clients in their health care, enhancing consumer satisfaction.
- It strengthens the client's commitment to achieving the identified goals.
- The use of the nursing process enables you as a nurse to have more control over your practice during child care.
- This enhances the opportunity for nurses to use knowledge, expertise, and intuition constructively and dynamically to increase the likelihood of a successful client outcome.
- The use of the nursing process provides a common language (nursing diagnosis) for practice, unifying the nursing profession.
- In addition, the structure of the process provides a format for documenting the client's response to all aspects of the planned care.
- The use of the nursing process provides a means of assessing nursing's economic contribution to client care.
- The nursing process supplies a vehicle for the quantitative and qualitative measurement of nursing care that meets the goal of cost-effectiveness and still promotes holistic care towards child health.

Steps in Nursing Process

In nursing practices, this process is one of the foundations of practice. It offers a framework for thinking through problems and provides some organization to a nurse's critical thinking skills. It's important to point out that this process is flexible and not rigid. It is a tool to use in nursing care, but one that should allow for creativity and thinking outside of the nursing process table.

Nursing Process which Stand for 'ADPIE'

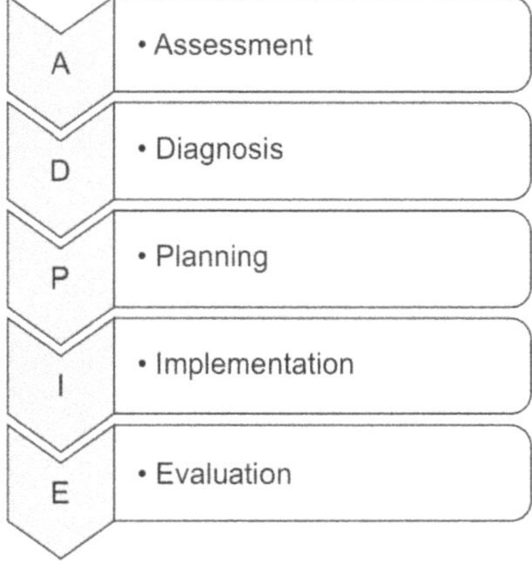

Assessment Phase

The first step of the nursing process is assessment. During this phase, the nurse gathers information about a patient's psychological, physiological, sociological, and spiritual status. This data can be collected in a variety of ways. Generally, nurses will conduct a patient interview. Physical examinations, referencing a patient's health history, obtaining a patient's family history, and general observation can also be used to gather assessment data. Patient interaction is generally the heaviest during this evaluative phase.

Diagnosing Phase

The diagnosing phase involves a nurse making an educated judgment about a potential or actual health problem with a patient. Multiple diagnoses are sometimes made for a single patient. These assessments not only include an actual description of the problem (e.g. sleep deprivation) but also whether or not a patient is at risk of developing further problems. These diagnoses are also used to determine a patient's readiness for health improvement and whether or not they may have developed a syndrome. The diagnoses phase is a critical step as it is used to determine the course of treatment.

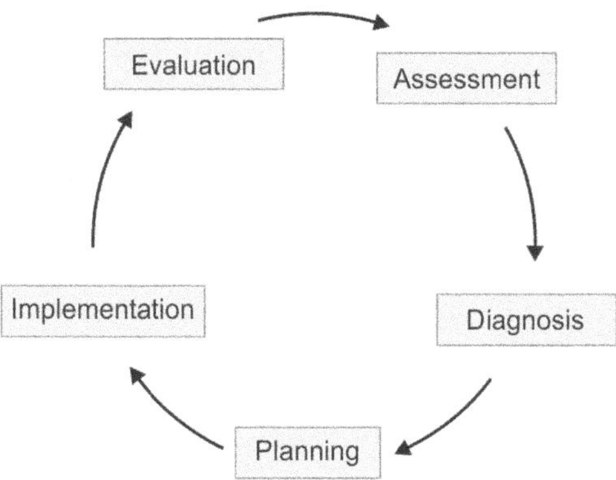

Planning Phase

In this phase once a client and nurse agree on the diagnoses, a plan of action can be developed. If multiple diagnoses need to be addressed, the head nurse will prioritize each assessment and devote attention to severe symptoms and high risk factors. Each problem is assigned a clear, measurable goal for the expected beneficial outcome. For this phase, nurses generally refer to the evidence-based Nursing Outcome Classification, which is a set of standardized terms and measurements for tracking patient wellness. The Nursing Interventions Classification may also be used as a resource for planning.

Implementing Phase

The implementing phase is where the nurse follows through on the decided plan of action. This plan is specific to each patient and focuses on achievable outcomes. Actions involved in a nursing care plan include monitoring the patient for signs of change or improvement, directly caring for the patient or performing necessary medical tasks, educating and instructing the patient about further health management, and referring or contacting the patient for follow-up. Implementation can take place over the course of hours, days, weeks, or even months.

Evaluation Phase

In this once all nursing intervention actions have taken place, the nurse completes an evaluation to determine of the goals for patient wellnesses have been met. The possible patient outcomes are generally described under three terms: patient's condition improved, patient's condition stabilized, and patient's condition deteriorated, died, or discharged. In the event the condition of the patient has shown no improvement, or if the wellness goals were not met, the nursing process begins again from the first step.

EVALUATION CRITERIA FOR MEDICAL CARE PLAN

Name of Child :...   Total Marks: 25

Ward :..   IP/No :...

Diagnosis :..

S. No.	Content	Score	Marks obtained
1.	**Child Profile and Assessment:**		
	• Identification data	1	
	• History collection	1	
	• Nutritional assessment	1	
	• Physical examination	2	
	• Immunization status	2	
	• Investigations	1	
	• Medication	2	
2.	**Nursing Management**		
	• Identification of needs and problems	2	
	• List out and prioritizing the nursing diagnosis	2	
	• Goals	1	
	• Implementation	5	
	• Evaluation	1	
3.	**Health Education**	2	
4.	**Summary and Conclusion**	1	
5.	**Bibliography**	1	
Total Marks		**25**	

Signature of Student   **Incharge Teacher**   **Signature of the HOD**

MEDICAL CARE PLAN

ON

CHILD WITH ....

Identification Data

Name of the Child	: Baby/Master ....
Chronological Age	:
Developmental Stage	:
Sex/Gender	: Male/Female ....
Date of Admission	:
IP Number	:
Ward	:
Bed Number	:
Diagnosis	:
Informant	: Mother/Father/others ....
Address	: ....
	: ....
	: ....
Date of care started	: ....
Date of care ended	: ....

History Collection

Chief Complaints:

....
....
....
....
....

Socioeconomic Background of the Family:

....
....
....
....
....

Family Health History:

....
....
....
....
....

Family Tree:

[ ] – Male

( ) – Female

/// – Child

Past Medical History:

....
....
....

Present Medical History:

....
....
....

Birth History:

Antenatal history:

....
....
....

Intranatal history:

....
....
....

Postnatal history:

....
....
....

Nutritional history:

Food habits : ....
....

Feeding skill : ....
....

Likable food : ....
....

Dislikable food : ....
....

24 Hours recall : ....
....

Malnutrition Assessments

$$\frac{\text{Actual weight} \times 100}{\text{Expected weight}} \quad =............................. \times 100$$

$$= ....$$

$$= ....\%$$

Degree of malnutrition: **Mild/Moderate/Severe**

Personal History

Habits : ....
....
....

Elimination : ....
....
....

Play activity : ....
....
....

Immunization History

Date	Recommended age	Vaccine	Dose	Route	Remarks given/not given
	At birth	BCG (0.05 till one month age)	0.1 mL	ID	
		OPV (zero dose)	2 drops	Oral	
		Hepatitis B-1	0.5 mL	IM	
	6 weeks	OPV-1 + IPV-1 with OPV-1	2 drops	Oral	
		DPTw-1/DPTa-1 dose	0.5 mL	IM	
		Hepatitis B-2 dose	0.5 mL	IM	
		Hib Vaccine-1 dose	0.5 mL	IM	
	10 weeks	OPV-2+ IPV-2 with OPV-2	2 drops	Oral	
		DPTw-2/DPTa-2 dose	0.5 mL	IM	
		Hib vaccine-2 dose	0.5 mL	IM	
	14 weeks	OPV-3 + IPV-2 with OPV-3	2 drops	Oral	
		DPTw-3/DPTa-2 dose	0.5 mL	IM	
		Hepatitis B-3 dose	0.5 mL	IM	
		Hib Vaccine-3 dose	0.5 mL	IM	
	9 months	Measles	0.5 mL	Sub	
		Vitamin – A (1 episode)	1 mL	Oral	
	15 to 18 months	OPV-4 + IPV-booster 1 with OPV-4	2 drops	Oral	
		DPT booster-1 or DPTa- B1	0.5 mL	IM	
		Hib vaccine booster	0.5 mL	IM	
		MMR-1 dose	0.5 mL	Sub	
	2 years	Typhoid vaccine	0.5 mL	IM	
	5 years	OPV-5 dose	2 drops	Oral	
		DPT booster-2 dose	0.5 mL	IM	
		MMR-2 dose	0.5 mL	Sub	
	10 years	TT	0.5 mL	IM	

Physical Examination

Physical features	Theory/book picture	Clinical picture
General appearance • Level of consciousness • Posture • Grooming • Body build • Gait • Activity	: Conscious/semi-conscious/unconscious : Normal/kyphosis/lordosis/scoliosis : Well groomed/dirty : Endomorphic/mesomorphic/ectomorphic : Any limp/unsteady gait/normal gait : Bedridden/bed rest/active.	
Vital signs • Temperature • Pulse • Respiration • Blood pressure	:……………..°C/°F :……………...Beats/minute :……………...Breath/minute :………./…….Mm/Hg	Normal/abnormal
Skin • Temperature • Color • Texture • Lesions • Sensation	: Normal/warm/cold and clammy : Normal/pallor/cyanosis/icterus/flushing : Smooth/wrinkling/flaking/hydrated/edema : No/papule/vesicle/ulcer : Normal/anesthesia/paresthesia/hypothesia	
Head and scalp • Head circumference • Scalp • Anterior Fontanelle • Posterior Fontanelle • Shape of Skull	: Normal/hydrocephalus/micro and macrocephalus : Lesion/cleanliness/infection/psoriasis/normal : Closed/not closed/not applicable : Closed/not closed/not applicable : Micro/macro shape/odd shape/not applicable	
Hair • Texture • Color • Dandruff • Pediculosis **Face** • Worried • Pale Color	: Normal/brittle/dry/oily/thin/alopecia : Normal/colored : No/yes : No/yes : No/yes : No/yes	
Eyes • Eyebrow • Eyelashes • Eyelids • Eyeballs • Conjunctiva • Sclera • Lens • Pupils • Visual power **Vision** • Eye movement • Eye discharge	: Symmetrical/asymmetrical/can not raise : Infection/stye/normal : Edema/lesions/normal : Normal/protruded/sunken : Healthy/moist/pale/watery : Normal/icterus/redness : Opaque/transparent : Dilated/constricted/reaction to light : Normal/blurred vision : Normal/strabismus : Absent/present	
Ears • Ear discharge • Tympanic membrane • Hearing ability	: Absent/present : Normal/perforated/lesion/bulging : Normal/hearing aids	
Nose • Crust or discharge • Nasal septum • Mucous membrane • Polyps • Sinus	: Absent/present : Normal/perforated/deviated to which side : Normal/swollen/epitasis : Absent/present : Absent/present	

Physical features	Theory/book picture	Clinical picture
Mouth • Breath • Throat • Tonsils • Teeth • Tongue • Mucus and gums • Lips	: Normal/halitosis : Normal/congested (short neck) : Normal/inflamed : Healthy/poorly aligned/dental caries/plaque : Pink/pale/moist/dry/coated/lesion/glossitis : Ulcer/gingivitis/bleeding/pus/normal : Redness/swelling/cyanosis/normal	
Neck • Movement • Lymph nodes • Thyroid gland	: Flexion/extension/normal : Normal/tender/palpable : Normal/enlarged	
Chest • Thorax • Breath sounds • Breast • Nipple • Heart beat • Heart sound	: Symmetry/shape (specify) : Normal/wheeze/grunting : Normal/mastitis/lump : Normal/cracked/secretion : Rate/rhythm/volume : Normal/murmur/gallops	
Axilla • Lymph node	: Not palpable/palpable/tenderness	
Abdomen • Inspection • Palpation • Percussion • Bowel sound (Auscultation)	: Skin rash/hernia/ascites/distension/normal : Tenderness/palpable organs (liver, spleen) : Presence of gas (dullness)/masses : Present/absent	
Genitals **Females:** • Mons pubis • External genitalia • Urinary pattern • Congenital anomalies **Males:** Mons pubis • Urinary pattern • Scrotum • Inguinal canal • Congenital anomalies	: Normal : Inflammation/edema/lesion/normal : Normal/burning/micturation/normal : Absent/present : Healthy/nits/lice : Normal/epispadias/hypospadias : Descended testis/undescended testis : Normal/hernia : Absent/present	
Rectum and anus • Congenital anomalies • Others	: Absent/present : Piles/polyps/melina/ulcer/excoriation/rash	

Impression

Baby/Master ....

....

....

....

....

....

INVESTIGATIONS

Blood Test

S. No.	Name of the investigation	Child findings	Normal values	Remarks
1.				
2.				
3.				
4.				
5.				
6.				
7.				
8.				
9.				
10.				

Urine Analysis

S. No.	Name of the Investigation	Child findings	Normal values	Remarks
1.				
2.				
3.				
4.				
5.				
6.				
7.				
8.				
9.				
10.				

Radiological Investigation

Name of the study	Impression
X-ray	
USG Scan	
CT Scan	
MRI Scan	

MEDICATION

S. No.	Drug name	Action	Dose/route	Indication	Side effects	Nursing responsibility

MEDICATION

S. No.	Drug name	Action	Dose/route	Indication	Side effects	Nursing responsibility

MEDICATION

S. No.	Drug name	Action	Dose/route	Indication	Side effects	Nursing responsibility

NURSING DIAGNOSIS: (Should be based on NANDA classification)

1. ....

2. ....

3. ....

4. ....

5. ....

6. ....

7. ....

8. ....

9. ....

10. ....

Nursing Care Plan/Nursing Process

Date	Nursing assessment	Nursing diagnosis	Goal	Nursing intervention	Nursing implementation	Evaluation
Day	Subjective Data: Objective Data:					

Nursing Care Plan/Nursing Process

Date	Nursing assessment	Nursing diagnosis	Goal	Nursing intervention	Nursing implementation	Evaluation
Day	Subjective Data: Objective Data:					

Nursing Care Plan/Nursing Process

Date	Nursing assessment	Nursing diagnosis	Goal	Nursing intervention	Nursing implementation	Evaluation
Day	Subjective Data: Objective Data:					

Nursing Care Plan/Nursing Process

Date	Nursing assessment	Nursing diagnosis	Goal	Nursing intervention	Nursing implementation	Evaluation
Day	Subjective Data: Objective Data:					

Nursing Care Plan/Nursing Process

Date	Nursing assessment	Nursing diagnosis	Goal	Nursing intervention	Nursing implementation	Evaluation
Day	Subjective Data: Objective Data:					

Health Education

Medication ....
....
....

Hygiene ....
....
....

Diet ....
....
....

Play/Exercise ....
....
....

Follow-up care ....
....
....

Prognosis

Day 1:
: ....
....
....

Day 2:
: ....
....
....

Day 3:
: ....
....
....

Summary:

....
....
....

Conclusion:

....
....
....
....

BIBLIOGRAPHY

It should be minimum 5 References of Textbook, Journals and Internet, etc.

1.

2.

3.

4.

5.

SURGICAL CARE PLAN

Evaluation Criteria for Surgical Care Plan

Name of child :...   Total Marks: 25

Ward :...   IP/No :...

Diagnosis :..

S. No.	Content	Score	Marks obtained
1.	**Child profile and assessment**		
	• Identification data	1	
	• History collection	1	
	• Nutritional assessment	1	
	• Physical examination	2	
	• Immunization status	2	
	• Investigations	1	
	• Medication	2	
2.	**Nursing management**		
	• Identification of needs and problems	2	
	• List out and prioritizing the nursing diagnosis	2	
	• Goals	1	
	• Implementation	5	
	• Evaluation	1	
3.	Prognosis and health education	2	
4.	Summary and conclusion	1	
5.	Bibliography	1	
	Total Marks	**25**	

Signature of Student   **Incharge Teacher**   **Signature of the HOD**

SURGICAL CARE PLAN
ON
CHILD WITH ....

Identification Data

Name of the Child	: Baby/Master ....
Chronological Age	:
Developmental Stage	:
Sex/Gender	: Male/Female ....
Date of Admission	:
IP Number	:
Ward	:
Bed Number	:
Diagnosis	:
Name of the Surgery	:
Date of the Surgery	:
Informant	: Mother/Father/others ....
Address	: ....
	: ....
	: ....
Date of care started	:
Date of care ended	:

History Collection

Chief complaints:

....

....

....

....

Socioeconomic background of the family:

....

....

....

....

Family health history:

....

....

....

....

Family Tree:

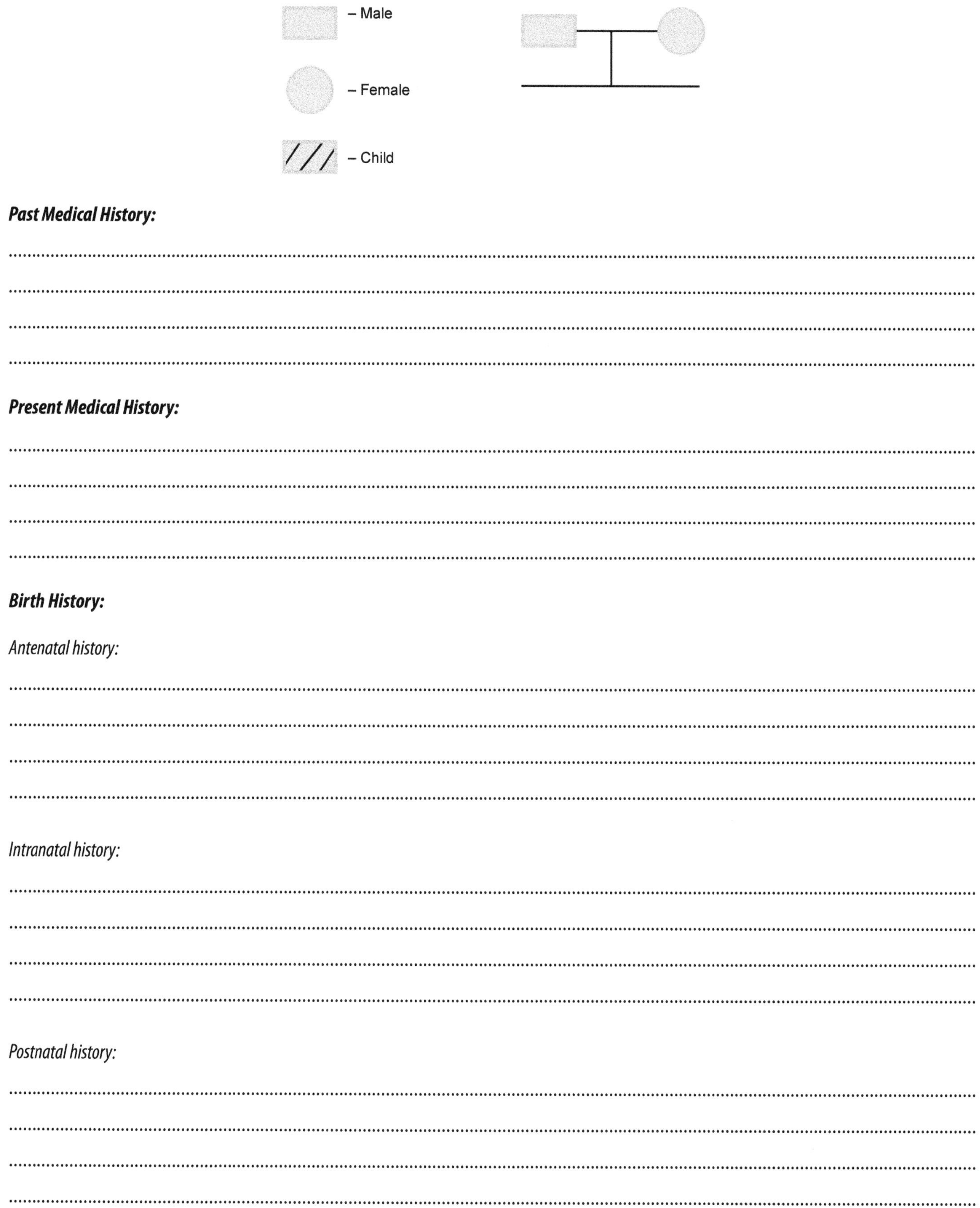

Past Medical History:

....
....
....
....

Present Medical History:

....
....
....
....

Birth History:

Antenatal history:

....
....
....
....

Intranatal history:

....
....
....
....

Postnatal history:

....
....
....
....

Nutritional History:

Food habits : ....

....

Feeding skill : ....

....

Likable food : ....

....

Dislikable food : ....

....

....

24 Hours recall : ....

....

....

Malnutrition Assessments:

$$\frac{\text{Actual weight} \times 100}{\text{Expected weight}} = \text{.............................} \times 100$$

$$= \text{...................................}$$

$$= \text{...................................}\%$$

Degree of malnutrition: **Mild/Moderate/Severe** [ ]

Personal History

Habits : ....

: ....

: ....

: ....

Elimination : ....

: ....

: ....

: ....

Play activity : ....

: ....

: ....

: ....

Immunization History

Date	Recommended age	Vaccine	Dose	Route	Remarks given/not given
	At birth	BCG (0.05 till one month age)	0.1 mL	ID	
		OPV (zero dose)	2 drops	Oral	
		Hepatitis B-1	0.5 mL	IM	
	6 weeks	OPV-1 + IPV-1 with OPV-1	2 drops	Oral	
		DPTw-1/DPTa-1 dose	0.5 mL	IM	
		Hepatitis B-2 dose	0.5 mL	IM	
		Hib vaccine-1 dose	0.5 mL	IM	
	10 weeks	OPV-2+ IPV-2 with OPV-2	2 drops	Oral	
		DPTw-2/DPTa-2 dose	0.5 mL	IM	
		Hib vaccine-2 dose	0.5 mL	IM	
	14 weeks	OPV-3 + IPV-2 with OPV-3	2 drops	Oral	
		DPTw-3/DPTa-2 dose	0.5 mL	IM	
		Hepatitis B-3 dose	0.5 mL	IM	
		Hib vaccine-3 dose	0.5 mL	IM	
	9 months	Measles	0.5 mL	Sub	
		Vitamin – A (1 episode)	1 mL	Oral	
	15 to 18 months	OPV-4 + IPV-booster 1 with OPV-4	2 drops	Oral	
		DPT booster-1 or DPTa- B1	0.5 mL	IM	
		Hib vaccine booster	0.5 mL	IM	
		MMR-1 dose	0.5 mL	Sub	
	2 years	Typhoid vaccine	0.5 mL	IM	
	5 years	OPV-5 dose	2 drops	Oral	
		DPT booster-2 dose	0.5 mL	IM	
		MMR-2 dose	0.5 mL	Sub	
	10 years	TT	0.5 mL	IM	

Physical Examination

Physical features	Theory picture	Child picture
General appearance • Level of consciousness • Posture • Grooming • Body build • Gait • Activity	: Conscious/semi conscious/unconscious : Normal/kyphosis/lordosis/scoliosis : Well groomed/dirty : Endomorphic/mesomorphic/ectomorphic : Any Limp/Unsteady gait/normal gait : Bedridden/bed rest/active.	
Vital signs • Temperature • Pulse • Respiration • Blood pressure	:................°C/°F :................Beats/minute :................Breath/minute :........./.......mm/Hg	Normal/abnormal
Skin • Temperature • Color • Texture • Lesions • Sensation	: Normal/warm/cold and clammy : Normal/pallor/cyanosis/icterus/flushing : Smooth/wrinkling/flaking/hydrated/edema : No/papule/vesicle/ulcer : Normal/anesthesia/paresthesia/hypothesia	

Contd...

Contd...

Physical features	Theory picture	Child picture
Head and scalp • Head circumference • Scalp • Anterior fontanelle • Posterior fontanelle • Shape of skull	 : Normal/hydrocephalus/micro and macrocephalus : Lesion/cleanliness/infection/psoriasis/normal : Closed/not closed/not applicable : Closed/not closed/not applicable : Micro/macro shape/odd shape/not applicable	
Hair • Texture • Color • Dandruff • Pediculosis	 : Normal/brittle/dry/oily/thin/alopecia : Normal/colored : No/yes : No/yes	
Face • Worried • Pale Color	 : No/yes : No/yes	
Eyes • Eyebrow • Eyelashes • Eyelids • Eyeballs • Conjunctiva • Sclera • Lens • Pupils • Visual power **Vision** • Eye movement • Eye discharge	 : Symmetrical/asymmetrical/can not raise : Infection/stye/normal : Edema/lesions/normal : Normal/protruded/sunken : Healthy/moist/pale/watery : Normal/icterus/redness : Opaque/transparent : Dilated/constricted/reaction to light : Normal/blurred vision : Normal/strabismus : Absent/present	
Ears • Ear discharge • Tympanic membrane • Hearing ability	 : Absent/present : Normal/perforated/lesion/bulging : Normal/hearing aids	
Nose • Crust or discharge • Nasal septum • Mucous membrane • Polyps • Sinus	 : Absent/present : Normal/perforated/deviated to which side : Normal/swollen/epitasis : Absent/present : Absent/present	
Mouth • Breath • Throat • Tonsils • Teeth • Tongue • Mucus and gums • Lips	 : Normal/halitosis : Normal/congested (short neck) : Normal/inflamed : Healthy/poorly aligned/dental caries/plaque : Pink/pale/moist/dry/coated/lesion/glossitis : Ulcer/gingivitis/bleeding/pus/normal : Redness/swelling/cyanosis/normal	
Neck • Movement • Lymph nodes • Thyroid gland	 : Flexion/extension/normal : Normal/tender/palpable : Normal/enlarged	
Chest • Thorax • Breath sounds • Breast • Nipple • Heart beat • Heart sound	 : Symmetry/shape (specify) : Normal/wheeze/grunting : Normal/mastitis/lump : Normal/cracked/secretion : Rate/rhythm/volume : Normal/murmur/gallops	

Contd...

Contd...

Physical features	Theory picture	Child picture
Axilla • Lymph node	: Not palpable/palpable/tenderness	
Abdomen • Inspection • Palpation • Percussion • Bowel sound (Auscultation)	: Skin rash/hernia/ascites/distension/normal : Tenderness/palpable organs (liver, spleen) : Presence of gas (dullness)/masses : Present/absent	
Genitalia *Females:* • Mons pubis • External genitalia • Urinary pattern • Congenital anomalies *Males:* Mons pubis • Urinary pattern • Scrotum • Inguinal canal • Congenital anomalies	 : Normal : Inflammation/edema/lesion/normal : Normal/burning/micturation/normal : Absent/present : Healthy/nits/lice : Normal/epispadias/hypospadias : Descended testis/undescended testis : Normal/hernia : Absent/present	
Rectum and anus • Congenital anomalies • Others	: Absent/present : Piles/polyps/melina/ulcer/excoriation/rash	

Impression

Baby/Master ....

....

....

....

....

....

....

....

....

....

....

....

....

....

....

Investigations

Blood Test

S. No.	Name of the investigation	Child findings	Normal values	Remarks
1.				
2.				
3.				
4.				
5.				
6.				
7.				
8.				
9.				
10.				

Urine Analysis

S. No.	Name of the investigation	Child findings	Normal values	Remarks
1.				
2.				
3.				
4.				
5.				
6.				
7.				
8.				
9.				
10.				

Radiological Investigation

Name of the study	Impression
X-ray	
USG Scan	
CT Scan	
MRI Scan	

MEDICATION

S. No.	Drug name	Action	Dose/route	Indication	Side effects	Nursing responsibility

MEDICATION

S. No.	Drug name	Action	Dose/route	Indication	Side effects	Nursing responsibility

MEDICATION

S. No.	Drug name	Action	Dose/route	Indication	Side effects	Nursing responsibility

Nursing Diagnosis

Preoperative Nursing Diagnosis

1. ....
....
....

2. ....
....
....

3. ....
....
....

4. ....
....
....

5. ....
....
....

6. ....
....
....

7. ....
....
....

8. ....
....
....

9. ....
....
....

10. ....
....
....

Preoperative Nursing Care Plan/Nursing Process

Date	Nursing assessment	Nursing diagnosis	Goal	Nursing intervention	Nursing implementation	Evaluation
Day	Subjective Data: Objective Data:					

Preoperative Nursing Care Plan/Nursing Process

Date	Nursing assessment	Nursing diagnosis	Goal	Nursing intervention	Nursing implementation	Evaluation
Day	Subjective Data: Objective Data:					

Preoperative Nursing Care Plan/Nursing Process

Date	Nursing assessment	Nursing diagnosis	Goal	Nursing intervention	Nursing implementation	Evaluation
Day	Subjective Data: Objective Data:					

Preoperative Nursing Care Plan/Nursing Process

Date	Nursing assessment	Nursing diagnosis	Goal	Nursing intervention	Nursing implementation	Evaluation
Day	Subjective Data: Objective Data:					

Preoperative Nursing Care Plan/Nursing Process

Date	Nursing assessment	Nursing diagnosis	Goal	Nursing intervention	Nursing implementation	Evaluation
Day	Subjective Data: Objective Data:					

Nursing Diagnosis

Postoperative Nursing Diagnosis

1. ....

2. ....

3. ....

4. ....

5. ....

6. ....

7. ....

8. ....

9. ....

10. ....

Postoperative Nursing Care Plan/Nursing Process

Date	Nursing assessment	Nursing diagnosis	Goal	Nursing intervention	Nursing implementation	Evaluation
Day	Subjective Data: Objective Data:					

Postoperative Nursing Care Plan/Nursing Process

Date	Nursing assessment	Nursing diagnosis	Goal	Nursing intervention	Nursing implementation	Evaluation
Day	Subjective Data: Objective Data:					

Postoperative Nursing Care Plan/Nursing Process

Date	Nursing assessment	Nursing diagnosis	Goal	Nursing intervention	Nursing implementation	Evaluation
Day	Subjective Data: Objective Data:					

Postoperative Nursing Care Plan/Nursing Process

Date	Nursing assessment	Nursing diagnosis	Goal	Nursing intervention	Nursing implementation	Evaluation
Day	Subjective Data: Objective Data:					

Postoperative Nursing Care Plan/Nursing Process

Date	Nursing assessment	Nursing diagnosis	Goal	Nursing intervention	Nursing implementation	Evaluation
Day	Subjective Data: Objective Data:					

HEALTH EDUCATION

Medication ....
....
....

Hygiene ....
....
....

Diet ....
....
....

Play/Exercise ....
....
....

Follow-up care ....
....
....

Prognosis

Day 1:
: ....
....
....

Day 2:
: ....
....
....

Day 3:
: ....
....
....

Summary:
....
....
....

Conclusion:
....
....
....

BIBLIOGRAPHY

It should be minimum 5 References of Textbook, Journals and Internet, etc.

1.

2.

3.

4.

5.

NURSING CASE STUDY

MEDICAL CASE STUDY-1

Evaluation Criteria for Medical Case Study-1

Name of child: ....

Ward: ....

Diagnosis: ....

Total Marks: 50

IP/No: ....

S. No.	Contents	Score	Marks obtained
1.	**Child profile and assessment:** • Identification data • History collection • Nutritional history • Physical examination • Immunization status • Investigations • Medication	 1 1 2 5 1 2 3	
2.	**Disease condition** • Definition • Etiology and risk factors • Pathophysiology • Clinical manifestation • Diagnostic evaluation • Management • Complication • Prognosis	 1 2 5 2 1 1 1 1	
3.	**Nursing management** 1. Identification of needs and problems 2. List out and prioritizing the nursing diagnosis 3. Goals 4. Implementation 5. Evaluation	 2 2 1 10 2	
4.	Health education	3	
5.	Summary and conclusion	1	
6.	Bibliography	1	
	Total Marks	**50**	

Signature of Student　　　　　　　　**Incharge Teacher**　　　　　　　　**Signature of the HOD**

MEDICAL CASE STUDY-1

ON

CHILD WITH ....

Identification Data

Name of the Child	: Baby/Master ....
Chronological Age	:
Developmental Stage	:
Sex/Gender	: Male/Female ....
Date of Admission	:
IP Number	:
Ward	:
Bed Number	:
Diagnosis	:
Informant	: Mother/Father/others ....
Address	: ....
	: ....
	: ....
Date of care started	: ....
Date of care ended	: ....

History Collection

Chief complaints:

....

....

....

....

Socioeconomic background of the family:

....

....

....

....

Family health history:

....

....

....

....

Family Tree:

– Male

– Female

/// – Child

Past Medical History:

....
....
....

Present Medical History:

....
....
....

Birth History:

Antenatal history:

....
....
....

Intranatal history:

....
....
....

Postnatal history:

....
....
....

Nutritional history:

Food habits : ....
....
....

Feeding skill : ....
....
....

Likable food : ....

....

....

Dislikable food : ....

....

....

24 hours recall : ....

....

....

Malnutrition Assessments:

$$\frac{\text{Actual weight} \times 100}{\text{Expected weight}} = \text{................................} \times 100$$

$$= \text{................................}$$

$$= \text{................................}\%$$

Degree of malnutrition: **Mild/Moderate/Severe** ☐

Personal History

Habits : ....

....

....

Elimination : ....

....

....

Play activity : ....

....

....

Immunization History

Date	Recommended age	Vaccine	Dose	Route	Remarks given/not given
	At birth	BCG (0.05 till one month age)	0.1 mL	ID	
		OPV (zero dose)	2 drops	Oral	
		Hepatitis B-1	0.5 mL	IM	
	6 weeks	OPV-1 + IPV-1 with OPV-1	2 drops	Oral	
		DPTw-1/DPTa-1 dose	0.5 mL	IM	
		Hepatitis B-2 dose	0.5 mL	IM	
		Hib vaccine-1 dose	0.5 mL	IM	
	10 weeks	OPV-2+ IPV-2 with OPV-2	2 drops	Oral	
		DPTw-2/DPTa-2 dose	0.5 mL	IM	
		Hib Vaccine-2 dose	0.5 mL	IM	

Date	Recommended age	Vaccine	Dose	Route	Remarks given/not given
	14 weeks	OPV-3 + IPV-2 with OPV-3	2 drops	Oral	
		DPTw-3/DPTa-2 dose	0.5 mL	IM	
		Hepatitis B-3 dose	0.5 mL	IM	
		Hib vaccine-3 dose	0.5 mL	IM	
	9 months	Measles	0.5 mL	Sub	
		Vitamin – A (1 episode)	1 mL	Oral	
	15 to 18 months	OPV-4 + IPV-booster 1 with OPV-4	2 drops	Oral	
		DPT booster-1 or DPTa- B1	0.5 mL	IM	
		Hib vaccine booster	0.5 mL	IM	
		MMR-1 dose	0.5 mL	Sub	
	2 years	Typhoid vaccine	0.5 mL	IM	
	5 years	OPV-5 dose	2 drops	Oral	
		DPT booster-2 dose	0.5 mL	IM	
		MMR-2 dose	0.5 mL	Sub	
	10 years	TT	0.5 mL	IM	

Physical Examination

Physical features	Theory picture	Child picture
General appearance • Level of consciousness • Posture • Grooming • Body build • Gait • Activity	: Conscious/semi conscious/unconscious : Normal/kyphosis/lordosis/scoliosis : Well groomed/dirty : Endomorphic/mesomorphic/ectomorphic : Any Limp/Unsteady gait/normal gait : Bedridden/bed rest/active	
Vital signs • Temperature • Pulses • Respiration • Blood pressure	:................°C/°F :................beats/minute :................breath/minute :........./.......mm/Hg	Normal/abnormal
Skin • Temperature • Color • Texture • Lesions • Sensation	: Normal/warm/cold and clammy : Normal/pallor/cyanosis/icterus/flushing : Smooth/wrinkling/flaking/hydrated/edema : No/papule/vesicle/ulcer : Normal/anesthesia/paresthesia/hypothesia	
Head and scalp • Head circumference • Scalp • Anterior fontanelle • Posterior fontanelle • Shape of skull	: Normal/hydrocephalus/micro and macrocephalus : Lesion/cleanliness/infection/psoriasis/normal : Closed/not closed/not applicable : Closed/not closed/not applicable : Micro/macro shape/odd shape/not applicable	
Hair • Texture • Color • Dandruff • Pediculosis	: Normal/brittle/dry/oily/thin/alopecia : Normal/colored : No/yes : No/yes	
Face • Worried • Pale Color	: No/yes : No/yes	

Physical features	Theory picture	Child picture
Eyes • Eyebrow • Eyelashes • Eyelids • Eyeballs • Conjunctiva • Sclera • Lens • Pupil's • Visual power **Vision** • Eye movement • Eye discharge	: Symmetrical/asymmetrical/can not raise : Infection/stye/normal : Edema/lesions/normal : Normal/protruded/sunken : Healthy/moist/pale/watery : Normal/icterus/redness : Opaque/transparent : Dilated/constricted/reaction to light : Normal/blurred vision : Normal/strabismus : Absent/present	
Ears • Ear discharge • Tympanic membrane • Hearing ability	: Absent/present : Normal/perforated/lesion/bulging : Normal/hearing aids	
Nose • Crust or discharge • Nasal septum • Mucous membrane • Polyps • Sinus	: Absent/present : Normal/perforated/deviated to which side : Normal/swollen/epitasis : Absent/present : Absent/present	
Mouth • Breath • Throat • Tonsils • Teeth • Tongue • Mucus and gums • Lips	: Normal/halitosis : Normal/congested (short neck) : Normal/inflamed : Healthy/poorly aligned/dental caries/plaque : Pink/pale/moist/dry/coated/lesion/glossitis : Ulcer/gingivitis/bleeding/pus/normal : Redness/swelling/cyanosis/normal	
Neck • Movement • Lymph nodes • Thyroid gland	: Flexion/extension/normal : Normal/tender/palpable : Normal/enlarged	
Chest • Thorax • Breath sounds • Breast • Nipple • Heart beat • Heart sound	: Symmetry/shape (specify) : Normal/wheeze/grunting : Normal/mastitis/lump : Normal/cracked/secretion : Rate/rhythm/volume : Normal/murmur/gallops	
Axilla • Lymph node	: Not palpable/palpable/tenderness	
Abdomen • Inspection • Palpation • Percussion • Bowel sound (auscultation)	: Skin rash/hernia/ascites/distension/normal : Tenderness/palpable organs (liver, spleen) : Presence of gas (dullness)/masses : Present/absent	
Genitalia *Females:* • Mons pubis • External genitalia • Urinary pattern • Congenital anomalies	 : Normal : Inflammation/edema/lesion/normal : Normal/burning/micturation/normal : Absent/present	

Physical features	Theory picture	Child picture
Males: Mons pubis • Urinary pattern • Scrotum • Inguinal canal • Congenital anomalies	: Healthy/nits/lice : Normal/epispadias/hypospadias : Descended testis/undescended testis : Normal/hernia : Absent/present	
Rectum and anus • Congenital anomalies • Others	: Absent/present : Piles/polyps/melina/ulcer/excoriation/rash	

Impression

Baby/Master ....
....
....
....

Investigations

Blood Test

S. No.	Name of the investigation	Child findings	Normal values	Remarks
1.				
2.				
3.				
4.				
5.				
6.				
7.				
8.				
9.				
10.				

Urine Analysis

S. No.	Name of the Investigation	Child findings	Normal values	Remarks
1				
2				
3				
4				
5				
6				
7				
8				
9				
10				

Radiological Investigation

Name of the study	Impression
X-ray	
USG scan	
CT scan	
MRI scan	

MEDICATION

S. No.	Drug name	Action	Dose/Route	Indication	Side effects	Nursing responsibility

MEDICATION

S. No.	Drug name	Action	Dose/Route	Indication	Side effects	Nursing responsibility

REVIEW OF ANATOMY AND PHYSIOLOGY

System: ....

Draw a diagram

Physiology:

....

....

....

....

....

....

....

....

....

....

....

....

....

....

DISEASE CONDITION

Topic name: ....

Definition

....

....

Causes

S. No.	Book View	Child View	Remarks
1.			
2.			
3.			
4.			
5.			
6.			
7.			
8.			
9.			
10.			

Types/Classification

1. ....

2. ....

3. ....

4. ....

5. ....

6. ....

7. ....

8. ....

Pathophysiology

Pathophysiology of ....

Signs and Symptoms

S. No.	Book view	Child view

182 Practical Casebook: Child Health Nursing for GNM and Post Basic BSc Nursing Students

Diagnostic Evaluation

S. No.	Book view	Child view	Remarks
S. No.	Book view	Child view	Remarks

Management

Medical Management

S. No.	Book view	Child view	Remarks Given/Not Given

Surgical Management (If any)

....
....
....
....
....
....
....
....
....
....
....
....
....
....

Diet Management

Book view	Child view	Remarks

Supportive Measures/Therapy (If any)

....
....
....
....

Nursing Management

Book view	Child View

Complications

Prognosis

NURSING DIAGNOSIS

1. ....

2. ....

3. ....

4. ....

5. ....

6. ....

7. ....

8. ....

9. ....

10. ....

Nursing Care Plan/Nursing Process

Date	Nursing assessment	Nursing diagnosis	Goal	Nursing intervention	Nursing implementation	Evaluation
Day	Subjective Data: Objective Data:					

Nursing Care Plan/Nursing Process

Date	Nursing assessment	Nursing diagnosis	Goal	Nursing intervention	Nursing implementation	Evaluation
Day	Subjective Data: Objective Data:					

Nursing Care Plan/Nursing Process

Date	Nursing assessment	Nursing diagnosis	Goal	Nursing intervention	Nursing implementation	Evaluation
Day	Subjective Data: Objective Data:					

Nursing Care Plan/Nursing Process

Date	Nursing assessment	Nursing diagnosis	Goal	Nursing intervention	Nursing implementation	Evaluation
Day	Subjective Data: Objective Data:					

Nursing Care Plan/Nursing Process

Date	Nursing assessment	Nursing diagnosis	Goal	Nursing intervention	Nursing implementation	Evaluation
Day	Subjective Data: Objective Data:					

Nursing Care Plan/Nursing Process

Date	Nursing assessment	Nursing diagnosis	Goal	Nursing intervention	Nursing implementation	Evaluation
Day	Subjective Data: Objective Data:					

BIBLIOGRAPHY

It should be minimum 5 References of Textbook, Journals and Internet, etc.

1.

2.

3.

4.

5.

SURGICAL CASE STUDY-1

Evaluation Criteria for Surgical Case Study

Name of child : ....   **Total Marks: 25**

Ward : ....   IP/No :...

Diagnosis : ....

S. No.	Content	Score	Marks obtained
1.	**Child profile and assessment:** • Identification data • History collection • Nutritional history • Physical examination • Immunization status • Investigations • Medication	 1 1 2 5 1 2 3	
2.	**Disease condition** • Definition • Etiology and risk factors • Pathophysiology • Clinical Manifestation • Diagnostic evaluation • Management • Complication • Prognosis	 1 2 1 2 1 1 1 1	
3.	**Nursing management** • Identification of needs and problems • List out and prioritizing the nursing diagnosis • Goals • Implementation • Evaluation	 2 5 1 10 2	
4.	Prognosis and health education	3	
5.	Summary and conclusion	1	
6.	Bibliography	1	
	Total Marks	**50**	

Signature of Student   **Incharge Teacher**   **Signature of the HOD**

SURGICAL CASE STUDY
ON

CHILD WITH ....

Identification Data

Name of the Child	: Baby/Master ....
Chronological Age	:
Developmental Stage	:
Sex/Gender	: Male/Female ....
Date of Admission	:
IP Number	:
Ward	:
Bed Number	:
Diagnosis	:
Name of the Surgery	:
Date of the Surgery	:
Informant	: Mother/Father/others ....
Address	: ....
	: ....
	: ....
Date of care started	:
Date of care ended	:

History Collection

Chief complaints:

....
....
....

Socioeconomic background of the family:

....
....
....

Family health history:

....
....
....
....

Family Tree:

- Male
- Female
/// – Child

Past Medical History:

....
....
....

Present Medical History:

....
....
....

Birth History:

Antenatal history:

....
....
....

Intranatal history:

....
....
....

Postnatal history:

....
....
....

Nutritional history:

Food habits : ....
....
....

Feeding skill : ....
....
....

Likable food: ....

....

Dislikable food: ....

....

24 Hours Recall: ....

....

Malnutrition Assessments:

$$\frac{\text{Actual weight} \times 100}{\text{Expected weight}} = \text{................................} \times 100$$

$$= \text{................................}$$

$$= \text{................................}\%$$

Degree of malnutrition: **Mild/Moderate/Severe** [________________]

Personal History

Habits : ....

....

....

Elimination : ....

....

....

Play activity : ....

....

Immunization History

Date	Recommended age	Vaccine	Dose	Route	Remarks given/not given
	At birth	BCG (0.05 till one month age)	0.1 mL	ID	
		OPV (zero dose)	2 drops	Oral	
		Hepatitis B-1	0.5 mL	IM	
	6 weeks	OPV-1 + IPV-1 with OPV-1	2 drops	Oral	
		DPTw-1/DPTa-1 dose	0.5 mL	IM	
		Hepatitis B-2 dose	0.5 mL	IM	
		Hib Vaccine-1 dose	0.5 mL	IM	
	10 weeks	OPV-2+ IPV-2 with OPV-2	2 drops	Oral	
		DPTw-2/DPTa-2 dose	0.5 mL	IM	
		Hib vaccine-2 dose	0.5 mL	IM	
	14 weeks	OPV-3 + IPV-2 with OPV-3	2 drops	Oral	
		DPTw-3/DPTa-2 dose	0.5 mL	IM	
		Hepatitis B-3 dose	0.5 mL	IM	
		Hib vaccine-3 dose	0.5 mL	IM	

Date	Recommended age	Vaccine	Dose	Route	Remarks given/not given
	9 months	Measles	0.5 mL	Sub	
		Vitamin – A (1 episode)	1 mL	Oral	
	15 to 18 months	OPV-4 + IPV-booster 1 with OPV-4	2 drops	Oral	
		DPT booster-1 or DPTa- B1	0.5 mL	IM	
		Hib vaccine booster	0.5 mL	IM	
		MMR-1 dose	0.5 mL	Sub	
	2 years	Typhoid vaccine	0.5 mL	IM	
	5 years	OPV-5 dose	2 drops	Oral	
		DPT booster-2 dose	0.5 mL	IM	
		MMR-2 dose	0.5 mL	Sub	
	10 years	TT	0.5 mL	IM	

Physical Examination

Physical features	Theory picture	Child picture
General appearance • Level of consciousness • Posture • Grooming • Body build • Gait • Activity	: Conscious/semi conscious/unconscious : Normal/kyphosis/lordosis/scoliosis : Well groomed/dirty : Endomorphic/mesomorphic/ectomorphic : Any limp/unsteady gait/normal gait : Bed ridden/bed rest/active.	
Vital signs • Temperature • Pulse • Respiration • Blood pressure	:................°C/°F :................Beats/minute :................Breath/minute :........./.......Mm/Hg	Normal/abnormal
Skin • Temperature • Color • Texture • Lesions • Sensation	: Normal/warm/cold and clammy : Normal/pallor/cyanosis/icterus/flushing : Smooth/wrinkling/flaking/hydrated/edema : No/papule/vesicle/ulcer : Normal/anesthesia/paresthesia/hypothesia	
Head and scalp • Head circumference • Scalp • Anterior fontanelle • Posterior fontanelle • Shape of skull	: Normal/hydrocephalus/micro and macrocephalus : Lesion/cleanliness/infection/psoriasis/normal : Closed/not closed/not applicable : Closed/not closed/not applicable : Micro/macro shape/odd shape/not applicable	
Hair • Texture • Color • Dandruff • Pediculosis	: Normal/brittle/dry/oily/thin/alopecia : Normal/colored : No/yes : No/yes	

Physical features	Theory picture	Child picture
Face • Worried • Pale color	: No/yes : No/yes	
Eyes • Eyebrow • Eyelashes • Eyelids • Eyeballs • Conjunctiva • Sclera • Lens • Pupils • Visual power **Vision** • Eye movement • Eye discharge	: Symmetrical/asymmetrical/can not raise : Infection/stye/normal : Edema/lesions/normal : Normal/protruded/sunken : Healthy/moist/pale/watery : Normal/icterus/redness : Opaque/transparent : Dilated/constricted/reaction to light : Normal/blurred vision : Normal/strabismus : Absent/present	
Ears • Ear discharge • Tympanic membrane • Hearing ability	: Absent/present : Normal/perforated/lesion/bulging : Normal/hearing aids	
Nose • Crust or discharge • Nasal septum • Mucous membrane • Polyps • Sinus	: Absent/present : Normal/perforated/deviated to which side : Normal/swollen/epitasis : Absent/present : Absent/present	
Mouth • Breath • Throat • Tonsils • Teeth • Tongue • Mucus and gums • Lips	: Normal/halitosis : Normal/congested (short neck) : Normal/inflamed : Healthy/poorly aligned/dental caries/plaque : Pink/pale/moist/dry/coated/lesion/glossitis : Ulcer/gingivitis/bleeding/pus//normal : Redness/swelling/cyanosis/normal	
Neck • Movement • Lymph nodes • Thyroid gland	: Flexion/extension/normal : Normal/tender/palpable : Normal/enlarged	
Chest • Thorax • Breath sounds • Breast • Nipple • Heart beat • Heart sound	: Symmetry/shape (specify) : Normal/wheeze/grunting : Normal/mastitis/lump : Normal/cracked/secretion : Rate/rhythm/volume : Normal/murmur/gallops	
Axilla • Lymph node	: Not palpable/palpable/tenderness	
Abdomen • Inspection • Palpation • Percussion • Bowel sound (auscultation)	: Skin rash/hernia/ascites/distension/normal : Tenderness/palpable organs (liver, spleen) : Presence of gas (dullness)/masses : Present/absent	

Physical features	Theory picture	Child picture
Genitalia **Females:** • Mons pubis • External genitalia • Urinary pattern • Congenital anomalies	: Normal : Inflammation/edema/lesion/normal : Normal/burning/micturation/normal : Absent/present	
Males: Mons pubis • Urinary pattern • Scrotum • Inguinal canal • Congenital anomalies	: Healthy/nits/lice : Normal/epispadias/hypospadias : Descended testis/undescended testis : Normal/hernia : Absent/present	
Rectum and anus • Congenital anomalies • Others	: Absent/present : Piles/polyps/melina/ulcer/excoriation/rash	

Impression:

Baby/Master ....
....
....

Investigations

Blood Test

S. No.	Name of the investigation	Child findings	Normal values	Remarks
1				
2				
3				
4				
5				
6				
7				
8				
9				
10				

Urine Analysis

S. No.	Name of the investigation	Child findings	Normal values	Remarks
1.				
2.				
3.				
4.				
5.				
6.				
7.				
8.				
9.				
10.				

Radiological Investigation

Name of the study	Impression
X-ray	
USG scan	
CT scan	
MRI scan	

MEDICATION

S. No.	Drug name	Action	Dose/Route	Indication	Side effects	Nursing responsibility

MEDICATION

S. No.	Drug name	Action	Dose/Route	Indication	Side effects	Nursing responsibility

MEDICATION

S. No.	Drug name	Action	Dose/Route	Indication	Side effects	Nursing responsibility

REVIEW OF ANATOMY AND PHYSIOLOGY

System: ....

Draw a diagram

Physiology:

....
....
....
....
....
....
....
....
....
....
....

DISEASE CONDITION

Topic name: ....

Definition

....

....

....

....

....

Causes

S. No.	Book view	Child view	Remarks
1.			
2.			
3.			
4.			
5.			
6.			
7.			
8.			
9.			
10.			

Types/Classification

1. ....

2. ....

3. ....

4. ....

5. ....

6. ....

7. ....

8. ....

Pathophysiology

Pathophysiology of ....

Signs and Symptoms

S. No.	Book view	Child view
S. No.	Book view	Child view

Diagnostic Evaluation

S. No.	Book view	Child view	Remarks
S. No.	Book view	Child view	Remarks

Management

Medical Management

S. No.	Book view	Child view	Remarks Given/Not Given

Medical Management

S. No.	Book view	Child view	Remarks Given/Not Given

Surgical Management (If any)

....
....
....
....
....
....
....
....
....
....
....
....

Diet Management

Book view	Child view	Remarks

Supportive Measures/Therapy (If any)

....
....
....
....
....

Nursing Management

Book view	Child view

Complications

Prognosis

Nursing Diagnosis

Preoperative Nursing Diagnosis

1. ....
   ....
   ....

2. ....
   ....
   ....

3. ....
   ....
   ....

4. ....
   ....
   ....

5. ....
   ....
   ....

6. ....
   ....
   ....

7. ....
   ....
   ....

8. ....
   ....
   ....

9. ....
   ....

10. ....
   ....

Preoperative Nursing Care Plan/Nursing Process

Date	Nursing assessment	Nursing diagnosis	Goal	Nursing intervention	Nursing implementation	Evaluation
Day	Subjective Data: Objective Data:					

Preoperative Nursing Care Plan/Nursing Process

Date	Nursing assessment	Nursing diagnosis	Goal	Nursing intervention	Nursing implementation	Evaluation
Day	Subjective Data: Objective Data:					

Preoperative Nursing Care Plan/Nursing Process

Date	Nursing assessment	Nursing diagnosis	Goal	Nursing intervention	Nursing implementation	Evaluation
Day	Subjective Data: Objective Data:					

Preoperative Nursing Care Plan/Nursing Process

Date	Nursing assessment	Nursing diagnosis	Goal	Nursing intervention	Nursing implementation	Evaluation
Day	Subjective Data: Objective Data:					

Preoperative Nursing Care Plan/Nursing Process

Date	Nursing assessment	Nursing diagnosis	Goal	Nursing intervention	Nursing implementation	Evaluation
Day	Subjective Data: Objective Data:					

Nursing Diagnosis

Postoperative Nursing Diagnosis

1. ....

2. ....

3. ....

4. ....

5. ....

6. ....

7. ....

8. ....

9. ....

10. ....

Postoperative Nursing Care Plan/Nursing Process

Date	Nursing assessment	Nursing diagnosis	Goal	Nursing intervention	Nursing implementation	Evaluation
Day	Subjective Data: Objective Data:					

Postoperative Nursing Care Plan/Nursing Process

Date	Nursing assessment	Nursing diagnosis	Goal	Nursing intervention	Nursing implementation	Evaluation
Day	Subjective Data: Objective Data:					

Postoperative Nursing Care Plan/Nursing Process

Date	Nursing assessment	Nursing diagnosis	Goal	Nursing intervention	Nursing implementation	Evaluation
Day	Subjective Data: Objective Data:					

Postoperative Nursing Care Plan/Nursing Process

Date	Nursing assessment	Nursing diagnosis	Goal	Nursing intervention	Nursing implementation	Evaluation
Day	Subjective Data: Objective Data:					

Postoperative Nursing Care Plan/Nursing Process

Date	Nursing assessment	Nursing diagnosis	Goal	Nursing intervention	Nursing implementation	Evaluation
Day	Subjective Data: Objective Data:					

HEALTH EDUCATION

Medication ....

....

....

Hygiene ....

....

....

Diet ....

....

....

Play/Exercise ....

....

....

Follow-up care ....

....

....

Prognosis

Day 1:

: ....

....

....

Day 2:

: ....

....

....

Day 3:

: ....

....

....

Summary:

....

....

....

Conclusion:

....

....

....

BIBLIOGRAPHY

It should be minimum 5 References of Textbook, Journals and Internet, etc.

1.

2.

3.

4.

5.

CASE PRESENTATION

Evaluation Criteria for Case Presentation

Name of Child   : ....   **Total Marks: 50**

Topic   : ....

Date and Time : ....../....../20......at...........to..

S. No.	Components	Score	Marks Obtained	Remarks
1.	Introduction of the child condition	2		
2.	Adequate content	6		
3.	Organization of the contents	5		
4.	Reliable client history	5		
5.	Knowledge on comparative study	5		
6.	Comprehensive explanation on critical areas and terminology	5		
7.	Clarity in speech	2		
8.	Modulation of voice	2		
9.	Confidence about topic	2		
10.	Using of appropriate AV Aids	4		
11.	Controlling the group members	2		
12.	Handling the questions	2		
13.	Evaluation of the groups	2		
14.	Time management	2		
15.	Personal appearance of student	2		
16.	Bibliography	2		
	Total Marks	**50**		

Overall Comments by the Teacher

....

....

....

....

Signature of Student   **Incharge Teacher**   **Subject Coordinator**

CASE PRESENTATION

ON

CHILD WITH..

Introduction

....
....
....
....
....

General Objective

....
....
....
....
....

Specific Objective

....
....
....
....
....

At the end of the case presentation the student nurse able to:

1. ....
2. ....
3. ....
4. ....
5. ....
6. ....
7. ....
8. ....
9. ....
10. ....

CASE PRESENTATION
ON

CHILD WITH..

Identification Data

Name of the Child   : Baby/Master ....

Chronological Age   :

Developmental Stage   :

Sex/Gender   : Male/Female ....

Date of Admission   :

IP Number   :

Ward   :

Bed Number   :

Diagnosis   :

Name of the Surgery   :

Date of the Surgery   :

Informant   : Mother/Father/others ....

Address   : ....

                                   : ....

                                   : ....

Date of care started   :

Date of care ended   :

History Collection

Chief complaints:

....
....
....
....

Socioeconomic background of the family:

....
....
....
....

Family health history:

....
....
....
....

Family Tree:

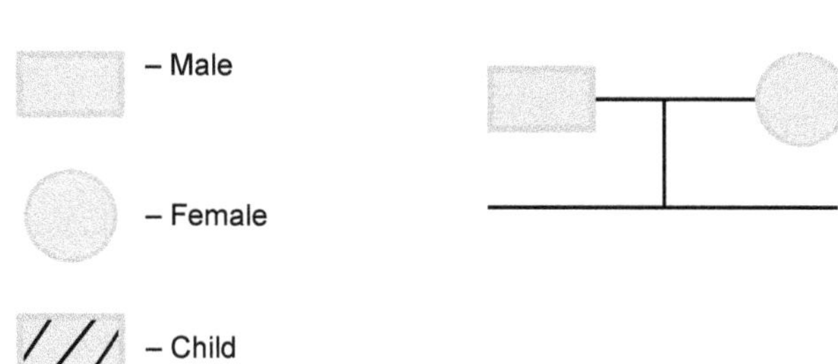

Past Medical History:

....
....
....

Present Medical History:

....
....
....

Birth History:

Antenatal history:

....
....
....

Intranatal history:

....
....
....

Postnatal history:

....
....
....

Nutritional history:

Food habits : ....
....
....

Feeding skill : ....
....
....

Likable food: ....

....

....

Dislikable food: ....

....

....

24 Hours recall: ....

....

....

Malnutrition Assessments:

$$\frac{\text{Actual weight} \times 100}{\text{Expected weight}} = ... \times 100$$

$$= ....$$

$$= ....\%$$

Degree of malnutrition: **Mild/Moderate/Severe** [   ]

Personal history

Habits : ....

....

....

Elimination: ....

....

....

....

Play activity: ....

....

....

....

Immunization History

Date	Recommended age	Vaccine	Dose	Route	Remarks Given/Not Given
	At birth	BCG (0.05 till one month age)	0.1 mL	ID	
		OPV (zero dose)	2 drops	Oral	
		Hepatitis B-1	0.5 mL	IM	
	6 weeks	OPV-1 + IPV-1 with OPV-1	2 drops	Oral	
		DPTw-1/DPTa-1 Dose	0.5 mL	IM	
		Hepatitis B-2 Dose	0.5 mL	IM	
		Hib Vaccine-1 Dose	0.5 mL	IM	

Date	Recommended age	Vaccine	Dose	Route	Remarks Given/Not Given
	10 weeks	OPV-2+ IPV-2 with OPV-2	2 drops	Oral	
		DPTw-2/DPTa-2 dose	0.5 mL	IM	
		Hib Vaccine -2 dose	0.5 mL	IM	
	14 weeks	OPV-3 + IPV-2 with OPV-3	2 drops	Oral	
		DPTw-3/DPTa-2 dose	0.5 mL	IM	
		Hepatitis B-3 dose	0.5 mL	IM	
		Hib vaccine-3 dose	0.5 mL	IM	
	9 months	Measles	0.5 mL	Sub	
		Vitamin – A (1 episode)	1 mL	Oral	
	15 to 18 months	OPV-4 + IPV-booster 1 with OPV-4	2 drops	Oral	
		DPT booster-1 or DPTa- B1	0.5 mL	IM	
		Hib Vaccine Booster	0.5 mL	IM	
		MMR-1 Dose	0.5 mL	Sub	
	2 years	Typhoid Vaccine	0.5 mL	IM	
	5 years	OPV-5 Dose	2 drops	Oral	
		DPT Booster-2 Dose	0.5 mL	IM	
		MMR-2 Dose	0.5 mL	Sub	
	10 years	TT	0.5 mL	IM	

Physical Examination

Physical features	Theory picture	Child picture
General appearance • Level of consciousness • Posture • Grooming • Body build • Gait • Activity	: Conscious/semi conscious/unconscious : Normal/kyphosis/lordosis/scoliosis : Well groomed/dirty : Endomorphic/mesomorphic/ectomorphic : Any limp/unsteady gait/normal gait : Bedridden/bed rest/active.	
Vital signs • Temperature • Pulse • Respiration • Blood pressure	:................°C/°F :................Beats/minute :................Breath/minute :........./.......Mm/Hg	Normal/abnormal
Skin • Temperature • Color • Texture • Lesions • Sensation	: Normal/warm/cold and clammy : Normal/pallor/cyanosis/icterus/flushing : Smooth/wrinkling/flaking/hydrated/edema : No/papule/vesicle/ulcer : Normal/anesthesia/paresthesia/hypothesia	
Head and scalp • Head circumference • Scalp • Anterior fontanelle • Posterior fontanelle • Shape of skull	: Normal/hydrocephalus/micro and macrocephalus : Lesion/cleanliness/infection/psoriasis/normal : Closed/not closed/not applicable : Closed/not closed/not applicable : Micro / macro shape/ odd shape/not applicable	

Physical features	Theory picture	Child picture
Hair • Texture • Color • Dandruff • Pediculosis	 : Normal/brittle/dry/oily/thin/alopecia : Normal/colored : No/yes : No/yes	
Face • Worried • Pale color	 : No/yes : No/yes	
Eyes • Eyebrow • Eyelashes • Eyelids • Eyeballs • Conjunctiva • Sclera • Lens • Pupils • Visual power **Vision** • Eye movement • Eye discharge	 : Symmetrical/asymmetrical/can not raise : Infection/stye/normal : Edema/lesions/normal : Normal/protruded/sunken : Healthy/moist/pale/watery : Normal/icterus/redness : Opaque/transparent : Dilated/constricted/reaction to light : Normal/blurred vision : Normal/strabismus : Absent/present	
Ears • Ear discharge • Tympanic membrane • Hearing ability	 : Absent/present : Normal/perforated/lesion/bulging : Normal/hearing aids	
Nose • Crust or discharge • Nasal septum • Mucous membrane • Polyps • Sinus	 : Absent/present : Normal/perforated/deviated to which side : Normal/swollen/epitasis : Absent/present : Absent/present	
Mouth • Breath • Throat • Tonsils • Teeth • Tongue • Mucus and gums • Lips **Neck** • Movement • Lymph nodes • Thyroid gland	 : Normal/halitosis : Normal/congested (short neck) : Normal/inflamed : Healthy/poorly aligned/dental caries/plaque : Pink/pale/moist/dry/coated/lesion/glossitis : Ulcer/gingivitis/bleeding/pus/normal : Redness/swelling/cyanosis/normal : Flexion/extension/normal : Normal/tender/palpable : Normal/enlarged	
Chest • Thorax • Breath sounds • Breast • Nipple • Heart beat • Heart sound	 : Symmetry/shape (specify) : Normal/wheeze/grunting : Normal/mastitis/lump : Normal/cracked/secretion : Rate/rhythm/volume : Normal/murmur/gallops	
Axilla • Lymph node	 : Not palpable/palpable/tenderness	
Abdomen • Inspection • Palpation • Percussion • Bowel sound (auscultation)	 : Skin rash/hernia/ascites/distension/normal : Tenderness/palpable organs (liver, spleen) : Presence of gas (dullness)/masses : Present/absent	

Physical features	Theory picture	Child picture
Genitals *Females:* • Mons pubis • External genitalia • Urinary pattern • Congenital anomalies *Males:* Mons pubis • Urinary pattern • Scrotum • Inguinal canal • Congenital anomalies	: Normal : Inflammation/edema/lesion/normal : Normal/burning/micturation/normal : Absent/present : Healthy/nits/lice : Normal/epispadias/hypospadias : Descended testis/undescended testis : Normal/hernia : Absent/present	
Rectum and anus • Congenital anomalies • Others	: Absent/present : Piles/polyps/melina/ulcer/excoriation/rash	

Impression

Baby/Master ....

....

....

Investigations

Blood Test

S. No.	Name of the investigation	Child findings	Normal values	Remarks
1.				
2.				
3.				
4.				
5.				
6.				
7.				
8.				
9.				
10.				

Urine Analysis

S. No.	Name of the Investigation	Child findings	Normal values	Remarks
1.				
2.				
3.				
4.				
5.				
6.				
7.				
8.				
9.				
10.				

Radiological Investigation

Name of the study	Impression
X-ray	
USG scan	
CT scan	
MRI scan	

MEDICATION

S. No.	Drug name	Action	Dose/route	Indication	Side effects	Nursing responsibility

MEDICATION

S. No.	Drug name	Action	Dose/route	Indication	Side effects	Nursing responsibility

MEDICATION

S. No.	Drug name	Action	Dose/route	Indication	Side effects	Nursing responsibility

REVIEW OF ANATOMY AND PHYSIOLOGY

System: ....

Draw a diagram

Physiology

....
....
....
....
....
....
....
....
....
....
....
....

Disease Condition

Topic name: ....

Definition

....

....

....

....

....

Causes

S. No.	Book view	Child view	Remarks
1.			
2.			
3.			
4.			
5.			
6.			
7.			
8.			
9.			
10.			

Types/Classification

1. ....

2. ....

3. ....

4. ....

5. ....

6. ....

7. ....

8. ....

Pathophysiology

Pathophysiology of ....

Signs and Symptoms

S. No.	Book view	Child view
S. No.	Book view	Child view

Diagnostic Evaluation

S. No.	Book view	Child View	Remarks

Management

Medical Management

S. No.	Book view	Child view	Remarks given/not given

Surgical Management (If any)

....
....
....
....
....
....
....
....
....
....

Diet Management

Book view	Child view	Remarks

Supportive Measures/Therapy (If any)

....
....
....
....
....

Nursing Management

S. No.	Book view	Child view
S. No.	Book view	Child view

Complications

Prognosis

Nursing Diagnosis

Preoperative Nursing Diagnosis

1. ....
....
....

2. ....
....
....

3. ....
....
....

4. ....
....
....

5. ....
....
....

6. ....
....
....

7. ....
....
....

8. ....
....
....

9. ....
....
....

10. ....
....
....

Preoperative Nursing Care Plan/Nursing Process

Date	Nursing assessment	Nursing diagnosis	Goal	Nursing intervention	Nursing implementation	Evaluation
Day	Subjective Data: Objective Data:					

Preoperative Nursing Care Plan/Nursing Process

Date	Nursing assessment	Nursing diagnosis	Goal	Nursing intervention	Nursing implementation	Evaluation
Day	Subjective Data: Objective Data:					

Preoperative Nursing Care Plan/Nursing Process

Date	Nursing assessment	Nursing diagnosis	Goal	Nursing intervention	Nursing implementation	Evaluation
Day	Subjective Data: Objective Data:					

Preoperative Nursing Care Plan/Nursing Process

Date	Nursing assessment	Nursing diagnosis	Goal	Nursing intervention	Nursing implementation	Evaluation
Day	Subjective Data: Objective Data:					

Preoperative Nursing Care Plan/Nursing Process

Date	Nursing assessment	Nursing diagnosis	Goal	Nursing intervention	Nursing implementation	Evaluation
Day	Subjective Data: Objective Data:					

Nursing Diagnosis

Postoperative Nursing Diagnosis

1. ....

   ....

   ....

2. ....

   ....

   ....

3. ....

   ....

   ....

4. ....

   ....

   ....

5. ....

   ....

   ....

6. ....

   ....

   ....

7. ....

   ....

   ....

8. ....

   ....

   ....

9. ....

   ....

   ....

10. ....

   ....

   ....

Postoperative Nursing Care Plan/Nursing Process

Date	Nursing assessment	Nursing diagnosis	Goal	Nursing intervention	Nursing implementation	Evaluation
Day	Subjective Data: Objective Data:					

Postoperative Nursing Care Plan/Nursing Process

Date	Nursing assessment	Nursing diagnosis	Goal	Nursing intervention	Nursing implementation	Evaluation
Day	Subjective Data: Objective Data:					

Postoperative Nursing Care Plan/Nursing Process

Date	Nursing assessment	Nursing diagnosis	Goal	Nursing intervention	Nursing implementation	Evaluation
Day	Subjective Data: Objective Data:					

Postoperative Nursing Care Plan/Nursing Process

Date	Nursing assessment	Nursing diagnosis	Goal	Nursing intervention	Nursing implementation	Evaluation
Day	Subjective Data: Objective Data:					

Postoperative Nursing Care Plan/Nursing Process

Date	Nursing assessment	Nursing diagnosis	Goal	Nursing intervention	Nursing implementation	Evaluation
Day	Subjective Data: Objective Data:					

HEALTH EDUCATION

Medication ....

....

....

Hygiene ....

....

....

Diet ....

....

....

Play/Exercise ....

....

....

Follow-up care ....

....

....

Prognosis

Day 1:

: ....

....

....

Day 2:

: ....

....

....

Day 3:

: ....

....

....

Summary:

....

....

....

Conclusion:

....

....

....

BIBLIOGRAPHY

It should be minimum 5 References of Textbook, Journals and Internet, etc.

1.

2.

3.

4.

5.

▉ HEALTH TALK

Evaluation Criteria for Health Talk

Name of Child   : ....   **Total Marks: 25**

Topic   : ....

Date and Time   : ...../...../20......at...........to.....................................

S. No.	Components	Score	Marks obtained	Remarks
1.	Introduction of the topic	1		
2.	Adequate content	4		
3.	Organization of the contents	2		
4.	Systematic presentation	2		
5.	Knowledge on topic	2		
6.	Comprehensive explanation on critical areas and terminology	2		
7.	Clarity in speech	1		
8.	Modulation of voice	1		
9.	Confidence about topic	1		
10.	Using of appropriate AV aids	3		
11.	Controlling the group members	1		
12.	Handling the questions	1		
13.	Evaluation of the groups	1		
14.	Time management	1		
15.	Personal appearance	1		
16.	Bibliography	1		
Total Marks		**25**		

Overall Comments by the Teacher ....

....

....

....

Signature of Student   **Incharge Teacher**   **Subject Coordinator**

HEALTH TALK

ON

CHILD WITH..

Subject	:	Child Health Nursing
Topic	:	....
Date	:	....
Time	:	....
Venue	:	....
Method of Evaluation	:	....
Teaching Aids	:	....
Name of Student Teacher	:	....
Name of the Evaluator	:	....
Designation of Evaluator	:	....

General Objective

....

....

....

....

....

....

Specific Objective

At the end of the Health talk session the student nurse will be able to:

1. ....

2. ....

3. ....

4. ....

5. ....

6. ....

7. ....

8. ....

9. ....

10. ....

Health Talk on ....

S. No.	Time	Specific Objective	Content	Teacher–Learner Activity	AV Aids	Evaluation

Health Talk on ....

S. No.	Time	Specific Objective	Content	Teacher–Learner Activity	AV Aids	Evaluation

Health Talk on ....

S. No.	Time	Specific Objective	Content	Teacher–Learner Activity	AV Aids	Evaluation

Health Talk on ....

S. No.	Time	Specific Objective	Content	Teacher–Learner Activity	AV Aids	Evaluation

Health Talk on ....

S. No.	Time	Specific Objective	Content	Teacher–Learner Activity	AV Aids	Evaluation

Health Talk on ....

S. No.	Time	Specific Objective	Content	Teacher–Learner Activity	AV Aids	Evaluation

Health Talk on ....

S. No.	Time	Specific Objective	Content	Teacher–Learner Activity	AV Aids	Evaluation

Health Talk on ....

S. No.	Time	Specific Objective	Content	Teacher–Learner Activity	AV Aids	Evaluation

OBSERVATION REPORT

NEONATAL INTENSIVE CARE UNIT (NICU AND PICU)

Introduction

Newborn babies constitute the foundation of life. Neonatal care is highly cost-effective because survival and productivity neonatology is the best developed subspecialty of pediatrics in India.

- Neonatal intensive care unit and environment
- Planning and organization of level
    - Level-I (basic care)
    - Level- II (intermittent care)
    - Level-III (special care)
    - Level-III (A) isolation neonatal care units.
- Equipment and personnel management.

Definition

Neonatal Intensive Care

Provided in a special or intensive care nursery for babies whose survival depends on highly specialized techniques including ventilation requires continuous skilled nursing expertise.

NEONATAL INTENSIVE CARE UNIT (NICU)

- It is also called as Intensive Care Nursery (ICN) A Special Care Baby Unit (SCBU).
- It is a unit of a hospital specializing in the care of ill or premature newborn infants.

Purpose of NICU

- To improve the clinical care of the critically ill neonates.
- To reduce the neonatal mortality and morbidly.
- To provide continuing in—service tearing of medical and nursing intense awareness about this specialization and retain interest among the nursing personnel.

Indications

- Critically ill babies receiving assisted ventilator viz. intermittent mandatory ventilations, constant positive airway pressure and in the first 24 hours following its withdrawal.
- Critically really ill babies, including those with recurrent opera requiring constant attention.
- Babies who have had major surgery, e.g. PDA ligation or their surgical conditions as required by the pediatric surgeon.
- Babies with severe prenatal asphyxia severe meconium aspirator syndrome.
- Babies with persistent hypothermia below 36°C.
- Infants weighing less than 1250 g or preterm deliveries below 30 weeks.
- Babies with convulsions.
- Babies receiving partial or total parenteral nutrition.
- Babies undergoing major medical procedures, such as article catheterization, peritoneal dialysis or exchange transfusions.

Equipments in the NICU

- Resuscitation set   6
- Open care system   4
- Incubators   2
- Infusion pumps   12–18
- Positive pressure ventilators   6
- Oxygen hoods, oxygen analyzers   6
- Heart rate apnea monitors I scope   6
- Phototherapy units   6

- Electronic weighing scale   1
- Pulse oximeter   6
- End, total CO_2 monitors   6
- Transcutaneous PO_2 and PCO_2 2-3
- Noninvasive BP monitors   1–2
- EC and monitor C defibullator   1
- Intracranial pressure monitor   1
- Portable radiographic machine   1
- Portable ultrasound machine   1
- Blood gas analyzer   1

Disposal Articles Required for NICU

- N catheters
- IV sets
- Microburette sets
- Bacterial filters
- Endotracheal tubes
- Suclow catheters
- Three way slop cocks
- Excavator tumbling
- Umbilical arteries/venous catheters
- Syringes
- Ventilator tubing
- Trocar and cannula.

Organization and Staffing

Medical Director/Intensivist Incharge

Preferably a pediatrician trained and experienced in critical care of newborn with following responsibilities:

- Establishing policies and protocols with the help of a group of experts including but not limited Pediatric consultants and subspecialists
- Nursing Director
- Administrator
- Laboratory and Blood Bank representatives
- Smooth functioning of PICU with implementation of policies and protocols including admission and Discharge criteria
- Quality assurance and improvement/member of audit committee.
- Advise administration regarding equipment needs
- Establishing teaching and training system of staff
- Maintaining PICU statistics for mortality and morbidity.

Staffing Requirement

Medical Staff

Round the clock post graduate level pediatrician in NICU with good airway and pediatric advanced life support skills.

Nursing Staff

Ventilated patients need one pediatric/ICU trained nurse by bed side. Very unstable patients (Hypotensive/Hypoxemic patient despite moderate support) may require two nurses by the bed side. Other unventilated/relatively stable patients (such as post operative patients and ones admitted for overnight observation may require only one nurse per 2-3 patients).

Ancillary Support Staff

- Physiotherapists
- Dieticians
- Technicians
- Radiographers
- Respiratory technicians

- Biomedical engineers
- Cleaning staff
- Secretarial/clerical staff
- Social worker
- Nursing director
- Administrator
- Laboratory and blood bank representatives
- Quality assurance and improvement/member of audit committee
- Advise administration regarding equipment needs
- Establishing teaching and training system of staff
- Maintaining PICU statistics for mortality and morbidity
- Smooth functioning of NICU with implementation of policies and protocols including admission and discharge criteria.

Admission Criteria

- Low birth weight babies
- Large size babies
- Malpresentation, fetal distress
- Birth asphyxia
- Birth injuries
- Neonatal infections
- Respiratory infections/distress
- Congenital malformation
- Rh/ABO isoimmunization
- Meconium aspiration syndrome
- Jaundice/anemia/cyanosis
- Infant of diabetic mother
- Chronic maternal diseases
- Neonatal convulsions
- Cyanotic heart diseases
- Tube parenteral nutrition
- Assisted ventilation
- Cardio pulmonary monitoring
- Unwell or unwilling mother
- Babies born by cesarean section and after forceps
- Any other baby who need special care/observation.

Criteria for Early Discharge from NICU (Before 48 Hours)

- Uncomplicated antepartum, intrapartum and postpartum course
- Vaginal delivery
- Singleton at 38–42 weeks (AFD)
- A stable and normal vital sign
- Physical examination reveals no abnormalities
- Passing urine/stool normally
- At least two uneventful, successful feedings
- No jaundice
- Parents able to feed baby properly, take care of cord and skin, able to recognize abnormal changes in color, behavior, feeding pattern of baby
- Mandatory prolonged follow up required:
- Birth asphyxia
- Malpresentation
- LBW
- Infant with congenital malformation
- Baby with jaundice/sepsis
- Severe illness
- Maternal psychiatric illness.

EVALUATION CRITERIA FOR OBSERVATION REPORT

Name of Unit   : ....   Total Marks: 25

Topic   : ....

Date and Time : ..../........./20...........at..............to............

S. No.	Components	Score	Marks obtained	Remarks
1.	Introduction of the unit	1		
2.	Objective of the unit	2		
3.	Organization pattern of the unit	2		
4.	Physical layout of the unit	4		
5.	Adequate knowledge on unit	1		
6.	Records details	2		
7.	Admission criteria	2		
8.	Available equipments	1		
9.	Team members of the unit	1		
10.	Emergency medication	2		
11.	Common procedures	1		
12.	Specific procedures	1		
13.	Discharge summary	2		
14.	Conclusion	1		
15.	Summary	1		
16.	Bibliography	1		
	Total Marks	**25**		

Signature of Student   **Incharge Teacher**   **Subject Coordinator**

OBSERVATION REPORT ON NICU/PICU

Name of Institute/Hospital   : ....

Address   : ....

   : ....

Name of Unit/Ward   : ....

Numbers of Beds   : ....

Date of Posting   : ....

Duration of Observation   : ....

Name of the Clinical Incharge   : ....

Introduce the Unit/Ward

....
....
....
....
....

Definition

....
....
....
....
....

Objective of the Unit

1. ....
2. ....
3. ....
4. ....
5. ....
6. ....
7. ....
8. ....
9. ....
10. ....

Organization Patterns of the Unit . . . .

LAYOUT OF NICU/PICU (PHYSICAL SETUP)

Admission criteria
1.
2.
3.
4.
5.
6.
7.
8.
9.
10.

Equipments used in NICU/PICU	
1.	11.
2.	12.
3.	13.
4.	14.
5.	15.
6.	16.
7.	17.
8.	18.
9.	19.
10.	20.

Health care team members	
Name of the staff	**Designation**
1.	
2.	
3.	
4.	
5.	
6.	
7.	
8.	
9.	
10.	
11.	
12.	
13.	
14.	
15.	
16.	
17.	
18.	
19.	
20.	

Emergency medicines	
1.	11.
2.	12.
3.	13.
4.	14.
5.	15.
6.	16.
7.	17.
8.	18.
9.	19.
10.	20.

List down the documents	
1.	11.
2.	12.
3.	13.
4.	14.
5.	15.
6.	16.
7.	17.
8.	18.
9.	19.
10.	20.

Common procedures practicing in the ward	
1.	11.
2.	12.
3.	13.
4.	14.
5.	15.
6.	16.
7.	17.
8.	18.
9.	19.
10.	20.

Special procedures
1.
2.
3.
4.
5.
6.
7.
8.
9.
10.

Discharge criteria
1.
2.
3.
4.
5.
6.
7.
8.
9.
10.
11.
12.
13.
14.
15.

Conclusion

Summary

Bibliography

1. ....
   ....
   ....
   ....

2. ....
   ....
   ....
   ....

3. ....
   ....
   ....
   ....

4. ....
   ....
   ....
   ....

5. ....
   ....
   ....
   ....

DRUG STUDY

Evaluation Criteria
for
Drug Study Presentation

Name of ward/unit   : ....   **Total Marks: 25**

Topic   : ....   **Duration:** ....

Date and time   : ..../........./20........at...........to................

S. No.	Components	Score	Marks obtained	Remarks
1.	Introduction of the drugs	1		
2.	Adequate content	3		
3.	Organization of the contents	2		
4.	Systematic presentation	2		
5.	Adequate knowledge on topics	2		
6.	Comprehensive explanation on critical areas and terminology	2		
7.	Clarity in speech	1		
8.	Modulation of voice	1		
9.	Confidence about topic	1		
10.	Using of appropriate AV Aids	2		
11.	Controlling the group members	1		
12.	Handling the questions	1		
13.	Evaluation of the groups	1		
14.	Time management	1		
15.	Personal appearance	1		
16.	Summarization	1		
17.	Bibliography	1		
Total Marks		**25**		

Overall Comments by the Teacher: ....

....

....

Signature of Student   **Incharge Teacher**   **Subject Coordinator**

DRUG STUDY PRESENTATION

Name of Ward/Unit :...   Date: ....

S. No.	Drug name/ pharmacological name	Action	Dose/route	Indication	Side effects	Nursing responsibility

DRUG STUDY PRESENTATION

Name of Ward/Unit :...

Date: ....

S. No.	Drug name/ pharmacological name	Action	Dose/route	Indication	Side effects	Nursing responsibility

DRUG STUDY PRESENTATION

Name of Ward/Unit :...   Date: ....

S. No.	Drug name/ pharmacological name	Action	Dose/route	Indication	Side effects	Nursing responsibility

DRUG STUDY PRESENTATION

Name of Ward/Unit :...........................

Date: ....

S. No.	Drug name/ pharmacological name	Action	Dose/route	Indication	Side effects	Nursing responsibility

Conclusion

Summary

Bibliography

1. ....
....

2. ....
....

3. ....
....

4. ....
....

5. ....
....

FIELD VISIT/EDUCATIONAL VISIT

S. No.	Name of the field visit	Field name and address	Date of visit
1.	Anganwadi school (or) under five clinic		
2.	School for mentally challenged children		
3.	School for blind/deaf and dumb children		
4.	Juvenile delinquency school		

Evaluation Criteria
for
Field Visit to Anganwadi School/Under-five Clinic

Name of field : .... **Total Marks: 25**

Address : ....

Duration: ....

Date and Time : ..../........./20..........at..............to...................

S. No.	Components	Score	Marks obtained	Remarks
1.	Introduction of the field	1		
2.	Vision and mission	2		
3.	Aims of field	2		
4.	Objective of the field	4		
5.	Organization pattern	1		
6.	Physical layout of the unit	2		
7.	Documents details	2		
8.	Admission criteria	1		
9.	Available facilities	1		
10.	Team members of the unit	2		
11.	Welfare services	1		
12.	Students interest on field visit	1		
13.	Punctuality	2		
14.	Summary	1		
15.	Conclusion	1		
16.	Bibliography	1		
	Total Marks	**25**		

Signature of Student **Incharge Teacher** **Subject Coordinator**

Field Visit

to

Anganwadi School/Under-Five Clinic

Name of Institute/School : ....

Address : ....

  : ....

Number of Students : ....

Date of Posting/Time : ....

Duration of field visit : ....

Name of the Tutor : ....

Introduction

....

....

....

....

....

....

Vision and Mission

Vision	Mission
Aims of the Anganwadi School/Under-Five Clinic	

Objective of the Anganwadi School/Under-Five Clinic

Physical Layout of the Anganwadi School / Under-Five Clinic

Organizational Structure of the Anganwadi School/Under-Five Clinic

Team members	
Name of the staff	Designation
1.	
2.	
3.	
4.	
5.	
6.	
7.	
8.	
9.	
10.	

Admission Criteria/Procedures

Common Facilities/Documents Details

Welfare Services

National welfare services	International services

Summary

Conclusion

Bibliography

1.
2.
3.
4.
5.

Evaluation Criteria
for
Field Visit to School for Mentally Challenged Children

Name of field : .... **Total Marks: 25**

Address : ....

Duration: ....

Date and time : ..../......../20.........at.............to...................

S. No.	Components	Score	Marks obtained	Remarks
1.	Introduction of the field	1		
2.	Vision and mission	2		
3.	Aims of field	2		
4.	Objective of the field	4		
5.	Organization pattern	1		
6.	Physical layout of the unit	2		
7.	Documents details	2		
8.	Admission criteria	1		
9.	Available facilities	1		
10.	Team members of the unit	2		
11.	Welfare services and rehabilitation	1		
12.	Students interest on field visit	1		
13.	Punctuality	2		
14.	Summary	1		
15.	Conclusion	1		
16.	Bibliography	1		
	Total Marks	**25**		

Signature of Student   **Incharge Teacher**   **Subject Coordinator**

Field Visit

School for Mentally Challenged Children

Name of institute/school : ....

Address : ....

  : ....

Number of students : ....

Date of posting/time : ....

Duration of field visit : ....

Name of the tutor : ....

Introduction

....

....

....

....

....

Vision and Mission

Vision	Mission

Aim of the Institute

Objectives of Institute

Physical Layout of School for Mentally Challenged Children

Organizational Structure of the Institute

Team members	
Name of the staff	**Designation**
1.	
2.	
3.	
4.	
5.	
6.	
7.	
8.	
9.	
10.	

Admission Criteria/Procedures

....
....
....
....
....
....
....
....
....

Common Facilities/Documents Details

....
....
....
....
....
....
....
....
....

Welfare Services

National welfare services	International services

Rehabilitation Measures

Summary

Bibliography

1.
2.
3.
4.
5.

Evaluation Criteria
for
Field Visit to School for Blind/Deaf and Dumb Children

Name of field : .... **Total Marks: 25**

Address : .... **Duration:** ....…..........

Date and Time : ..../......../20.........at.............to................

S. No.	Components	Score	Marks obtained	Remarks
1.	Introduction of the field	1		
2.	Vision and mission	2		
3.	Aims of field	2		
4.	Objective of the field	4		
5.	Organization pattern	1		
6.	Physical layout of the unit	2		
7.	Documents details	2		
8.	Admission criteria	1		
9.	Available facilities	1		
10.	Team members of the unit	2		
11.	Welfare services and Rehabilitation	1		
12.	Students interest on field visit	1		
13.	Punctuality	2		
14.	Summary	1		
15.	Conclusion	1		
16.	Bibliography	1		
	Total Marks	**25**		

Signature of Student **Incharge Teacher** **Subject Coordinator**

Field Visit

School for Blind/Deaf and Dumb Children

Name of Institute/School   : ....

Address   : ....

  : ....

Number of Students   : ....

Date of Posting/Time   : ....

Duration of Field Visit   : ....

Name of the Tutor   : ....

Introduction

....

....

....

....

....

Vision and Mission

Vision	Mission
Aim of the Institute	

Objectives of the Institute

Physical Layout of School for Blind/Deaf and Dumb Children

Organizational Structure of the Institute

Team Members	
Name of the staff	**Designation**
1.	
2.	
3.	
4.	
5.	
6.	
7.	
8.	
9.	
10.	

Admission Criteria/Procedures

....
....
....
....
....
....
....
....

Common Facilities/Documents Details

....
....
....
....
....
....
....
....
....
....

Welfare Services

National welfare services	International services

Rehabilitation Measures

Summary

Bibliography

1.

2.

3.

4.

5.

Evaluation Criteria
for
Field Visit to Juvenile Deliquency School

Name of field   : ....   **Total Marks: 25**

Address   : ....   **Duration:** ....

Date and time : ..../........../20.........at.............to................

S. No.	Components	Score	Marks obtained	Remarks
1.	Introduction of the field	1		
2.	Vision and mission	2		
3.	Aims of field	2		
4.	Objective of the field	4		
5.	Organization pattern	1		
6.	Physical layout of the unit	2		
7.	Documents details	2		
8.	Admission criteria	1		
9.	Available facilities	1		
10.	Team members of the unit	2		
11.	Welfare services and rehabilitation	1		
12.	Students interest on field visit	1		
13.	Punctuality of the student	2		
14.	Summary	1		
15.	Conclusion	1		
16.	Bibliography	1		
	Total Marks	**25**		

Signature of Student   **Incharge Teacher**   **Subject Coordinator**

Field Visit
to
Juvenile Deliquency School

Name of Institute/School   : ....

Address   : ....

    : ....

Number of Students   : ....

Date of Posting/Time   : ....

Duration of Field Visit   : ....

Name of the Tutor   : ....

Introduction

....

....

....

....

....

Vision and Mission

Vision	Mission

Aim of the Institute

Objectives of the Institute

Physical Layout of Juvenile Deliquency School

Organizational Structure of the Institute

Faculty Members	
Name of the staff	**Designation**
1.	
2.	
3.	
4.	
5.	
6.	
7.	
8.	
9.	
10.	

Admission Criteria/Procedures

Common Facilities/Documents Details

Welfare Services

National welfare services	International services

Rehabilitation Measures

Summary

Bibliography

1.
2.
3.
4.
5.

CLINICAL EVALUATION OF THE STUDENTS

Overall Clinical Evaluation of the Students

Name of student : .... **Ward/unit:** ....

Year of study : .... **Duration:** ....

Subject : .... **Total Marks:** ..../100

Objective 1: Evidence of ability in planning comprehensive child care based on assessment of client needs	Excellent [5]	Very good [4]	Good [3]	Average [2]	Poor [1]	Remarks
• Identifies the child needs • Sets priority • Recognizes the patient short and long term goal						
Objective 2: Evidence of ability to implement appropriate nursing intervention based on scientific principles						
• Explains the nursing action before implementation • Collaborates with the other team members as needed. • Applies scientific principles- that justify nursing action • Utilizes the available resources • Carriers out nursing procedure effectively • Demonstrate communication skill in the use of interpersonal relationship • Applies rehabilitative principles in the nursing intervention						
Objective 3: Evidence of teaching skill in patient situation						
• Identifies the learning needs of patient and family • Utilizes opportunities for teaching • Teaches according to the level of understanding of the patient and family • Uses illustrative materials—wherever required						
Objective 4: Evidence of reporting and recording information essential for continuity of care						
• Reports/records patients condition and nursing action accurately						
Objective 5: Evidence of demonstrating professionalism.						
• Punctuality • Maintain dress code • Demonstrate responsibility • Demonstrate leadership quality • Acceptance of criticism						
Total						

Signature of Student **Incharge Teacher** **Subject Coordinator**

ANNEXURE 1: NANDA-NURSING DIAGNOSIS

NANDA INTERNATIONAL—APPROVED NURSING DIAGNOSES

North American Nursing Diagnosis Association International, Nursing diagnoses: Definitions and Classification, Philadelphia, NANDA International.

Activity intolerance

Activity intolerance, risk for

Adjustment, impaired

Airway clearance, ineffective

Allergy response, latex

Allergy response, risk for latex

Anxiety

Anxiety,, death

Aspiration, risk for

Attachment, risk for impaired parent/infant/child

Autonomic dysreflexia body image

Disturbed body temperature

Imbalanced

Risk for bowel incontinence breast-feeding

Effective breast-feeding

Ineffective breast-feeding

Interrupted breathing pattern

Ineffective cardiac output

Decreased caregiver role strain

Risk for comfort

Impaired communication,

Impaired verbal communication

Readiness for enhanced conflict

Decisional conflict

Parental role confusion

Acute confusion

Chronic constipation, constipation

Perceived constipation

Risk for coping

Compromised family coping

Defensive coping

Disabled family coping

Ineffective coping

Ineffective community coping

Readiness for enhanced coping

Readiness for enhanced family denial

Ineffective dentition

Impaired development

Risk for delayed diarrhea disuse syndrome

Risk for diversional activity

Deficient energy field

Disturbed environmental interpretation syndrome

Impaired failure to thrive

Adult falls

Risk for family processes

Alcoholism dysfunctional family processes

Interrupted family processes

Readiness for enhanced fatigue fear fluid balance

Readiness for enhanced fluid volume

Deficient fluid volume excess fluid volume

Risk for deficient

Fluid volume

Risk for imbalanced

Gas exchange

Impaired

Grieving

Grieving, anticipatory

Grieving, dysfunctional

Growth, risk for disproportionate

Growth and development, delayed

Health maintenance, ineffective

Health-seeking behaviors

Home maintenance, impaired

Hopelessness

Hyperthermia

Hypothermia

Identity, disturbed personal

Incontinence, functional urinary

Incontinence, reflex urinary

Incontinence, stress urinary

Incontinence, total urinary

Incontinence, urge urinary

Incontinence, risk for urge urinary

Infant behavior, disorganized

Infant behavior, readiness for enhanced organized

Infant behavior, risk for disorganizedInfant feeding pattern, ineffective

Infection, risk for

Injury, risk for

Injury, risk for perioperative-positioning

Intracranial adaptive capacity, decreased

Knowledge, deficient

Knowledge of, readiness for enhanced

Loneliness, risk for

Memory, impaired

Mobility, impaired bed

Mobility, impaired physical

Mobility, impaired wheelchair

Nausea

Neglect, unilateral

Noncompliance

Nutrition, readiness for enhanced

Nutrition, less than body requirements imbalanced

Nutrition, more than body requirements imbalanced

Nutrition, more than body requirements, risk for imbalanced

Oral mucous membrane, impaired

Pain, acute

Pain, chronic

Parenting, impaired

Parenting, readiness for enhanced

Parenting, risk for impaired

Peripheral neurovascular dysfunction, risk for

Poisoning, risk for

Post-trauma syndrome

Post-trauma syndrome, risk for

Powerlessness

Powerlessness, risk for

Protection, ineffective

Rape-trauma syndrome,

Rape-trauma syndrome: compound reaction

Rape-trauma syndrome: silent reaction

Relocation stress syndrome

Relocation stress syndrome, risk for

Role performance, ineffective

Self-care deficit, bathing/hygiene

Self-care deficit, feeding

Self-care deficit, feeding

Self-care deficit, feeding

Self-care deficit, toileting

Self-concept, readiness for enhanced

Self-esteem, chronic low

Self-esteem, situational low

Self-esteem, risk for situational low

Self-mutilation

Self-mutilation, risk for

Sensory perception, disturbed

Sexual dysfunction

Sexuality patterns, ineffective

Skin integrity, impaired

Skin integrity, risk for impaired

Sleep, readiness for enhanced

Sleep deprivation

Sleep pattern, disturbed

Social interaction, impaired

Social isolation

Sorrow, chronic

Spiritual distress

Spiritual distress, risk for

Spiritual well-being, readiness for enhanced

Sudden infant death syndrome, risk for

Suffocation, risk for

Suicide, risk for

Surgical recovery, delayed

Swallowing, impaired

Therapeutic regimen management, effective

Therapeutic regimen management, ineffective

Therapeutic regimen management, ineffective community

Therapeutic regimen management, ineffective family

Therapeutic regimen management, readiness for enhanced

Thermoregulation, ineffective

Thought processes, disturbed

Tissue integrity, impaired

Tissue perfusion, ineffective

Transfer ability, impaired

Trauma, risk for

Urinary elimination, impaired

Urinary elimination, readiness for enhanced

Urinary retention

Ventilation, impaired spontaneous

Ventilatory weaning response, dysfunction

Violence, risk for other-directed

Violence, risk for self-directed

Walking, impaired

Wandering

ANNEXURE 2: COMMON LABORATORY NORMAL VALUE

COMMON LABORATORY TESTS

Common Laboratory Tests and Test Results

Test/specimen	Age/gender/reference	Normal ranges	
		Conventional units	**International units (SI)**
Acetaminophen Serum or plasma	Therapeutic concentration Toxic concentration	10–30 µg/mL >200 µg/ML	66-200 µmol/L > 1300 µmol/L
Ammonia nitrogen Plasma or serum	Newborn 0-2 wk >1 mo Thereafter	90-150 µg/dL 79-129 µg/dL 29-70 µg/dL 0-50 µg/dL	64-107 µmol/ 56-92 µmol/L 21-50 µmol/L 0-35.7 µmol/L
Antistreptolysin O titer (ASO) Serum	2-4 yr School-age children	<160 Todd units 170-330 Todd units	
Base excess Whole blood	Newborn Infant Child Thereafter	(−10)-(−2) mEq/L (−7)-(−1) mEq/L (−4)-(+2) mEq/L (−3)-(+3) mEq\L	(−10)-(-2) mmol/L (−7)-(-1) mmol/L (−4)-(+2) mmol/L (−3)-(+3) mmol/L
Bicarbonate (HCO_3) Serum	Arterial Venous	21-28 mEq/L 22-29 mEq/L	21-28 mmol/L 22-29 mmol/L
Bilirubin, total serum		Premature Full Term (mg/dL) (mg/dL)	Premature Full Term (µmol/L) (µmol/L)
	Cord	<2.0 <2.0	<34 <34
	0-1d	<8.0 <6.0	<137 <103
	1-2d	<12.0 <8.0	<205 <137
	2-5d	<16.0 <12.0	<274 <205
	Thereafter	<20.0 <10.0	<340 <171
Bilirubin, direct conjugated serum Bleeding time blood from skin puncture		0.0-0.2 mg/dL	0-3.4 µmol/L
	Normal	2-7 min	2-7 min
Simplate (G-D)	Borderline	7-11 min 2.75-8 min	7-11 min 2.75-8 min
Blood volume Whole blood	Male Female	52-83 mL/kg 50-75 mL/kg	0.052-0.083 L/kg 0.050-0.075 L/kg
C-reactive protein Serum	Cord 2-12 yr	52-1330 ng/mL 67-1800 ng/mL	52-1330 µg/L 67-1800 µg/L
Calcium, ionized serum, plasma, or whole blood	Cord Newborn, 3-24 hr 24-48 hr Thereafter	5.0-6.0 mg/dL 4.3-5.1 mg/dL 4.0-4.7 mg/dL 4.8-4.92 mg/dL or 2.24-2.46 mEq/L	1.25-1.50 mmol/L 1.07-1.27 mmol/L 1.00-1.17 mmol/L 1.12-1.23 mmol/L
Calcium, total Serum	Cord Newborn, 3-24 yr 24-48 hr 4-7d Child Thereafter	9.0-11.5 mg/dL 9.0-10.6 mg/dL 7.0-12.0 mg/dL 9.0-10.9 mg/dL 8.8-10.8 mg/dL 8.4-10.2 mg/dL	2.25-2.88 mmol/L 2.3-2.65 mmol/L 1.75-3.0 mmol/L 2.25-2.73 mmol/L 2.2-2.70 mmol/L 2.1-2.55 mmol/L

Test/specimen	Age/gender/reference	Normal ranges	
		Conventional units	**International units (SI)**
Carbon dioxide, partial pressure (PCO_2) Whole blood, arterial	Newborn Infant Male Female	27-40 mm Hg 27-41 mm Hg 35-48 mm Hg 32-45 mm Hg	3.6-5.3 kPa 3.6-5.5 kPa 4.7-6.4 kPa 4.3-6.0 kPa
Carbon dioxide, total (tCO_2) Serum or plasma	Cord Premature (1 wk) Newborn Infant, child Thereafter	14-27 mEq/L 14-22 mEq/L 13-22 mEq/L 20-28 mEq/L 23-30 mEq/L	14-22 mmol/L 14-27 mmol/L 13-22 mmol/L 20-28 mmol/L 23-30 mmol/L
Cerebrospinal fluid (CSF) Pressure volume	Child Adult	70-180 mm water 60-100 mL 100-160 mL	70-180 mm water 0.06-0.10 L 0.10-0.16 L
Chloride Serum or plasma Sweat	Cord Newborn Thereafter Normal (homozygote) Marginal (e.g., asthma, Addison disease, malnutrition) Cystic fibrosis	96-104 mEq/L 97-110 mEq/L 98-106 mEq/L <40 mEq/L 45-60 mEq/L >60 mEq/L	96-104 mmol/L 97-110 mmol/L 98-106 mmol/L <40 mmol/L 45-60 mmol/L >60 mmol/L
Cholesterol, total Serum or plasma test	Acceptable Borderline High	<170 mg/dL 170-199 mg/dL ≥ 200 mg/dL	<4.4 mmol/L 4.4-5,1 mmol/L ≥ 5.2 mmol/L
Clotting time (Lee-White) White blood		5-8 min (glass tubes) 5-15 min (room temp) 30 min (silicone tube)	5-8 min 5-15 min 30 min
Creatine kinase (CK, CPK) Serum	Cord blood 5-8 hr 24-33 hr 72-100 hr Adult	70-380 U/L 214-1175 U/L 130-1200 U/L 87-725 U/L 5-130 U/L	70-380 U/L 214-1175 U/L 130-1200 U/L 87-725 U/L 5-130 U/L
Creatinine Serum	Cord Newborn Infant Child Adolescent Adult: Male Female	0.6-1.2 mg/dL 0.3-1.0 mg/dL 0.2-0.4 mg/dL 0.3-0.7 mg/dL 0.5-1.0 mg/dL 0.6-1.2 mg/dL 0.5-1.1 mg/dL	53-106 µmol/L 27-88 µmol/L 18-35 µmol/L 27-62 µmol/L 44-88 µmol/L 53-106 µmol/L 44-97 µmol/L
24 hours urine test	Premature Full term 1.5-7 yr 7-15 yr	8.1-15.0 mg/kg/24 hour 10.4-19.7 mg/kg/24 hour 10-15 mg/kg/24 hour 5.2-41 mg/kg/24 hour	72-133 µmol/kg/24 hour 92-174 µmol/kg/24 hour 88-133 µmol/kg/24 hour 46-362 µmol/kg/24 hour
Creatinine clearance (endogenous) Serum or plasma and urine	Newborn <40 yr: Male Female	40-65 mL/min/1.73 m² 97-137 mL/min/1.73m² 88-128 mL/min/1.73 m²	
Digoxin Serum, plasma; collect at least 12 hour after dose	Therapeutic cone procedure on CHF Arrhythmias	0.8-1.5 ng/mL 1.5-2.0 ng/mL	1.0-1.9 nmol/L 1.9-2.6 nmol/L
Serum, plasma; collect at least 12 hours after dose of any therapeutic drugs	Toxic concentration Child Adult	>2.5 ng/mL >3.0 ng/mL	>3.2 nmol/L >3.8 nmol/L

Test/specimen	Age/gender/reference	Normal ranges	
		Conventional units	**International units (SI)**
Eosinophil count Whole blood, capillary blood		50-250 cells/mm³ (µL)	50-250 × 10⁶ cells/L
Erythrocyte (RBC) count Whole blood	Cord 1-3 day 1 wk 2 wk 1 mo 2 mo 3-6 mo 0.5-2 yr 2-6 yr 6-12 yr 12-18 yr: Male Female	3.9-5.5 million/mm³ 4.0-6.6 million/mm³ 3.9-6,3 million/mm³ 3.6-6.2 million/mm³ 3.0-5,4 million/mm³ 2.7-4.9 million/mm³ 3.1-4.5 million/mm³ 3.7-53 million/mm³ 3.9-5.3 million/mm³ 4.0-5.2 million/mm³ 4.5-5.3 million/mm³ 4.1-5.1 million/mm³	3.9 - 5.5 × 10¹² cells/L 4.0 - 6.6 × 10¹² cells/L 3.9 - 6.3 × 10¹² cells/L 3.6 - 6.2 × 10¹² cells/L 3.0 - 5.4 × 10¹² cells/L 2.7 - 4.9 × 10¹² cells/L 3.1 - 4.5 × 10¹² cells/L 3.7 - 5 3 × 10¹² cells/L 3.9 - 5.3 × 10¹² cells/L 4.0 - 5.2 × 10¹² cells/L 4 5 - 5.3 × 10¹² cells/L 4.1 - 5.1 × 10¹² cells/L

Erythrocyte sedimentation rate (ESR)
Whole blood
Westergren (modified)
Wintrobe
	Child
	<50 yr: Male
	              Female
	Child
	Adult: Male
	             Female
		0-10 mm/hour
		0-15 mm/hour
		0-20 mm/hour
		0-13 mm/hour
		0-9 mm/hour
		0-20 mm/hour
			0-10 mm/hour
			0-15 mm/hour
			0-20 mm/hour
			0-13 mm/hour
			0-9 mm/hour
			0-20 mm/hour

Fibrinogen Plasma	Newborn Thereafter	125-300 mg/dL 200-400 mg/dL	1.25-3.00 g/L 2.00-4.00 g/L
Galactose Serum	Newborn Thereafter	0-20 mg/dL < 5 mg/dL	0-1.11 mmol/L <0.2S mmol/L
Urine	Newborn Thereafter	≤ 60 mg/dL ≤ 14 mg/24hr	≤ 3.33 mmol/L < 0.08 nmol/d
Glucose Serum	Cord Newborn, 1 d Newborn, >1 d Child Thereafter	45-96 mg/dL 40-60 mg/dL 50-90 mg/dL 60-100 mg/dL 70-105 mg/dL	2.5-5.3 mmol/L 2.2-3.3 mmol/L 2.8-5.0 mmol/L 3.3-5.5 mmol/L 3.9-5.8 mmol/L
Whole blood CSF Urine (quantitative) (qualitative) Glucose tolerance test (GTT), oral Serum	Adult Adult	65-95 mg/dL 40-70 mg/dL <0.5 g/d Negative	3.6-5.3 mmol/L 2.2-3.9 mmol/L <2.8 mmol/d Negative

Test/specimen	Age/gender/reference	Normal	Diabetic	Normal	Diabetic
Oral glucose tolerance test (OGTT) Adult : 75 g Child: 1.75 g/kg of ideal weight up to maximum of 75 g	Fasting 60 min 90 min 120 min	70-150 mg/dL 120-170 mg/dL 100-140 mg/dL 70-120 mg/dL	≥ 126 mg/dL ≥ 200 mg/dL ≥ 200 mg/dL ≥ 200 mg/dL	3.9-5.8 mmol/L 6.7-9.4 mmol/L 5.6-7.8 mmol/L 3.9-6.7 mmol/L	≥ 7.0 mmol/L ≥ 11 mmol/L ≥ 11 mmol/L ≥ 11 mmol/L

Test/specimen	Age/gender/reference	Conventional units	International units (SI)
Growth hormone (hGH, somatotropin) Plasma	1 d 1 wk 1-12 mo Fasting child/adult	5-53 ng/mL 5-27 ng/mL 2-10 ng/mL <0.7-6.0 ng/mL	5-53 µg/L 5-27 µg/L 2-10 µg/L <0.7-6.0 µg/L
Hematocrit (HCT, Hct) Whole blood	1 d (cap) 2 d 3 d 2 mo 6-12 yr 12-18 yr: Male Female	48%-69% 48%-75% 44%-72% 28%-42% 35%-45% 37%-49% 36%-46%	0.48-0.69 vol. fraction 0.48-0.75 vol. fraction 0.44-0.72 vol. fraction 0.28-0.42 vol. fraction 0.35-0.45 vol. fraction 0.37-0.49 vol. fraction 0.36-0.46 vol. fraction

Test/specimen	Age/gender/reference	Normal ranges	
		Conventional units	International units (SI)
Hemoglobin (Hb) Whole blood	1-3 d (cap) 2 mo 6-12 yr 12-18 yr: Male Female	14.5-22.5 g/dL 9.0-14.0 g/dL 11.5-15.5 g/dL 13.0-16.0 g/dL 12.0-16.0 g/dL	2.25-3.49 mmol/L 1.40-2.17 mmol/L 1.78-2.40 mmol/L 2.02-2.48 mmol/L 1.860-2.48 mmol/L
Hemoglobin F Whole blood	1d (cap) 5 d 3 wk 6-9 wk	63%-92% HbF 65%-88% HbF 55%-85% HbF 31%-75% HbF	0.63-0.92 mass fraction HbF 0.65-0.88 mass fraction HbF 0.55-0.85 mass fraction HbF 0.31-0.75 mass fraction HbF
	3-4 mo 6 mo Adult	<2%-59% HbF <2%-9% HbF <2.0% HbF	<0.02-0.59 mass fraction HbF <0.02-0.09 mass fraction HbF <0.02 mass fraction HbF
Immunoglobulin A (IgA) Serum	Cord blood 1-3 mo 4-6 mo 7 mo-1yr 2-5 yr 6-10 yr Adult	1.4-3.6 mg/dL 1.3-53 mg/dL 4.4-84 mg/dL 11-106 mg/dL 14-159 mg/dL 33-236 mg/dL 70-312 mg/dL	14-36 mg/L 13-530 mg/L 44-840 mg/L 110-1060 mg/L 140-1590 mg/L 330-2360 mg/L 700-3120 mg/L
Immunoglobulin D (IgD) Serum	Newborn Thereafter	None detected 0-8 mg/dL	None detected 0-80 mg/L
Immunoglobulin E (IgE) Serum	Male Female	0-230 IU/mL 0-170 IU/mL	0-230 kIU/L 0-170 kIU/L
Immunoglobulin G (IgG) Serum	Cord blood 1 mo 2-4 mo 5-12 mo 1 -5 yr 6-10 yr Adult	636-1606 mg/dL 251-906 mg/dL 176-601 mg/dL 172-1069 mg/dL 345-1236 mg/dL 608-1572 mg/dL 639-1349 mg/dL	6.36-16.06 g/L 2.51-9.06 g/L 1.76-6.01 g/L 1.72-10.69 g/L 3.45-12.36 g/L 6.08-15.72 g/L 6.39-13.49 g/L
Immunoglobulin M (IgM) Serum	Cord blood 1-4 mo 5-9 mo 10 mo-1 yr 2-8 yr 9-10 yr Adult	6.3-25 mg/dL 17-105 mg/dL 33-126 mg/dL 41-173 mg/dL 43-207 mg/dL 52-242 mg/dL 56-352 mg/dL	63-250 mg/L 170-1050 mg/L 330-1260 mg/L 410-1730 mg/L 430-2070 mg/L 520-2420 mg/L 560-3520 mg/L

Iron
Serum
	Newborn
	Infant
	Child
	Thereafter:
	      Male
	      Female
	Intoxicated child
	Fatally poisoned child
		100-250 µg/dL
		40-100 µg/dL
		50-120 µg/dL
		
		65-170 µg/dL
		50-170 µg/dL
		280-2550 µg/dL
		>1800 µg/dL
			18-45 µmol/L
			7-18 µmol/L
			9-22 µmol/L
			12-30 µmol/L
			9-30 µmol/L
			50.12-456.5 µmol/L
			>322.2 µmol/L

Iron-binding capacity, total (TIBC)	Infant Thereafter	100-400 µg/dL 250-400 µg/dL	17.90-71.60 µmol/L 44.75-71.60 µmol/L
Lead Whole blood Urine, 24 hour	Child	<10 µg/dL <80 µg/dL	<0.48 µmol/L <0.39 µmol/L

Test/specimen	Age/gender/reference	Normal ranges		
		Conventional units		**International units (SI)**
Leukocyte count (WBC count) Whole blood		× 1000 cells/mm³ (µL)		× 10⁹ cells/L
	Birth	9.0-30.0		9.0-30.0
	24 hour	9,4-34.0		9.4-34.0
	1 mont	5.0-19.5		5.0-19.5
	1-3 yr	6.0-17.5		6.0-17.5
	4-7 yr	5.5-15.5		5,5-15.5
	8-13 yr	4.5-13.5		4.5-13.5
	Adult	4.5-11.0		4.5-11.0
		× 1000 cells/mm³ (µL)		× 10⁹ cells/L
CSF	Premature	0-25 mononuclear		0-25
		0-10 polymorphonuclear		0-10
		0-1000 RBC		0-1000
	Newborn	0-20 mononuclear		0-20
		0-10 polymorphonuclear		0-10
		0-800 RBC		0-800
	Neonate	0-5 mononuclear		0-5
		0-10 polymorphonuclear		0-10
		0-50 RBC		0-50
	Thereafter	0-5 mononuclear		0-5
Leukocyte differential count Whole blood	Myelocytes Neutrophils ("bands")	0%	0 cells/mm³ (µL)	Number fraction 0
	Neutrophils ("segs")	3%-5%	150-400 ceils/ mm³ (µL)	Number fraction 0.03-0.05
	Neutrophils ("segs")	54%-62%	3000-5800 cells/mm³ (µL)	Number fraction 0.54-.0.62
	Lymphocytes	25%-33%	1500-3000 cell/mm³ (µL)	Number fraction 0.25-0.33
	Monocytes	3%-7%	285-500 cells/ mm³ (µL)	Number fraction 0.03-0.07
	Eosinophils Basophils	1%-3%	50-250 cells/ mm³ (µL)	Number fraction 0.01-0.03
		0%-0.75%	15-50cells/ mmˢ (µL)	Number fraction 0-0.0075
Mean corpuscular hemoglobin (MCH) Whole blood	Birth	31-37 pg/cell		0.48-0.57 fmol/cell
	1-3 day (cap)	31-37 pg/cell		0.48-0.57 fmol/cell
	1 wk-1 mo	28-40 pg/cell		0.43-0.62 fmol/cell
	2 mo	26-34 pg/cell		0.40-0.53 fmol/cell
	3-6 mo	25-35 pg/cell		0.39-0.54 fmol/cell
	0.5-2 yr	23-31 pg/cell		0.36-0.48 fmol/cell
	2-6 yr	24-30 pg/cell		0.37-0.47 fmol/cell
	6-12 yr	25-33 pg/cell		0.39-0.51 fmol/cell
	12-18 yr	25-35 pg/cell		0,39-0.54 fmol/cell
	18-49 yr	26-34 pg/cell		0.40-0.53 fmol/cell
Mean corpuscular hemoglobin concentration (MCHC) Whole blood	Birth	30%-36% Hb/cell or g Hb/dL RBC		4.65-5.58 mmol Hb/L RBC
	1-3 day (cap)	29%-37% Hb/cell or g Hb/dL RBC		4.50-5.74 mmol Hb/L RBC
	1-2 wk	28%-38% Hb/cell or g Hb/dL RBC		4.34-5.89 mmol Hb/L RBC
	1-2 mo	29%-37% Hb/cell or g Hb/dL RBC		4.50-5.74 mmol Hb/L RBC
	3 mo-2 yr	30%-36% Hb/cell or g Hb/dL RBC		4.65-5.58 mmol Hb/L RBC
	2-18 yr	31%-37% Hb/cell or g Hb/dL RBC		4:81-5.74 mmol Hb/L RBC
	>18 yr	31%-37% Hb/cell or g Hb/dL RBC		4.81-5.74 mmol Hb/L RBC

Test/specimen	Age/gender/reference	Normal ranges	
		Conventional units	International units (SI)
Mean corpuscular volume (MCV) Whole blood	1-3 d (cap) 0.5-2 yr 6-12 yr 12-18 yr: Male Female	95-121 μm^3 70-86 μm^3 77-95 μm^3 78-98 μm^3 78-102 μm^3	95-121 fL 70-86 fL 77-95 fL 78-98 fL 78-102 fL
Osmolality Serum urine, random	Child, adult	275-295 mOsm/kg H_2O 50-1400 mOsm/kg H_2O, depending on fluid intake; after 12-hour fluid restriction: >850 mOsm/kg H_2O	
Urine, 24 hour Oxygen, partial pressure (PO_2) Whole blood, arterial	Birth 5-10 min 30 min >1 hour 1 day Thereafter (decreased with age)	=300-900 mOsm/kg H_2O 8-24 mm Hg 33-75 mm Hg 31-85 mmHg 55-80 mm Hg 54-95 mm Hg 83-108 mm Hg	1.1-3.2 kPa 4.4-10.0 kPa 4.1-11.3 kPa 7.3-10.6 kPa 7.2-12.6 kPa 11-14.4 kPa
Oxygen saturation (SaO_2) Whole blood, arterial	Newborn Thereafter	85%-90% 95%-99%	Fraction saturated 0.85-9.90 Fraction saturated 0.95-0.99
Partial thromboplastin time (PTT) Whole blood (Na citrate) Nonactivated Activated		60-85 sec (Platelin) 25-35 sec (differs with method)	60-85 sec 25-35 sec
pH Whole blood, arterial	Premature Birth, full term 5-10 min 30 min > 1 hr 1 d Thereafter Must be corrected for body temperature	7.35-7.50 7.11-7.36 7.09-7.30 7.21-7.38 7.26-7.49 7.29-7.45 7.35-7.45	H^+ concentration 31-44 nmol/L 43-77 nmol/L 50-81 nmol/L 41-61 nmol/L 32-54 nmol/L 35-51 nmol/L 35-44 nmol/L
Urine, random Stool	Newborn/neonate Thereafter	5-7 4.5-8 7.0-7 5	0.1-10 $\mu mol/L$ 0.01-32 $\mu mol/L$ (average $\approx$ 1.0 $\mu mol/L$) 31-100 nmol/L
Phenylalanine Serum	Premature Newborn Thereafter	2.0-7.5 rng/dL 1.2-3.4 mg/dL 0.8-1.8 rng/dL	120-450 $\mu mol/L$ 70-120 $\mu mol/L$ 50-110 $\mu mol/L$ 6-12 $\mu mol/day$
Urine, 24 hour	10 day-2 wk 3-12 yr Thereafter	1 2 mg/day 4-18 mg/day Trace-17 mg/day	24 110 $\mu mol/day$ Trace-103 $\mu mol/day$
Plasma volume Plasma	Male Female	25-43 $\mu mlAg$ 78-45 mL/kg	0.025-0.043 L/kg 0.028-0.045 L/kg
Platelet count (thrombocyte count) Whole blood (EDTA)	Newborn (after 1 wk, same as adult) Adult	84-478 $\times 10^3$/mm^3 (μl) 150-400 $\times 10^3$/mm^3 (μl)	84-478 $\times 10^9$/L 150-400 $\times 10^9$/L

Test/specimen	Age/gender/reference	Normal ranges	
		Conventional units	**International units (SI)**
Potassium Serum Plasma (heparin) Urine, 24 hr	Newborn Thereafter	3.0 6.0 mEq/L 3.5-5.0 mEq/L 3.4-4.5 mEq/L 2.5-125 mEq/day; varies with diet	3.0-6.0 mmol/L 3.5-5.0 mmol/L 3.4-4.5 mmol/L 2.5-125 mmol/L
Protein Serum, total	Premature Newborn 1-7 yr 8-12 yr 13-19 yr	4.3-7.6 g/dL 4.6-7.4 g/dL 6.1-7.9 g/dL 6.4-8.1 g/dL 6.6-8.2 g/dL	43-76 g/L 46-74 g/L 61-79 g/L 64-81 g/L 66-82 g/L
Total Urine, 24 hr CSF		1-14 mg/dL 50-80 mg/day (at rest) <250 mg/day after intense exercise Lumbar: 8-32 mg/dL	10-140 mg/L 50-80 mg/day <250 mg/day after intense exercise 80-320 mg/L
Prothrombin time (PT) One-stage (Quick)	In general	11-15 sec (varies with type of thromboplastin)	11-15 sec
Whole blood (Na citrate) Two-stage modified (Ware and Seegers)	Newborn	Prolonged by 2-3 sec	Prolonged by 2-3 sec
Whole blood (Na citrate) RBC count: See Erythrocyte count Red blood cell volume Whole blood	 Male Female	18-22 sec 20-36 mL/kg 19-31 mL/kg	18-22 sec 0.020-0.036 L/kg 0.019-0.031 L/kg
Reticulocyte count Whole blood	Adults	0.5%-1.5% of erythrocytes or 25,000-75,000.mm^3 (µl)	0.005-0.015 (number fraction) or 25,000-75,000 × 10^6/L
Capillary	1 day 7 days 1-4 weeks 5-6 weeks 7-8 weeks 9-10 weeks 11-12 weeks	0.4%-6.0% <0.1%-1.3% <0.1%-1.2% <0.1%-2.4% <0.1%-2.9% <0.1%-2.6% 0.1%-1.3%	0.004-0.060 (number fraction) <0.001-0.013 (number fraction) <0.001-0.012 (number fraction) <0.001-0.024 (number fraction) <0.001-0.029 (number fraction) <0.001-0.026 (number fraction) 0.001-0.013 (number fraction)
Salicylates Serum, plasma	Therap cone Toxic cone	15-30 mg/dL >30 mg/dL	1.1-2.2 mmol/L >18.5 mmol/L
Sedimentation rate: See Erythrocyte sedimentation rate Sodium Serum or plasma	Newborn Infant Child Thereafter	134-146 mEq/L 139-146 mEq/L 138-145 mEq/L 136-146 mEq/L	134-146 mmol/L 139-146 mmol/L 138-145 mmol/L 40-220 mmol/L
Urine, 24 hr Sweat	Normal Indeterminate Cystic fibrosis	40-220 mEq/L (diet dependent) <40 mEq/L 45-60 mEq/L >60 mEq/L	40-220 mmol/L <40 mmol/L 45-60 mmol/L >60 mmol/L
Specific gravity Urine, random	Adult After 12-hr fluid restriction	1.002-1.030 >1.025	1.002-1.030 >1.025
Theophylline Serum, plasma	Therap. cone. Bronchodilator Premature apnea Toxic cone.	10-20 µg/mL 5-10 µg/mL >20 µg/mL	56-110 µmol/L 28-56 µmol/L >110 µmol/L
Thrombin time Whole blood (Na citrate)		Control time ±2 sec when control is 9-13 sec	Control time ±2 sec when control is 9-13 sec

Test/specimen	Age/gender/reference	Normal ranges	
		Conventional units	**International units (SI)**
Thyroxine, total (T,) Serum	Cord Newborn	8-13 µg/dL 11.5-24 (lower in low-birth-weight infants)	103-168 nmol/L 148-310 nmol/L
	Neonate Infant 1-5 yr 5-10 yr Thereafter Newborn screen (filter paper)	9-18 µg/dL 7-15 µg/dL 7.3-15 µg/dL 6.4-13.3 µg/dL 5-12 µg/dL 6.2-22 µg/dL	116-232 nmol/L 90-194 nmol/L 94-194 nmol/L 83-172 nmol/L 65-155 nmol/L 80-284 nmol/L
Triglycerides (TG)		Mg/dl	g/L
Serum blood, after ≥12-hour fast	Cord blood 0-5 yr 6-11 yr 12-15 yr 16-19 yr	**Male** **Female** 10-98 10-98 30-86 32-99 31-108 35-114 36-138 41-138 40-163 40-128	**Male** **Female** 0.10-0.98 0.10-0.98 0.30-0.86 0.32-0.99 0.31-1.08 0.35-1.14 0.36-1.38 0.41-1.38 0.40-1.63 0.40-1.28
Triiodothyronine, free Serum	Cord 1-3 day 6 wk Adults (20-50 yr)	20-240 pg/dL 200-610 pg/dL 240-560 pg/dL 230-660 pg/dL	0.3-3.7 pmol/L 3.1-9.4 pmol/L 3.7-8.6 pmol/L 3.5-10.0 pmol/L
Triiodothyronine, Total (T_3 – RIA) Serum	Cord Newborn 1-5 yr 5-10 yr 10-15 yr Thereafter	30-70 ng/dL 72-260 ng/dL 100-260 ng/dL 90-240 ng/dL 80-210 ng/dL 115-190 ng/dL	0.46-1.08 nmol/L 1.16-4 nmol/L 1.54-4 nmol/L 1.39-3.70 nmol/L 1.23-3.23 nmol/L 1.77-2.93 nmol/L
Urea nitrogen Serum or plasma	Cord Premature (1 wk) Newborn Infant/child Thereafter	21-40 mg/dL 3-25 mg/dL 3-12 mg/dL 5-18 mg/dL 7-18 mg/dL	7.5-14.3 mmol/L 1.1-9 mmol/L 1.1-4.3 mmol/L 1.8-6.4 mmol/L 2.5-6.4 mmol/L
Urea volume Urine, 24 hour	Newborn Infant Child Adolescent Thereafter : Male Female	50-300 mL/d 350-550 mL/d 500-1000 mL/d 700-1400 mL/d 800-1800 mL/d 600-1600 mL/d (varies with Intake and other factors)	0.050-0.3 L/day 0.350-0.5 L/day 0.500-1 L/day 0.700-1.4 L/day 0.800-1.8 L/day 0.600-1.6 L/day

ABBREVIATION USED IN LABORATORY TESTS

Abbreviation	Term
Cap	capillary
CHF	congestive heart failure
Conc	Concentration
CSF	cerebrospinal fluid
d	day; diem
EDTA	ethylene diamine tetra acetate
g	gram
m	meter
hr	hour
L,l	liter
mEq	milliequivalent
min	minute
mm	millimeter
mm^3	cubic millimeter
mo	month
mol	mole
mOsmol	milliosmole
sec	second
SI	International system of units
Therap	Therapeutic
U	International unit of enzyme activity
vol	volume
wk	week
yr	year
>	greater than
≥	greater than or equal to
<	less than
≤	less than or equal to
±	plus/minus
≈	approximately equal to

PREFIXES DENOTING DECIMAL FACTORS

Prefix	Symbols	Amount
deci	d	one tenth (10^{-1})
centi	c	one hundredth (10^{-2})
milli	m	one thousandth (10^{-3})
micro	μ	one millionth (10^{-6})
nano	n	one billionth (10^{-9})
pico	p	one trillionth (10^{-12})
femto	f	one quadrillionth (10^{-15})

ANNEXURE 3: COMMON DRUGS USED IN PEDIATRIC UNITS

CONCENTRATED DRUGS USED IN NICU

Drugs	Concentration used in NICU
Aminophylline	5 mg per mL
Caffeine base	10 mg/mL caffeine citrate 20 mg/mL
Dobutamine	0.05 to 3.5 mg/mL
Dopamine	0.05 to 3.5 mg/mL
Fentanyl	1.05 to 15.0 mg/mL
Heparin	0.05 to 2.0 units/mL

Drugs	Concentration used in NICU
Indomethacin	0.05 to 1.0 mg/mL
Morphine	0.01 to 2.0 mg/mL
Prostaglandin (PGEI)	3.0 to 6.0 mg/mL
Sodium bicarbonate	6.5 mm^2/mL
Parenteral nutrition	-
Intralipid	20%

DRUG CONTINUALLY USED IN NEONATOLOGY

Drug	Dose	Route	Frequency
Amikacin	15 mg/kg/day	IV	6 hourly
Caffeine	2 mg/kg/day	Orally	Daily
Calcium of gluconate	5 mL	IV very slow	State
Calcium Sandoz	1 mL	Orally	6 hourly
Cefotaxime	100 mg/kg/day	IV	6 hourly
Ceftriaxone	50 mg/kg/day	IM	Daily
Cloxacillin	100 mg/kg/day	IV	6 hourly
Dexamethasone	2 mg/kg/day	IV	6 hourly
Diazepam (Valium)	1 mg	Rectally Er slow ZY	Start
Erythromycin	40 mg/kg/day	Orally or ZY	6 hourly
Ferrous Lactate (Ferro drops)	0.3 mL (term)	Orally	Daily
Folate	1 mg	Orally	Daily
Furosemide (Lasix)	1 mg/kg	Orally or IV	Stat
Gentamicin	7.5 mg/kg/day	IV	6 hourly
Indomethacin (Indcid)	0.2 mg/kg/day	IV	8 hourly × 3
Isoniazid (INH)	10 mg/kg/day	Orally	Daily
Kanamycin	15 mg/kg/day	IV	6 hourly
Lanoxin	0.01 mg/kg/day	Orally	12 hourly
Liprocil	1 mL	Orally	6 hourly
Magnesium sulphate	0.05 mL	1 M 1 sat	
Multivitamin doses	0.3 mL (term) orally	Orally	Daily
Multivitamin drops	0.6 mL (Preterm)	Orally	Daily
Naloxone (Narcan)	0.1 mg/kg (0.25 mL/kg)	IV, IM or VIO ETT	Stat
Paraldehyde	0.3 mL/kg	IMI	Stat
Penicillin – G	50,000 u/kg/day	IV	6 hourly
Penicillin Procaine	50,000 u/kg/day	Orally	12 hourly
Phenobarbitone	5 mg/kg/.day	Orally	12 hourly
Phenytoin	5 mg/kg/day	Orally	12 hourly
Prostaglandins E2 (prostin)	¼ tablet	Orally	Hourly
Theophylline	4-8 mg/kg/day	Orally	6 hourly
Tobramycin	10 mg/kg/day	IV	6 hourly

S. No.	Drugs	Dose	Route and frequency	Action	Side effects	Nurses' responsibility
1.	Inj Amikacin	Inj 250 mg Inj 500 mg	Q 12 hrs Q 2 hrs	(Antibacterial) Amikacin is active against a wide range of gram negative and gram positive organisms including strains resistant to other antimicrobials. Amikacin exerts third generation cephalosporin's.	• Bone marrow suppression • Vestibular auditory toxicity	• Watch for vital signs • Check for the renal function test
2.	Inj. Aminophylline	Inj 25 mg T 100 mg	IV 1 POq – 6 – 8 hours	(Antiasthmatics/bronchodilators) Theophylline directly relaxes bronchial smooth muscle and also pulmonary blood vessels. It increase in intracellular cyclic amp through inhibition of phosphodiesterase.	• GI upset, arrhythmias, seizures, tachycardia	• Watch for heart rate and blood glucose level
3.	Inj. Albumin	10%	Q 12 hr	(Plasma expanders) It is highly soluble. Ellipsoidal protein, accounting for 70 – 80% of the colloid osmotic pressure of plasma. It regulating volume of circulating blood. It is also a transport protein in circulation for naturally occurring therapeutic and toxic materials.	• Chills, fever, pulmonary edema	• Watch for the BP • Vital sign also
4.	Inj Ciprofloxacin	IV 500 mg	Q 12 hr	(Antibacterial) Anti-infective. It is bactericidal against enteropathogens like shigella, salmonella. It is against both bacteria and protozoa.	• Constipation • Diarrhea • Joint pain	• Check the anthropometry assessment
5.	Inj Dexamethasone	4 mg	Q 6 hrs	(Corticosteroid) Glucocorticoids. Action is primarily anti-inflammatory with very little sodium retaining property. Wide spread metabolic effects and modification of immune responses can occur. Prolonged use of corticosteroids can cause suppression of the pituitary adrenal axis which may result in secondary adrenocortical insufficiency.	• Hypokalemia	• Watch for the BP
6.	Tab Diazepam	Tab 5 mg Syp 2 mL	Q 15 – 30 min	(Anxiolytic) It has the typical activity spectrum of benzodiazepines encompassing muscular relaxation. Sleep modifying and anti convulsant effects. Has no peripheral autonomics blocking action.	• Hyperbilirubinemia	• Watch for respiration
7.	Tab Digoxin	T 0.25 mg	Q 8 – 24 hrs in 2 doses	(Vasodilators and antiarrhythemics) Cardiac glycoside. It increases the course of myocardial contraction and slows the heart rate. It will increase the cardiac output.	• Bradycardia • Vomiting • Poor feeding • Hypokalemia	• Check for • S potassium levels
8.	Inj Dobutamine	250 mg	IV	(Inotropic agents) Drugs used in CHF. It is a direct acting inotropic agent whose primary action results from stimulation of the beta – 1 receptors of the heart while producing relatively mild chronoscopic effects. It increases the stroke volume and cardiac output.		• Check for the vital signs
9.	Inj. Dopamine	250 mg	IV	(Inotropic agents) Antishock drug. Increase heart rate and force of contraction. At higher rates vasoconstriction in skeletal muscles and a rise in BP.	• Pulmonary hyper tension antidote regitine	• Check for the BP and pulse pressure
10.	Tab. Enalapril	2.5 mg/5 g	Oral	(Antihypertensive) Inotropic agents.	• Hypotension • Oliguria • Hyperkalemia	• Monitor the electrolytes and heart rate and blood pressure of the child

S. No.	Drugs	Dose	Route and frequency	Action	Side effects	Nurses' responsibility
11.	Syp Erythromycin	125 g/5 mL	Q 8 h or Q 6th as advised the doctor	(Antimicrobial). Primarily bacteriostatic against a wide range of organisms. It is used as an alternative to penciling in patients allergic to the latter group.	• Cholestasis jaundice	• Check the CBC and LFT test
12.	Tab. Funcornazone	50 mg	Per oral Q 72 hr Q 48 hrs	(Antifungal). Found effective infections especially in candidiasis and cryptococcosis associated with immunosuppression as in AIDS or cancer therapy.	• Vomiting, diarrhea • Skin disorder	• Watch for the renal function and LFT
13.	Inj Gentamicin	10 mg 20 mg	Q 12 hrs	(Antibacterial). Active against a wide range of aerobic gram negative and some gram positive organisms including E-coli.	• Vestibular and auditory toxicity associated with high peak levels	• Watch for the S peak levels 30 min after IV in fusion
14.	Inj Heparin	0.5–10 mL of IV	IV	(Anticoagulant). It increase the incisory action of antithrombin III on factors XIIa, IXa, Xa and thrombin the major result being inhibition of the conversion of prothrombin to thrombin. It inhibits platelet function.	• Fever vomiting • Thrombocytopenia	• PTT – 1.5 – 2.5 times • CT 20 – 30 min platelet count every time check
15.	Tab Lorazepam Inj Lorazepam	T 2 mg In 2 mg/ml	Oral IM	(Sedatives). It has no appreciable effect on respiratory or cardio vascular systems. It results of facilitative effect on GABA activity	• CNS depression • Bradycardia • Circulatory collapse • Constipation • Respiratory depression • Hyper magnesia	• Check the BP, CA, Mg, knee joint reflects
16.	Inj. Metronidazole Tab. Metronidazole	In 500 mg T 200, 400 mg	Q 12 hrs once	(Antibacterial). Effective against a wide range of organisms including giardia. Active against gardnerella and campylobacter.	• Diarrhea • Leukemia • Thrombocytopenia	• Check the vital signs and conscious level
17.	Inj Midazolam	0.3 mg/kg dose	Intravenous Infusion IM	(Muscle relaxant) It is a short acting benzodiazepine with rapid onset of action, recovery and non painful induction and lack of venous irritation. It is a sedative and muscle relaxant.	• Respiratory distress • Apnea • Cardiac arrest • Bradycardia • Seizures reported 4–11 days after therapy	• Watch for the respiratory rate and blood pressure
18.	Tab Penicillin Syp Penicillin	T – 125 mg T 250 g Syp 25 mg/ 5ml	Oral Oral	(Antibacterial). It constitutes one of the most important groups of antibiotics. These are bactericidal and act by interfering with the synthesis of bacterial peptidoglycans cell wall.	• Bone marrow suppression • Hemolytic anemia • Nephritis	• Watch for the blood pressure
19.	In Phenytoin Tab. Phenytoin	15–20 mg 50 mg 100 mg	IV 1 mg, 1 mg, 1 min divided in 10 mg/kg Oral	(Anticonvulsant). Acting on the motor cortex, phenytoin prevents spread of seizure activity. Reduces brain stem activity responsible for the tonic phase of convulsion.	• Hypotension • Hyperglycemia • Dermatitis • Cardiovascular collapse	• Check BUN and creatinine
20.	Inj Potassium chloride	0.5–1 mg/1kg	T 8 mg Syp 1.5 mg/1.5 mL Oral and IV	(Diuretic) and corticosteroid therapy.	• Bradycardia • Hypotension • Peaked T waves in ECG	• Take the ECG

S. No.	Drugs	Dose	Route and frequency	Action	Side effects	Nurses' responsibility
21.	Inj Ranitidine Tab. Ranitidine	2–4 mg T 150 mg	Q 8–12 hrs Oral or IM or IV	(H_2 Antagonist). It is stimulated gastric acid secretion through competitive blockage of H_2 receptors.	• Vomiting • Diarrhea • Pruritus • Stomatitis	• Give more fluid and educate the patient avoid chilly foods
22.	In Taxim Tab. Taximo	250 mg/ 1500 mL 100 mg	Oral	(Antibacterial). Highly activity against gram negative bacteria and a variety of betalactamase producing organisms.	• Tachycardia • Arrhythmias • Hypertension	• Watch for the ECG monitor and check the blood pressure
23.	Tab. vitamin C and B12	Pre mature 40 mg Full term 60 mg	Per oral	(Antiasthmatics). A beta adrenoceptor against with a selective action on beta receptors. It will reduction in airways and pulmonary resistance, main effect is bronchodilator.	• Vomiting, diarrhea	• Give more fluids

MODEL MEDICAL CARE PLAN ON CHILD WITH LATE ONSET NEONATAL SEPSIS (LONS)

Identification Data

Name of the Child	: B/O Ruchi
Chronological Age	: 23 days
Developmental Stage	: Newborn
Sex/Gender	: Male/Female: Female
Date of Admission	: 16/5/2015
IP Number	: 1055
Ward	: Neonatal Intensive Care Unit (NICU)
Bed Number	: 4
Diagnosis	**: Late onset neonatal sepsis (LONS)**
Informant	: Mother/Father/others: Father
Address	: Nepalganj, Nepal
Date of care started	: 16/5/2015
Date of care ended	: 18/5/2015

History Collection

Chief Complaints

The child baby of Ruchi was admitted to Vivekananda polyclinic hospital with the complaints of such as:

- Difficulty in breathing : 10 days
- Cold and clammy skin : 5 days
- Irregular breathing pattern : 3 days
- Reduced activity-lethargic : 2 days
- Abnormal eye movements : 1 day

Socioeconomic Background of the Family

The **Baby of Ruchi's** father is a breadwinner and head of the family and his occupation is carpenter, she belongs to nuclear and low socioeconomic family and they are living in their own house. It is having all the facilities like Tap water supply, electricity, open drainage, toilet, etc. Their monthly income of family is ₹ 2000 only. Her family members maintaining good relationship with the society.

Family Health History

There is no significant of communicable and hereditary illness present in her family members.

Family Tree

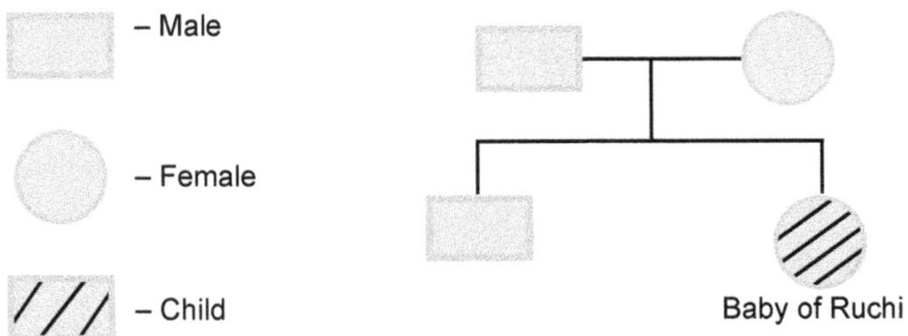

Past Medical History

There is no significant of past medical history of the child.

Present Medical History

The B/O Ruchi is admitted in Vivekananda Polyclinic Hospital on 8/11/2015 at 10.30 am with the complaints of difficulty breathing, cold and clammy skin, irregular respiration pattern, reduced activity, lethargy and poor cry. After the investigation doctor has been diagnosed as a case of late onset neonatal sepsis.

Birth History

Antenatal History

Her mother underwent to three antenatal checkups and she has taken two doses of Tetanus Toxoid. During antenatal period there is no any other complication.

Intranatal History

She is not a prime baby and delivered through lower caesarian section, soon after birth cried and she had respiratory difficulty problem.

Postnatal History

She is receiving breast milk and there is complication of respiratory difficulty means irregular respiration.

Nutritional History

Food habits   :   There is no any specific food habit, only exclusive breastfeeding

Feeding skill   :   Orogastric tube feeding

Likable food   :   No likable foods only breast milk

Dislikable food   :   No any dislikable food

24 Hours recall   :   200 mL of breast milk feeding per day

Malnutrition Assessments

$$\frac{\text{Actual weight} \times 100}{\text{Expected weight}} = 2.7/3 \times 100$$

$$= 270/3$$

$$= 90\%$$

Degree of malnutrition: **Mild/Moderate/Severe** | No malnutrition |

Personal History

Habits   :   There is no any specific habit of playing, only onlooker playing.

Elimination   :   Urine output-150 mL per 24 hours.

Play activity   :   No playing activities only movement of hands and legs

Immunization History

Date	Recommended age	Vaccine	Dose	Route	Remarks Given/Not Given
8/11/15	At birth	BCG (0.05 till one month age)	0.1 mL	ID	Given
		OPV (zero Dose)	2 drops	Oral	Given
		Hepatitis B-1	0.5 mL	IM	Given
	6 weeks	OPV-1 + IPV-1 with OPV-1	2 drops	Oral	-
		DPTw-1/DPTa-1 Dose	0.5 mL	IM	-
		Hepatitis B-2 Dose	0.5 mL	IM	-
		Hib Vaccine-1 Dose	0.5 mL	IM	-
	10 weeks	OPV-2+ IPV-2 with OPV-2	2 drops	Oral	-
		DPTw-2/DPTa-2 Dose	0.5 mL	IM	-
		Hib Vaccine-2 Dose	0.5 mL	IM	-
	14 weeks	OPV-3 + IPV-2 with OPV-3	2 drops	Oral	-
		DPTw-3/DPTa-2 Dose	0.5 mL	IM	-
		Hepatitis B-3 Dose	0.5 mL	IM	-
		Hib Vaccine-3 Dose	0.5 mL	IM	-
	9 months	Measles	0.5 mL	Sub	-
		Vitamin–A (1 Episode)	1 mL	Oral	-
	15 to 18 Months	OPV-4 + IPV-Booster 1 with OPV-4	2 drops	Oral	-
		DPT Booster-1 or DPTa–B1	0.5 mL	IM	-
		Hib Vaccine Booster	0.5 mL	IM	-
		MMR-1 Dose	0.5 mL	Sub	-
	2 years	Typhoid Vaccine	0.5 mL	IM	-
	5 years	OPV-5 Dose	2 drops	Oral	-
		DPT Booster-2 Dose	0.5 mL	IM	-
		MMR-2 Dose	0.5 mL	Sub	-
	10 years	TT	0.5 mL	IM	-

PHYSICAL EXAMINATION

Physical features	Theory picture	Child picture
General Appearance		
• Level of consciousness	: Conscious/Semi Conscious/Unconscious	Conscious
• Posture	: Normal/Kyphosis/Lordosis/Scoliosis	Normal
• Grooming	: Well Groomed/Dirty	Well Groomed
• Body build	: Endomorphic/Mesomorphic/Ectomorphic	Mesomorphic
• Gait	: Any Limp/Unsteady Gait/Normal Gait	Normal Gait
• Activity	: Bedridden/Bed rest/Active.	Bedridden
Vital Signs		Normal/Abnormal
• Temperature	: 36.5 °C/97.5 °F	Normal 36.5 °C
• Pulse	: 126 Beats/Minute	126 Beats/Minute
• Respiration	: 40 Breath/Minute	40 Breaths/Minute
• Blood pressure	: 60/40 mm/Hg	60/40 mm Hg
Skin		
• Temperature	: Normal/Warm/Cold and Clammy	Cold and Clammy
• Color	: Normal/Pallor/Cyanosis/Icterus/Flushing	Normal
• Texture	: Smooth/Wrinkling/Flaking/Hydrated/Edema	Smooth and slight cyanosis
• Lesions	: No/Papule/Vesicle/Ulcer	No lesions
• Sensation	: Normal/Anesthesia/Paresthesia/Hypothesia	Normal
Head and Scalp		
• Head circumference	: Normal/Hydrocephalus/Micro and macrocephalus	Normal
• Scalp	: Lesion/Cleanliness/Infection/Psoriasis/Normal	Cleanliness
• Anterior Fontanelle	: Closed/Not closed/Depressed/Not Applicable	Not Closed
• Posterior Fontanelle	: Closed/Not closed/Depressed/Not Applicable	Not Closed
• Shape of Skull	: Micro/Macro shape/Odd shape/Not Applicable	Odd shape
Hair		
• Texture	: Normal/Brittle/Dry/Oily/Thin/Alopecia	Normal
• Color	: Normal/Colored	Normal
• Dandruff	: No/Yes	No
• Pediculosis	: No/Yes	No
Face		
• Worried	: No/Yes	No
• Pale Color	: No/Yes	No
Eyes		
• Eyebrow	: Symmetrical/Asymmetrical/Can not Raise	Symmetrical
• Eyelashes	: Infection/Stye/Normal	Normal
• Eyelids	: Edema/Lesions/Normal	Normal
• Eyeballs	: Normal/protruded/sunken	Normal
• Conjunctiva	: Healthy/moist/pale/watery	Healthy
• Sclera	: Normal/icterus/redness	Normal
• Lens	: Opaque/transparent	Transparent
• Pupils	: Dilated/constricted/reaction to light	Reaction to light
• Visual power	: Normal/blurred vision	
Vision		
• Eye movement	: Normal/strabismus	Normal
• Eye discharge	: Absent/present	Present
• Eye tears	: Absent/present	Present
Ears		
• Ear discharge	: Absent/present	Absent
• Tympanic membrane	: Normal/perforated/lesion/bulging	Normal
• Hearing ability	: Normal/hearing aids	Normal
Nose		
• Crust or discharge	: Absent/present	Absent
• Nasal septum	: Normal/perforated/deviated to which side	Normal
• Mucous membrane	: Normal/swollen/epitasis	Normal
• Polyps	: Absent/present	Absent
• Sinus	: Absent/present	Absent

Physical features	Theory picture	Child picture
Mouth • Breath • Throat • Tonsils • Teeth • Tongue • Mucus and gums • Lips	 : Normal/Halitosis : Normal/Congested (Short Neck) : Normal/Inflamed/Swollen : Healthy/Poorly Aligned/Dental Caries/Plaque : Pink/Pale/Moist/Dry/Coated/Lesion/Glossitis : Ulcer/Gingivitis/Bleeding/Pus/Normal : Redness/Swelling/Cyanosis/Normal	 Normal Normal Normal Absent Coated Normal Normal
Neck • Movement • Lymph nodes • Thyroid gland	 : Flexion/Extension/Normal : Normal/Tender/Palpable : Normal/Enlarged	 Normal Normal Normal
Chest • Thorax • Breath sounds • Breast • Nipple • Heart beat • Heart sound	 : Symmetry/Shape (Specify) : Normal/Wheeze/Grunting : Normal/Mastitis/Lump : Normal/Cracked/Secretion : Rate/Rhythm/Volume : Normal/Murmur/Gallops	 Symmetrical Wheeze Normal Normal 142 beats/minute Normal
Axilla • Lymph node	 : Not Palpable/Palpable/Tenderness	 Not Palpable
Abdomen • Inspection • Palpation • Percussion • Bowel sound (Auscultation)	 : Skin Rash/Hernia/Ascites/Distension/Normal : Tenderness/Palpable Organs (Liver, Spleen) : Presence of Gas (Dullness)/Masses : Present/Absent	 Normal Palpable organs Masses Present
Genitals **Females:** • Mons pubis • External genitalia • Urinary pattern – Congenital anomalies **Males:** • Mons pubis • Urinary pattern • Scrotum • Inguinal canal • Congenital anomalies	 : Normal : Inflammation/Edema/Lesion/Normal : Normal/Burning/Micturation/Normal : Absent/Present : Healthy/Nits/Lice : Normal/Epispadias/Hypospadias : Descended Testis/Undescended Testis : Normal/Hernia : Absent/Present	 Normal Normal Normal Absent - - - -
Rectum and Anus • Congenital anomalies • Others	 : Absent/Present : Piles/Polyps/Melina/Ulcer/Excoriation/Rash	 Absent -
Impression: **The Baby of Ruchi is having the distended abdomen and increased respiratory rate and slight bluish discoloration of the skin.**		

INVESTIGATIONS

Blood Test

S. No.	Name of the Investigation	Child findings	Normal values	Remarks
1.	Hemoglobulin	15.9 gm/dl	14–22 gm/dl	Normal
2.	Platelets	3.19 lac/Cumm	1.5–4 lac/Cumm	Normal
3.	Packed Cell Volume (PCV)	48%	32–44%	**Above Normal**
4.	Blood Urea	22 mg%	12–45 mg%	Normal
5.	Serum Creatinine	0.5 mg%	0.1–1.5%	Normal
6.	Serum Calcium	8.6 mg%	8.7–11.0%	**Below Normal**
7.	SGOT (AST)	56 IU/Lit	35–40 IU/Lit	**Above Normal**
8.	SGPT (ALT)	13 IU/Lit	40 IU/Lit	**Below Normal**

Urine Analysis

S. No.	Name of the investigation	Child findings	Normal values	Remarks (Not yet done/Not suggested)
1.				
2.				
3.				
4.				
5.				
6.				
7.				
8.				
9.				
10.				

Radiological Investigation

Name of the study	Impression
X-ray	Not recommended the X-ray
USG Scan	Not recommended the USG scan
CT Scan	Not recommended the CT Scan
MRI Scan	Not recommended the MRI scan

Medication

S. No.	Drug name	Action	Dose/route	Indication	Side effects	Nursing responsibility
1.	Trade name—Inj. Rantac Pharmacological name—Inj Ranitidine Hydrochloride	A potent antiulcer drug that competitively and reversibly inhibits histamine action at H_2 receptor sites on parietal cells.	1 mL once a day Route-(IV) Intravenous	• Duodenal ulcer • Gastroesophageal Reflex Disease • Gastric Ulcer • Treatment of pathologic GI hypersecretion conditions (Zollinger-Ellison syndrome systemic mastocytosis and post operative hypersecretion) • heartburn	• CNS-Headache, Malaise, Dizziness, Somnolence, Insomnia • Vertigo, Mental Confusion • Agitation • Depression • Hallucination in elderly patients. **Cardiovascular:** • Tachycardia • Bradycardia (rare) **Gastrointestinal:** • Constipation • Nausea • Abdominal pain • Diarrhea. **Others:** • Rash • Decrease WBC counts • Thrombocytopenia • Anaphylaxis	• Simultaneous administration of food does not appear to reduce oral ranitidine absorption or serum concentration. • Store tablets in light resistant, tightly capped container at 15-30°C (59-86°F) in a dry place. • Follow the 7 rights of the patients. • Long-term ranitidine therapy may lead to vitamin B12 deficiency. • Creatinine clearance is monitored if renal dysfunctions present or suspected
2.	Trade name—Inj Amitax Pharmacological name—Inj Amikacin sulphate	Appears to inhibit protein synthesis in bacterial cell and is usually bacterial.	IV/IM-10 mg/kg loading dose then 7.5 mg/kg	• Primarily for short term treatment of serious infections of respiratory tract, bones, joints, skin and soft tissues • CNS(including meningitis) • Peritonitis • Burns • Recurrent urinary tract infections.	• CNS-Neurotoxicity • Drowsiness • Unsteady gait • Weakness • Tremors • ENT-toxicity • High frequency hearing loss • Complete hearing loss • Tinnitus • Gastrointestinal-Nausea • Vomiting.	• Monitor drip rate carefully. • Discard solution that appear discolored or that contain particulate matter. • Store at 15-30°c unless otherwise directed. • Verify correct IV concentration and rate of infusion • Culture and sensitivity tests should be performed before initial dose. • Monitor drip rate carefully. A rapid rise in serum amikacin level can cause respiratory depression and other sign of toxicity. • Follow the seven rights of patients. • Color of solution may vary from color to light straw color or very pale yellow. • Monitor or report any changes in intake/output.

S. No.	Drug name	Action	Dose/route	Indication	Side effects	Nursing responsibility
3	Trade name—Calcium Sandoz Pharmacological name— Calcium Gluconate	Regulating the excitation threshold of nerves and muscles, cardiac function (rhythm, tonicity, contractility)	PO—1–2 gm bd	• Neonatal tetany • Hyperparathyroidism • Vitamin D Deficiency • Alkalosis	• Hypercalcemia • Tingling sensation • Tissue irritation • Burning	• IV Calcium should be administered slowly • Solution must be diluted • IV cannula should be properly working • Monitor the lab values of calcium • Monitor for hypocalcemia and Hypercalcemia • Follow the seven rights of the patients • Adequate dilution of • Calcium gluconate must be mentioned • Intake/output chart must be maintained • Before and after every of dosage cannula care • must be given • Laboratory values must be monitored regularly

Nursing Diagnosis: (Should be based on NANDA Classification)

1. Ineffective breathing pattern related to inflammatory process as evidenced by excessive secretion and increased respiratory.
2. Hyperthermia related to infectious process as evidenced by increased body temperature 102°F.
3. Fluid volume deficits related to poor feeding as evidenced by weight loss.
4. Imbalance nutrition less than body requirement related to poor feeding as evidenced by poor sucking reflex.
5. Constipation related to decrease peristalsis movement as evidenced by abdominal distension.
6. Anxiety related to hospitalization of the baby as evidenced by anxious patients.
7. Risk for infection related to intravenous cannulation and other invasive diagnostic procedure.
8. Parental knowledge deficit regarding treatment and follow-up care.

Nursing Care Plan/Nursing Process

	Nursing assessment	Nursing diagnosis	Goal	Nursing intervention	Nursing implementation	Evaluation
Day 1	**Subjective Data:** Child parents complaining that baby is having • Breathing problem • Irritability • Restlessness **Objective Data:** • By observing the baby • Child respiratory rate =50 breaths/min. • Wheezing sound was noticed. • SpO_2: 85%	Ineffective breathing pattern related to inflammatory process.	To improve the normal breathing status of the baby.	• Assess the breathing pattern of the baby • Provide comfortable position to the baby. • To provide oxygen therapy • To provide medication according to the doctor's prescription.	Baby respiratory rate is increased and pattern is irregular. Respiratory rate = 50 breaths/min Prompt–up position is provided to the baby. Oxygen is provided at the rate of 2 mL/hour Medications are provided to the baby according to the doctor's order. Neb Asthalin 0.5 mg/1.5 mL NS	Respiratory distress was reduced and maintained the normal breathing status. Respiration: 40 breath per minutes Skin Color is pink

Nursing Care Plan/Nursing Process

	Nursing assessment	Nursing diagnosis	Goal	Nursing intervention	Nursing implementation	Evaluation
Day 2	**Subjective Data** The child mother says that • Poor feeding • Irritable cry • Vomiting • Restlessness **Objective Data** By observing the child • Refusal of feeding • Cry • I/O chart :…… • Baby has taken • 60 mL/5 hourly	• Imbalance • Nutritional status • Less than body requirement • Related to poor • Feeding	To maintain the normal nutritional status of the baby	• To assess the nutritional status of the baby • To provide feeding on time • To administer intravenous fluid to the child. • To maintain the intake/output chart of the child. • To monitor the weight of the child daily.	To assess the nutritional status of the baby. Weight:______________ Malnutrition status: ______% **Anthropometric assessment** Head circumference:……… Chest circumference :…….. Mid arm circumference:…… • Feeding is given on time (whenever baby is needed) Breast milk: 60 mL/5 hourly • Intravenous fluid ISOP is given at the rate of 2ml/hour through IV pump. Intake/output of the child is maintained. Urine–80 mL/day Stool–2 times/day • Weight monitored 24 hourly Weight = 2 kg	The child normal nutritional status was maintained. The child is maintained Intake: ………............. Urine: 120 mL/day

Nursing Care Plan/Nursing Process

	Nursing assessment	Nursing diagnosis	Goal	Nursing intervention	Nursing implementation	Evaluation
Day 3	**Subjective Data:** The child parents says that • Poor feeding • Vomiting • Restlessness • Irritable crying **Objective Data:** • By the observation child having the complaints of : • Refusal of feeding • Vomiting • Restlessness • Irritable crying • I/O chart:...... • Weight :.......	Fluid volume deficit related to poor feeding.	To maintain the normal fluid electrolyte balance.	• To assess the condition of the child. • Administer IV fluids as prescribed rate. • Give feeding at adequate time. • Maintain intake/output chart of the baby. • Monitoring of the baby Weight every 24 hours. • Provide play therapy	• Child dehydration level is assessed.(Mild dehydration) • Vital signs: • Temperature:................ • Pulse:...................... • Respiration :............... • Blood Pressure :........... • Fluid ISOP is administered at the rate of 7ml/hour. • 30 mL feed (milk-EBM+ lactogen) is given as per doctors orders. • Intake and output chart was maintained • Intake :............. • Output :............. • Weight-2.45 kg . • Therapeutic play was given to the baby, e.g. rattle play	The baby normal fluid and electrolyte status was maintained As evidenced by Weight :........... Intake :............. Output :............

Nursing Care Plan/Nursing Process

	Nursing assessment	Nursing diagnosis	Goal	Nursing intervention	Nursing implementation	Evaluation
Day 4	**Subjective Data:** The child parents told that: • Fever • Irritability • Restlessness **Objective Data:** By the observation of baby • Fever 101°F • Irritability • Crying • Mild Dehydration	Hyperthermia relater to infectious process as evidenced by increased body temperature	To maintain the normal body temperature of the baby	• To check the body temperature of the baby. • To reduce the extra clothing's of the baby • To provide sponging to the baby To provide cool and calm • Environment to the baby • To administer antipyretic to the baby according to doctor's order	• Body temperature of the baby is 101 ºF • Baby extra clothing's are removed • Sponging is provided to the baby. • Normal lukewarm water • Up to 15 minutes • Cool and calm environment is provided to the baby. • Room temperature: 285 °C • Antipyretic is administered According to doctor's order Inj. Febrinil–2 mL once a day	The baby normal temperature was maintained. As evidenced by temperature : 98.8°F

Nursing Care Plan/Nursing Process

	Nursing assessment	Nursing diagnosis	Goal	Nursing intervention	Nursing implementation	Evaluation
Day 5	**Subjective Data:** The child parents says that • Fear of child health condition • Lack of knowledge about diseases condition **Objective Data:** Parents are looking anxious • Worried • Confused • Dull face	Parental anxiety related to hospitalization of the newborn	To reduce the anxiety of the Parents	To assess the level of anxiety among newborn child parents. To provide the adequate knowledge about diseases condition. To find out the main reason of anxiety. To explain the procedures to the parents of baby. To involve the parents while caring of baby.	There is mild level of anxiety among parents. The adequate knowledge was provided by health education Using the flash card Parents are worried about that baby prognosis is good or not. Procedures are explained to the parents and told what all the benefits are. Parents are involved while cared the baby like feeding, massaging.	Parent's anxiety is reduced.

HEALTH EDUCATION

Medication

- Provide the health education to child's mother.
- Do not skip the medications.
- Give medications on time.
- After completion of medications.
- If baby developed any side effect immediately informed to consultant.

Hygiene

- Educate the child mother to maintain the personal hygiene of the baby.
- Provide baby bathing with lukewarm water.
- Provide hygienic environment to the baby through clean room, clean cloths.
- Educate the mother regarding importance of hand washing.

Diet

- Educate the mother to give exclusive breastfeeding.
- Use katori and spoon for feeding.
- Clean the utensils before feeding with boiled water.

Play/Exercise

- Educate the child family members to play with child.
- Ask them to provide baby massage for proper growth and development.
- Ask them to encourage the play and exercises.

Follow-up Care

- Teach the family members that after the completion of medication inform consultant.
- If any complication noted ask them to inform consultant immediately.
- Explain the treatment and follow-up care details.

Prognosis

- **Day 1:** Baby is admitted with the complaints of respiratory difficulty, lethargic activity, cold and calmly skin and poor feeding.
- **Day 2:** Medication and nursing care is given according to doctor's order and sign and symptoms reduced.
- **Day 3:** Baby take feeding properly, increased activity, respiratory rate become normal.

Summary

At the time of admission baby had a complaints of difficulty in breathing, restlessness, fever, vomiting, poor feeding etc. after that she was undergone medical investigation after that doctors has diagnosed as **Late Onset Neonatal Sepsis (LONS)**. She was treated with antibiotic, antipyretics and saline. After that her health status has been improved.

Conclusion

The Baby of RUCHI 23 days old admitted in Neonatal Intensive Care Unit (NICU). I make medical care plan on her condition. She is admitted under the Dr HK Pandey with the diagnosis of Late onset neonatal sepsis. Now she is better from previous stage.

BIBLIOGRAPHY

1. Parul Dutta. A Textbook of Pediatric Nursing, Jaypee Brothers Medical Publishers (P) Ltd, Third Edition. Page no. 490, 486, 482
2. Rimple Sharma. Essential of Pediatric Nursing, Jaypee Brothers Medical Publishers (P) Ltd, Page no. 460, 471.
3. Mosby. 2013 Nursing Drug Reference, 26th Edition, Page No. 924-926
4. Available at: emedicine.medscape.com/article/978352
5. Available at: https://www.nlm.nih.gov/medlineplus/enccy/article/007303.htm

ANNEXURE 5: PEDIATRIC ANTIDOTES DRUGS LIST

Name of antidote	Indication	Mode of action
Acetylcysteine (mucomyst)	Acetaminophen/tylenol/paracetamol	Restores depleted glutathione stores and protects against renal and hepatic failure
Activated charcoal	Non-specific poisons except cyanide, iron, lithium, caustics and alcohol	Absorption of drug in the gastric and intestinal tracts. Interrupts the enterohepatic cycle with multiple dose
Albuterol inhaler, insulin and glucose, $NaHCO_3$, kayexalate	Potassium	
Anticholinesterase agents	Neuromuscular blockade (paralytics)	
Atropine sulfate or pralidoxime	Anticholinesterase	Competitive inhibition of muscarinic receptors
Benzylpenicillin	Amanita phalloides (death cap mushroom)	Not known; partial protection against acute hepatic failure; may displace amatoxin from protein-binding sites allowing increased renal excretion; may also inhibit penetration of amatoxin to hepatocytes
Calcium salts	Fluoride ingestion	Rapidly complexes with fluoride ion
Deferoxamine	Iron	Deferoxamine acts by binding free iron in the bloodstream and enhancing its elimination in the urine
Digibind digoxin immune fab	Digoxin	Binds molecules of digoxin, making them unavailable for binding at their site of action on cells in the body
Dimercapol, edetate calcium, disodium,	Lead	Chelation of lead ions and endogenous metals (e.g., zinc, manganese, iron, copper)
Diphenhydramine (benadryl)	Extrapyramidal symptoms (EPS)	A potent antagonist to acetylcholine in muscarinic receptors
Flumazenil	Benzodiazepines	Reverses the effects of benzodiazepines by competitive inhibition at the benzodiazepine binding site on the gabaareceptor
Fomepizole	Ethylene glycol	A competitive inhibitor of the enzyme alcohol dehydrogenase found in the liver. This enzyme plays a key role in the metabolism of ethylene glycol and methanol
Glucagon	Beta blockers and calcium channel blockers	Stimulates the formation of adenyl cyclase causing intracellular increase in cycling AMP and enhanced glycogenolysis and elevated serum glucose concentration
Glucose (dextrose 50%)	Insulin reaction	Dextrose (the monosaccharide glucose) is used, distributed and stored by body tissues and is metabolized to carbon dioxide and water with the release of energy
Heparin	Ergotamine	Reverses hypercoagulable state by interacting with antithrombin III. Used in combination with vasodilator phentolamine or nitroprusside to prevent local thrombosis and ischemia
Hydroxocobalamin	Cyanide	Forms cyanocobalamin, a non-toxic metabolite that is easily excreted through the kidneys
Leucovorin calcium	Fluorouracil	
	Methotrexate	Protects the healthy cells from the effects of methotrexate while allowing methotrexate to enter and kill cancer cells
Magnesium sulfate	Calcium gluconate	
Mesna	Cyclophosphamide	A "chemoprotectant" drug that reduces the undesired effects of certain chemotherapy drugs
Methylene blue	Chemical producing severe methemoglobinemia. Ifosamide-induced encephalopathy	Reduces methemoglobin to hemoglobin

Name of antidote	Indication	Mode of action
Nalmefene or naloxone	Opioid analgesics	Prevents or reverses the effects of opioids including respiratory depression, sedation and hypotension
Naloxone (narcan)	Narcotics	Naloxone is believed to antagonize opioid effects by competing for the μ, κ and σ opiate receptor sites in the CNS, with the greatest affinity for the μ receptor
Neostigmine	Anticholinergics	Anticholinesterase which causes accumulation of acetylcholine at cholinergic receptor sites
Nitrite, sodium and glyceryl trinitrate	Cyanide	Oxidizes hemoglobin to methemoglobin which binds the free cyanide and can enhance endothelial cyanide detoxification by producing vasodilation
Penicillamine	Copper, gold, lead, mercury, zinc, arsenic	Chelation of metal ions
Phentolamine (regitine)	Dopamine	Regitine produces an alpha-adrenergic block of relatively short duration. It also has direct, but less marked, positive inotropic and chronotropic effects on cardiac muscle and vasodilator effects on vascular smooth muscle
Phyostigmine or $NaHCO_3$	Tricyclic antidepressants	A reversible anticholinesterase which effectively increases the concentration of acetylcholine at the sites of cholinergic transmission
Phytomenadione (vitamin K)	Coumadin/Warfarin	Bypasses inhibition of vitamin K epoxide reductase enzyme
Protamine sulfate	Heparin	Protamine that is strongly basic combines with acidic heparin forming a stable complex and neutralizes the anticoagulant activity of both drugs
Pyridoxine	Isoniazid, theophylline, monomethyl hydrazine. Adjunctive therapy in ethylene glycol poisoning	Reverses acute pyridoxine deficiency by promoting GABA synthesis. Promotes the conversion of toxic metabolite glycolic acid to glycine
Snake anti-venin	Cobra bite	Neutralizes venom by binding with circulating venom components and with locally deposited venom by accumulating at the bite site
Sodium bicarbonate	Iron	Prevents conversion of ferrous to ferric
	Cardiotoxic drug affecting fast sodium channel (TCA, cocaine)	Decreases affinity of cardiotoxic drugs to the fast sodium channel
	Weak acids	Promotes ionization of weak acids
	Chlorine gas inhalational poisoning	Neutralization of hydrochloric acid formed when chlorine gas reacts with water in the airways
Sodium thiosulphate	Cyanide	Replenishes depleted thiosulphate stores by acting as sulfur donor necessary for the conversion of CN-O to thiocyanate through the action of sulfur transferase enzyme rhodanese
Thiamine	Alcohol, Wernicke-Korsakoff syndrome	Reverses acute thiamine deficiency
	Adjunctive in ethylene glycol	Enhances detoxification of glyoxylic acid
Vitamin C	Chemicals causing methemoglobinemia in patients with G6PD deficiency	Reduces methemoglobin to hemoglobin

EU GSPR Authorised Reprsentative
Logos Europe, 9 rue Nicolas Poussin
1700, La Rochelle, France
Phone: +33 (0) 6 67 93 73 78
E-mail: contact@logoseurope.eu

www.ingramcontent.com/pod-product-compliance
Ingram Content Group UK Ltd.
Pitfield, Milton Keynes, MK11 3LW, UK
UKHW051942150726
7214IPUK00020B/385